SURGICAL COMPLICATIONS IN ORAL IMPLANTOLOGY

Etiology, Prevention, and Management

SURGICAL COMPLICATIONS IN ORAL IMPLANTOLOGY

Etiology, Prevention, and Management

Louie Al-Faraje, DDS

Founder and Director
California Implant Institute
San Diego, California

With contributions by
James L. Rutkowski, DMD, PhD
Christopher Church, MD

Quintessence Publishing Co, Inc

Chicago, Berlin, Tokyo, London, Paris, Milan, Barcelona,
Istanbul, Moscow, New Delhi, Prague, São Paulo, and Warsaw

Library of Congress Cataloging-in-Publication Data

Al-Faraje, Louie.
  Surgical complications in oral implantology : etiology, prevention, and
management / Louie Al-Faraje.
      p. ; cm.
  Includes bibliographical references.
  ISBN 978-0-86715-506-8 (hardcover)
  1. Dental implants–Complications. I. Title.
  [DNLM: 1. Dental Implantation–adverse effects. 2. Maxillary Sinus-
-surgery. 3. Oral Surgical Procedures, Preprosthetic–adverse effects. WU
640]
  RK667.I45A44 2011
  617.6'93–dc22
                                2011006601

© 2011 Quintessence Publishing Co, Inc

Quintessence Publishing Co, Inc
4350 Chandler Drive
Hanover Park, IL 60133
www.quintpub.com

Editor: Lisa C. Bywaters
Design: Ted Pereda
Production: Sue Robinson

Printed in China

CONTENTS

Part III Postoperative Complications

Complications

Part IV Complications Associated with Lateral Window Sinus Elevation

Preoperative Complications

Intraoperative Complications

Early Postoperative Complications

Part V Pharmacology: Prevention and Management of Pain, Infection, and Drug-Related Complications

Appendices

To Abu al-Qasim Al-Zahrawi (aka Abulcasis), 936–1013 CE

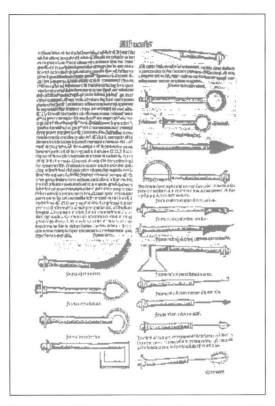

Page from a 1531 Latin translation by Peter Argellata of Al-Zahrawi's treatise on surgical and medical instruments.

A pioneer in all fields of surgery, Al-Zahrawi conceived and developed innumerable surgical techniques and instruments and, in 1000 CE, published the first surgical encyclopedia, *Kitab Al Tasrif* (*The Method of Medicine*), which spanned 30 volumes. For his monumental accomplishments and contributions to surgery, he earned the title Father of Modern Surgery. His way of thinking and his practice of surgery inspired many subsequent surgeons to achieve greatness and provided a beacon of light in the dark ages of Europe. In his many papers and manuals, he describes various operations and procedures that had never before been recorded. He wrote detailed descriptions of many surgical techniques, including cautery and wound management. Some have described him as the first plastic surgeon, notably for his attention to and methods of incision and use of silk thread suture to achieve good cosmesis. He devised about 200 surgical instruments, among them the surgical needle, scalpels, curettes, retractors, spoons, sounds, hooks, rods, and specula.

The street in Córdoba where his house still stands is named Calle Abulcasis in his memory. In 1977, the Spanish Tourist Board commemorated it in his honor with a bronze plaque that reads: "This was the house where lived Abu al-Qasim Al-Zahrawi."

CONTRIBUTORS

Christopher Church, MD

Director
Loma Linda Sinus and Allergy Center

Associate Professor
Department of Otolaryngology–Head and Neck Surgery
Loma Linda University School of Medicine
Loma Linda, California

James L. Rutkowski, DMD, PhD

Clinical Instructor
Department of Restorative Dentistry
School of Dental Medicine
University at Buffalo
The State University of New York
Buffalo, New York

Private Practice
Clarion, Pennsylvania

PREFACE

The use of dental implants to restore missing teeth has steadily increased over the past three decades. It is perhaps not surprising, then, that the number of implant-related complications has grown as well. Numerous clinical studies involving dental implants have revealed encouraging outcomes; however, there is an element of risk associated with all clinical procedures, and these encouraging results may have given rise to unrealistic expectations. Despite careful planning, there is always a potential for surgical complications. Nevertheless, carrying out routine tasks with care and attention, choosing minimally invasive techniques when indicated, recognizing evidence of a developing problem, and giving prompt attention will reduce postoperative complications.

The successful outcome of any surgical procedure requires attention to a series of patient-related and procedure-dependent parameters. Sound knowledge of surgical anatomy and experience and training in the fundamentals of internal medicine are important prerequisites for predictable implant surgery. Also, adequate presurgical planning, appropriate quality and quantity of available bone, a well-executed surgical technique, good primary stability, a sufficient healing period, and detailed postoperative instructions are all factors that play a vital role in the success of dental implant surgery and osseointegration. Aging, changing health conditions, wear and tear, and inadequate professional maintenance are important variables influencing prognosis.

This book is designed as a self-instruction guide to the diagnosis and management of surgery-related complications and to the development of a protocol that allows for the early detection of potential surgical complications and how to avoid them. It is a well-documented fact that early detection of complications that are amenable to rescue therapies may reverse the fate of a failing implant or bone grafting procedure.

The evidence-based methods of complications management described in this book are not meant to preclude the clinical judgment of experienced clinicians but rather should be applied to either support or prompt them to rethink their chosen methods of therapy on the basis of existing evidence.

ACKNOWLEDGMENTS

I would like to express sincere gratitude to my parents, Omar Al-Faraje and Nadia Al-Rifai, for their extraordinary sacrifices for too many years. Thank you for your unconditional love and support.

Also to my wife Rana, my lifelong companion and "book widow." Her support was invaluable as I was hunched over my computer, sometimes for 12 hours a day. And to our children—Nadia, Omar, and Tim—who contributed immensely to this book by sacrificing their precious time with "Papa."

In addition, I would like to thank my teachers at each of the medical institutions I attended. I was indeed fortunate to have had outstanding anatomical, clinical, and surgical training at the medical institutes in Russia, the Ukraine, and the United States.

Three special individuals have profoundly influenced my career:

Dr Nizar Al-Tair, my dental mentor, who spent countless hours challenging my knowledge and skills to deliver excellence and to be my best.

Dr Igor Persidsky, who taught me how to connect patients' medical problems with their dental needs and to think like a dental surgeon with internal medicine in mind. I treasure our years of friendship.

Dr Dewhirst Floyd, who gave me a helping hand and believed in me. This book would not have seen the light without his support during my early years in the dental field.

Finally, I would like to thank all of my students at the California Implant Institute. It is always a pleasure and an honor to share with you my knowledge and expertise in implant dentistry. For the last few years, my greatest professional joy has been interacting with my students and colleagues at the California Implant Institute.

I also would like to express my gratitude to Dr Christopher Church and Dr James Rutkowski for their contributions to this textbook.

Special thanks to Lisa Bywaters and her editorial team at Quintessence Publishing Company. Their tremendous support throughout the project allowed the creation of this modern, easy-to-consult textbook.

Identifying Preoperative Conditions That Could Lead to Complications

Inadequate or Excessive Vertical Restorative Space

Vertical restorative space, or *crown-height space*, is the distance from the crest of the residual alveolar ridge to the occlusal plane of a planned restoration or to the opposing dentition. The amount of this space will influence your choice of prosthesis, restorative material, and surgical technique; therefore, it should be carefully measured intraorally or on properly articulated diagnostic wax-ups or master casts before surgery.[1–8] Soft tissue thickness should also be assessed prior to surgery; thick soft tissue may yield greater vertical space than anticipated.

If the vertical restorative space is not considered until the implants have integrated and the patient is ready for restoration, the prosthetic outcome may be unacceptable. For example, the patient may require a different type of prosthesis than originally planned, need additional surgical procedures to correct the problem, or experience subsequent prosthetic failure, such as repeated porcelain or acrylic fracture.

Vertical space requirement for fixed restorations

Single-unit fixed restoration

In treatment planning a single-unit fixed restoration to replace a posterior tooth, the minimum vertical space needed for a cement-retained crown is 9 mm from the crestal bone to the occlusal plane of the opposing dentition or 6 mm from the soft tissue to the occlusal plane (Fig 1-1).

Components of the needed space are 3 mm cement, ceramic/metal substructure, and occlusal porcelain + 5 mm abutment height – 1 mm abutment height typically below the soft tissue level + 2 mm peri-implant soft tissue = 9 mm. This space is reduced to 8 mm for a cement-retained prosthesis with a metal occlusal surface and 5 to 6 mm for a screw-retained prosthesis (Table 1-1). For an anterior crown, the space required is 1 to 2 mm greater to accommodate the longer abutment necessary for proper retention.

Ideally, the implant should be positioned 3 mm below the most apical point of the free gingival margin.[9] Placement of the crown-abutment interface 1 mm below the most apical point of the free gingival margin will maintain the peri-implant biologic width (usually 2 mm).

Multi-unit fixed prosthesis

Space requirements for a multi-unit fixed prosthesis also vary by material. If the crown-height space is less than 15 mm, porcelain is the restorative material of choice rather than acrylic resin, which requires bulk for strength. If the space is 15 mm or greater, a hybrid prosthesis should be considered.

Vertical cantilever

Vertical cantilever, or the ratio of crown to implant, should be taken into consideration in the fabrication of a fixed implant-supported prosthesis.

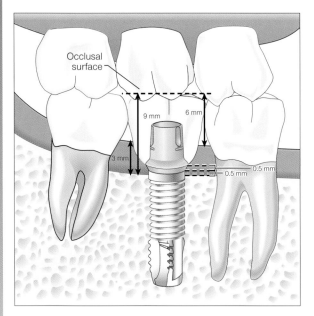

Fig 1-1 Vertical restorative space requirement for posterior single fixed cement-retained implant restoration with 3-mm-thick soft tissue.

Table 1-1	Minimum vertical space requirement (mm) from crestal bone to opposing dentition			
	Cement-retained		**Screw-retained**	
Dimension	**Porcelain crown**	**Metal crown**	**Porcelain crown**	**Metal crown**
Implant platform to bone	0.5	0.5	0.5	0.5
Abutment collar height	0.5	0.5	0.5	0.5
Abutment height	5.0	5.0	3.0	3.0
Cement space	0.5	0.5	NA	NA
Ceramic core or metal substructure	0.5	NA	NA	NA
Porcelain occlusal material	2.0	NA	2.0	NA
Metal occlusal material	NA	1.5	NA	1.0
Total	9.0	8.0	6.0	5.0

Vertical space requirement for removable restorations

The two types of removable implant prostheses are bar-retained and low-profile independent attachments (eg, ball and Locator [Zest] attachments).

Bar-retained overdenture

The bar-retained overdenture requires a minimum of 17 mm of crown-height space depending on the type of attachment used. The space is divided as follows: 3 mm bone to soft tissue + 1 mm soft tissue to bar (necessary for proper hygiene; Fig 1-2) + 5 mm bar height. The remaining 8 mm is the minimum required thickness for acrylic resin from the superior edge of the bar to the incisal edges of the denture teeth.

Ball- or Locator-retained overdenture

A ball- or Locator-retained overdenture requires a minimum of 14 mm crown-height space, or 3 to 4 mm less than that needed for a bar overdenture. The space is divided as follows: 3 mm bone to soft tissue + 2.5 to 3.5 mm abutment height + 8 mm acrylic resin thickness between the top of the ball Locator abutment and the incisal edges of the denture teeth (Fig 1-3).

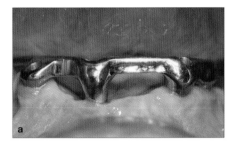 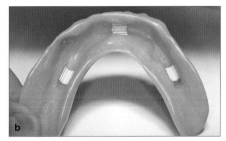 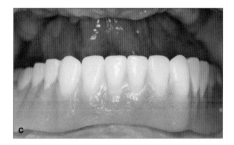

Fig 1-2 *(a to c)* Cast bar overdenture. A distance of 1 mm or more is maintained between the lower border of the bar and the soft tissues for adequate hygiene access.

Fig 1-3 *(a to e)* Ball-retained overdenture. These ball attachments have a higher profile than the Locator abutments, but this is acceptable in this scenario because there is adequate vertical restorative space.

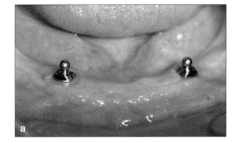 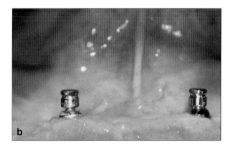

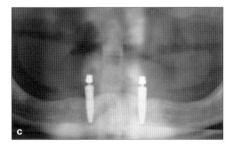 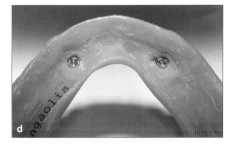 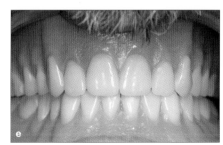

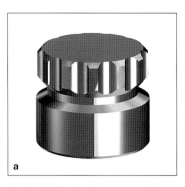 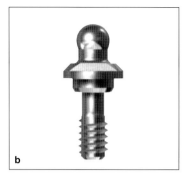 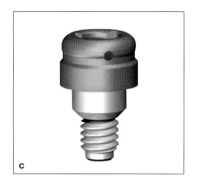

Fig 1-4 *(a)* The ball abutment. *(b)* The ball abutment cap. *(c)* The low-profile Locator abutment.

Solutions for deficient vertical space

One or more of the following can be used to gain a satisfactory clinical result:

- Removal of hard tissue (alveoloplasty).
- Surgical removal of soft tissue.
- Use of a different abutment type, which can result in a gain of 1 mm or more of available vertical dimension. The Locator abutment has a height of approximately 2 mm, whereas ball attachments are 4 to 6 mm in height (Fig 1-4). The Locator abutment thus offers an advantage in clinical situations with limited vertical space.
- Selection of a different type of prosthesis, which can also result in a gain of 1 mm or more in available vertical height. As noted above, placement of a screw-retained rather than a cement-retained restoration or placement of a fixed instead of a removable prosthesis reduces space requirements considerably. In the presence of minimal bone resorption, fixed ceramic restorations will best accommodate limited interarch space; however, the cost of these prostheses is greater.

- Incorporation of a metal framework into an implant-supported complete denture. This step is recommended to provide sufficient strength while reducing vertical space requirements by 2 mm or more.
- Reduction of the amount of space between the framework and tissue to the minimum required. This can be accomplished in some cases without compromising hygiene access.
- Use of an alloy with a relatively high elastic modulus, such as a type IV extra-hard high-noble alloy. This may allow the fabrication of a framework with reduced occlusogingival dimension without compromising strength. The recommended occlusogingival dimension for type IV extra-hard high-noble alloy is 3.5 mm, compared with 6 mm for low-gold high-palladium alloys.[10]
- Orthodontic intrusion of teeth. This might be indicated if the vertical restorative space is compromised because of hypereruption of the opposing teeth.
- Fabrication of a traditional (non-implant-supported) fixed or removable prosthesis. This might be preferred over implant treatment in some clinical situations.

Solutions for excessive vertical space

Excessive vertical restorative space leads to excessive vertical cantilever. Solutions to this problem include:

- Use of surgical techniques to increase the height of the available bone, including block grafting, guided bone regeneration with barrier membrane or titanium mesh, or distraction osteogenesis

- Placement of traditional (non–implant-supported) partial or complete removable dentures.

COMPLICATION 2	Inadequate Horizontal Restorative Space

A minimum amount of horizontal space must be maintained between implants or between implants and natural teeth to prevent unnecessary bone loss or compromised esthetics that can result from invading that space.

The *horizontal restorative space* refers to the mesiodistal distance between implants, between an implant and a natural tooth, and between natural teeth.

Implant-to-implant space requirement

The distance between two implants, or *interimplant distance*, should be a minimum of 3 mm. When this distance is maintained, vertical bone loss resulting from crestal bone remodeling during establishment of the biologic width at the implant-abutment interface will have a minimal lateral or horizontal component. In a study by Tarnow et al,[11] horizontal bone loss around implants at the crest was only 0.45 mm when the interimplant distance was greater than 3 mm and 1.04 mm when it was less than 3 mm.

The clinical significance of this phenomenon is that crestal bone loss increases the distance between the interproximal contact of the adjacent implant restorations and the crestal bone. This distance may determine whether the interdental papilla is present or absent, which has implications for both hygiene and esthetics.

It is important to note that for fixed-detachable, spark-erosion, and overdenture types of implant prostheses, the distance between implants can be less or much more than 3 mm; the 3-mm guideline applies primarily to the fixed partial denture-type of implant prosthesis.

Calculating ideal implant-to-implant space

There are three ways of calculating an ideal mesiodistal space between implants.

1. Width of implant crowns
The first formula, which is based on the width of the planned implant crowns, requires a diagnostic wax-up and is ideal for determining the space between implant centers (Fig 1-5):

$$\frac{\text{Width of crown 1}}{2} + \frac{\text{Width of crown 2}}{2}$$

2. Papillary fill of interproximal space
The second method is less accurate; however, in most cases the result is close to the ideal distance between implants, which will vary in proportion to the diameter of the implants used (Fig 1-6):

$$R1 + R2 + 3 \text{ mm (where R = implant radius)}$$

This method is based on the fact that, as discussed above, the horizontal distance between implants influences the appearance of the papillae,[12] and a 3-mm interimplant distance most closely correlates with adequate papillary fill of the interproximal space.[13]

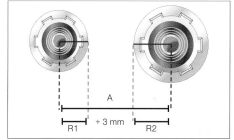

Fig 1-6 The distance between the centers of two adjacent implants (A) is calculated by adding 3 mm to the sum of implant 1 radius (R1) and implant 2 radius (R2).

3. Standard distance
The third method is to allow a standard distance of 7 to 8 mm between narrow platform and regular platform implants and 8 to 9 mm between two regular platform implants or one regular and one wide platform implant. These distances are acceptable for restoration with a fixed prosthesis (Fig 1-7).

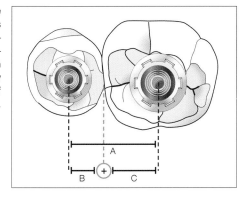

Fig 1-5 The distance between the centers of two adjacent implants (A) is calculated by adding B (width of crown 1 divided by 2) and C (width of crown 2 divided by 2).

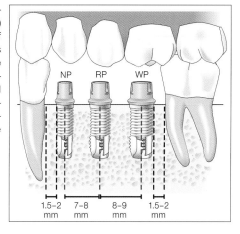

Fig 1-7 Standard distance (center-to-center) between implants of different diameters and optimal distance (edge-to-edge) between implants and natural teeth. NP, narrow platform; RP, regular platform; WP, wide platform.

Implant-to–natural tooth space requirement

Calculating ideal implant-to–natural tooth space

There are two ways of calculating an ideal mesiodistal space between an implant and a natural tooth.

1. Width of implant crown

The first approach is similar to the first method described for calculating the mesiodistal space between implants, ie, it is based on the width of the planned implant crown (Fig 1-8):

$$\frac{\text{Width of crown}}{2}$$

2. Standard distance

The second method is to place the edge of the implant 1.5 to 2.0 mm away from the adjacent root surface.[14] Therefore, the following formula can be used:

$$1 \text{ to } 2 \text{ mm} + R \ \text{(where R = implant radius)}$$

This distance will prevent vertical bone resorption at the adjacent tooth; moreover, if bone loss occurs around the implant, it will not affect the adjacent tooth and vice versa (see Fig 1-7).

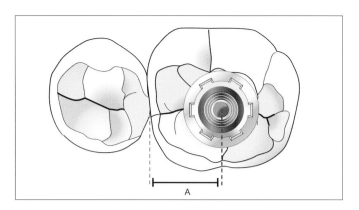

Fig 1-8 An optimal way of calculating the distance between an implant and a natural tooth. Distance A is half of the width of the future implant crown.

Case examples

Figure 1-9 illustrates a case of incorrect implant positioning. An implant to replace the missing mandibular right first molar was placed 3 to 4 mm distal to the mandibular right second premolar so as to avoid damaging the premolar's distally inclined root. As a result, the prosthesis has a large and biomechanically undesirable mesial cantilever. The proper course of action in this case would have been to adjust the root position of the second premolar by orthodontic intervention before implant placement. Figure 1-10 shows a case with ideal implant-tooth and interimplant distances.

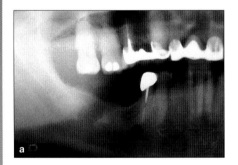
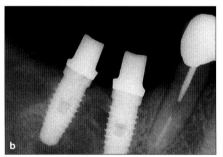
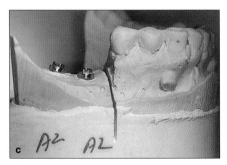
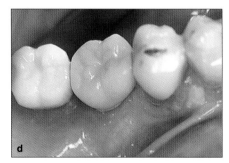

Fig 1-9 *(a to d)* The distance between the second premolar and the mesial implant is greater than ideal to avoid the inclined root. The result was an undesirable mesial cantilever of the implant prosthesis, which could have been avoided if the inclined root had been straightened using orthodontic treatment before implant placement.

Fig 1-10 *(a to d)* Clinical case with optimal distance of 3 mm between implants (edge-to-edge) and 2 mm between implants and natural teeth (edge-to-edge).

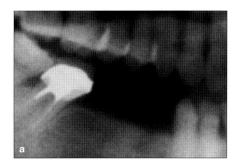
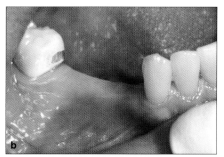
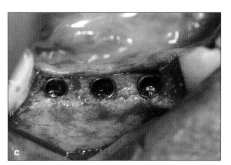
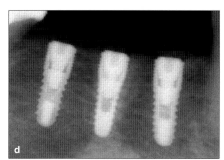

Tooth-to-tooth space requirement

Anterior teeth

The minimum mesiodistal space required for treating loss of a single tooth in the anterior area with a dental implant is the implant diameter + 1.5 mm to the adjacent root on either side (ie, 3 mm). For example, a minimum distance of 6.5 mm is required for a 3.5-mm narrow platform implant, 7.5 mm if the implant diameter is 4.5 mm, and 8.5 mm if the implant diameter is 5.5 mm (Fig 1-11).

It is important to note that the distance of implant diameter + 3 mm is adequate for osseointegration but not necessarily ideal esthetically. Because the abutment diameter is usually wider than the diameter of the implant, 1 mm or more additional space is preferable for a more esthetic emergence profile of the implant crown. Alternatively, a smaller-diameter implant can be used.

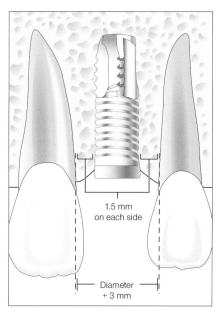

Fig 1-11 The minimum recommended distance for implant placement between two teeth is the diameter of the planned implant + 3 mm.

Posterior teeth

As in the anterior area, the mesiodistal distance of implant diameter + 3 mm between two natural posterior teeth is acceptable for placement of an implant. However, in the posterior region, there is often a problem of too much rather than not enough space. Although the natural molar is multirooted, it should be replaced by only a single implant. The placement of two implants to replace one missing molar is not recommended because it is surgically challenging, difficult to restore, and esthetically unacceptable to most patients. Moreover, the prosthesis must be configured such that an opening can be maintained between the implants for hygiene purposes, creating a so-called *tunneled molar*. Figure 1-12 demonstrates such a case.

If the alveolar ridge is wide (> 7 mm), a 5- or 6-mm-diameter implant should be used to replace one molar. Otherwise, one of the methods described below can be used for space management.

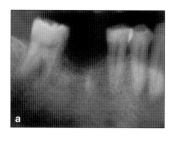
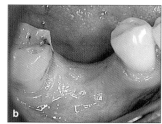
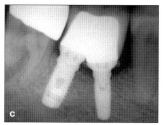
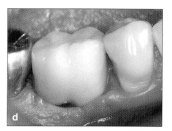

Fig 1-12 *(a to d)* Restoration of a missing mandibular molar using two implants. Note that space is maintained between the two implants for hygiene access under the prosthesis.

Management of horizontal restorative space problems

Orthodontic treatment

If the edentulous area is not ideal for implant placement because of space concerns, orthodontic treatment can be initiated to increase or decrease the edentulous area. This may be especially helpful when space is excessive. Without such treatment, the restoration may be substantially wider than the diameter of the implant. The resulting torque, or *moment of force*, on the implant will increase as a factor of the magnitude and off-axis distance of occlusal forces applied (torque = force × distance; Fig 1-13), which has negative implications for the long-term outcome of the implant.

Enameloplasty

If only a small gain is needed in the mesiodistal dimension, enameloplasty may be adequate.

Smaller-diameter implants

Selective use of implants with a smaller diameter at the implant-abutment interface may be beneficial in some scenarios. Figure 1-14 shows replacement of a molar using a smaller-diameter (3.5-mm) implant, which is acceptable if the occlusal table on the crown is also small.

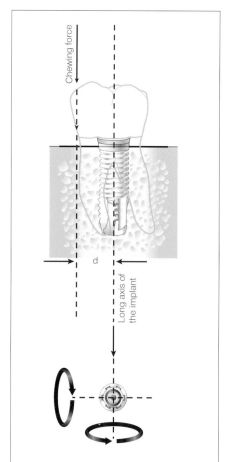

Fig 1-13 Chewing forces applied at a distance *(d)* from the long axis of an implant will increase the moment of force applied onto the implant and cause bending in all directions.

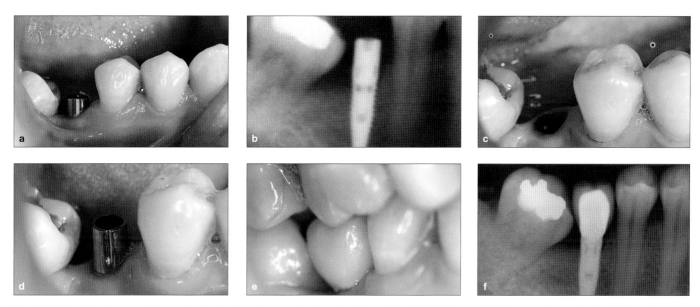

Fig 1-14 *(a to e)* Replacement of a missing first molar with a smaller-diameter (3.5-mm) implant. This is acceptable because the mesiodistal distance between the second premolar and the second molar is reduced as a result of mesial shifting of the second molar. Therefore, the occlusal table of the implant prosthesis can be considerably smaller than that of a normal-sized molar.

Narrow-diameter implants

For more substantial space deficiencies, narrow-diameter (1.8- to 3.0-mm) one- or two-piece implants have been used successfully for compromised horizontal restorative spaces for many years and are well documented in the literature[15–17] (Fig 1-15). However, it is crucial to carefully assess biomechanical risk factors before using narrow-diameter implants.

Features

- A reduced diameter at the neck of these implants makes it possible to conserve crucial millimeters of space when horizontal intertooth restorative space is compromised.
- A one-piece design eliminates the microgap between implant platform and abutment found in two-piece implants. Less crestal bone loss is observed around one-piece implants over time.

Indications

For the last 10 years, applications for narrow-diameter implants have included:

- Stabilization of full-arch dentures
- Single tooth replacement in compromised intertooth space situations
- Single tooth replacement in compromised interroot space situations
- Orthodontic anchorage
- Minimally invasive surgery as indicated

Fig 1-15 *(a to f)* A narrow (< 6-mm) lateral incisor space was restored using a narrow-diameter (3-mm) implant. This allowed sufficient space on each side of the implant for the papillae.

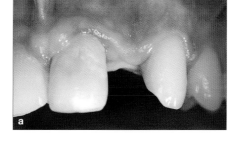
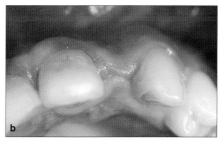
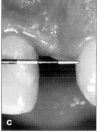
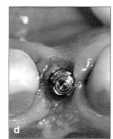
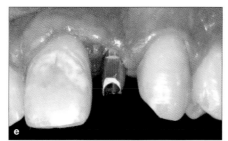
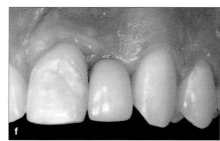

Limited Jaw Opening and Interarch Distance

Limited jaw opening

The patient's ability to open should be assessed before the intraoral examination begins. Normal opening is 40 mm from maxillary to mandibular incisal edge.[18]

If mouth opening is less than 40 mm, the implant surgeon may encounter difficulty when placing implants in the posterior region of the mouth. A specially designed ruler (Fig 1-16) can be used for this purpose.

Placement of implants in the posterior region when mouth opening is limited can result in excessively angulated implants. Figure 1-17 illustrates such a case. The distal implant could not be restored and therefore was left submerged and not put into function.

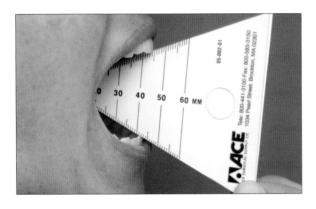

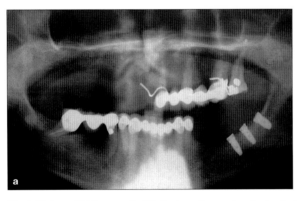

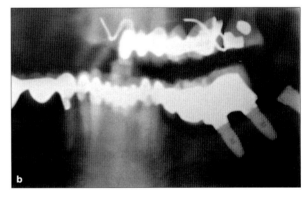

Fig 1-16 A specially designed ruler is used to assess mouth opening for implant placement in the posterior region.

Fig 1-17 *(a and b)* As a result of limited mouth opening, the implants were placed with incorrect angulation. The distal implant could not be properly restored from a biomechanical perspective and was therefore submerged.

Interarch distance

Hypererupted opposing teeth could interfere with implant placement even if jaw opening is adequate. In such a scenario, the occlusal plane of the hypererupted teeth should be corrected by enameloplasty or orthodontic intrusion. Furthermore, excessive coronal height of a tooth adjacent to the edentulous area may require the use of a drill extension; however, the patient's limited opening may interfere with use of the extension. When it is not possible to use implant handpieces to place implants in the correct position and angulation, implant placement is contraindicated.

Inadequate Alveolar Width for Optimal Buccolingual Positioning

Posterior ridge deficiency

As previously noted, endosseous root-form implants distribute occlusal loads best when the forces are applied along the long axis of the implant body. When implants are placed in the posterior region, the center of the implant (during surgery, the pilot hole) should correspond to the central fossa of the planned implant restoration. This is easy to achieve if the implants are being placed in an immediate extraction site or in edentulous areas where minimal resorption has taken place

(ie, recent extraction sites). Figure 1-18 illustrates a case of immediate implant placement. The alveolar ridge exhibited no buccolingual resorption at the time of implant placement, allowing the implant to be placed in an ideal position. When the implant body is located under the central fossa of the planned restoration, the occlusion can also be ideal, with the buccal cusp of the implant restoration overlapping the buccal cusps of the mandibular teeth.

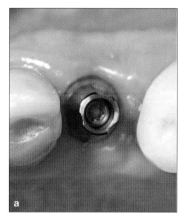 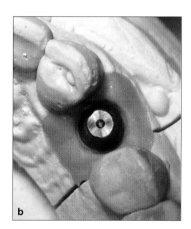 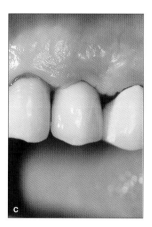 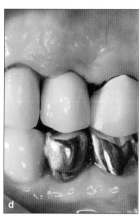

Fig 1-18 *(a to d)* The implant was placed immediately following tooth extraction in an optimal buccolingual position because there was adequate width of the alveolar ridge. The result is an implant prosthesis with ideal occlusion (ie, its buccal cusp overlaps the opposing mandibular buccal cusp).

In resorbed alveolar ridges where buccolingual bone loss compromises correct implant positioning, attaining axial loading requires the implant to be positioned lingually or palatally unless a bone augmentation procedure is performed. If no bone grafting procedure is to be performed to augment the width of the alveolar ridge, implants should be centered buccolingually in available bone and the restoration placed in either a cusp-to-cusp or reverse articulation (Fig 1-19), depending on the severity of the bone loss. Such positioning of the restoration will prevent buccal cantilever forces on the implant and minimize consequent damage to the implant from offset occlusal load forces. Figure 1-20 shows a patient with severe resorption in the posterior right quadrant of the maxilla. The patient declined veneer block bone grafting to augment the width of the alveolar ridge. The wax-up shows that reverse articulation is necessary if axial loading is to be maintained on the implants. A sinus elevation bone graft was performed with delayed implant placement, and clinical photos show the definitive prosthesis in reverse articulation.

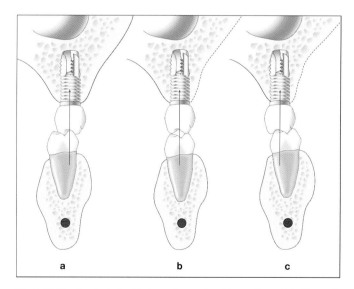

Fig 1-19 The implant should always be centered buccolingually in the available alveolar ridge unless a simultaneous bone grafting procedure is to be performed to increase alveolar width. However, the location of the implant prosthesis should be modified so that buccal cantilever of the implant prosthesis is avoided and occlusal forces are directed along the long axis of the implant. Therefore, depending on the location of the implant relative to the opposing dentition, the restoration may be in ideal occlusion *(a)*, cusp-to-cusp contact *(b)*, or even in reverse articulation *(c)*.

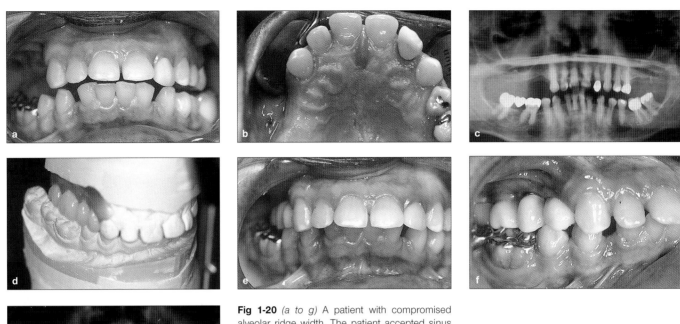

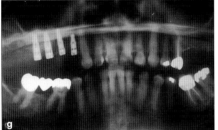

Fig 1-20 (a to g) A patient with compromised alveolar ridge width. The patient accepted sinus elevation treatment but declined veneer block augmentation to increase the width of the alveolar ridge. The result is the placement of implants in the middle of the available alveolar ridge with the implant prosthesis in a crossbite position to eliminate the buccal extension (cantilever) on the implant crowns.

Anterior ridge deficiency

Unlike buccolingual positioning in the posterior region (where the implant is placed under the central fossa of the planned restoration), the position of the implant in the anterior region depends on the type of prosthesis to be fabricated: screw-retained or cement-retained (Fig 1-21).

If the definitive restoration is to be cement-retained, the implant should be centered (and its pilot hole drilled) under the incisal edge of the planned implant crown. This is because the cement-retained abutment must be large enough to gain adequate retention. Centering the implant under the cingulum will make the cement-retained crown very bulky. However, the opposite is true if a screw-retained prosthesis is planned; that is, the implant should be centered under the cingulum of the planned crown. This is because the access hole for the abutment screw should not compromise esthetics. Cement-retained versus screw-retained implant prostheses are discussed further in complication 39 (see part 3).

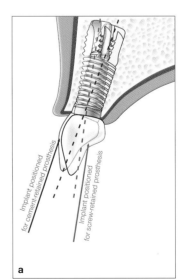

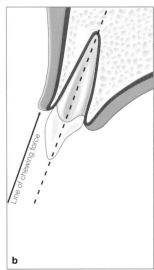

Fig 1-21 (a) In the anterior region, the buccolingual position of the implant depends on the type of prosthesis planned. For a screw-retained implant prosthesis, the position of the center of the implant is under the cingulum of the future crown (to provide for screw access without compromising esthetics); however, for a cement-retained prosthesis, the center of the implant is located under the incisal edge of the future crown. (b) The latter situation is better from a biomechanical point of view because the chewing forces are directed at the incisal edges and therefore will be along the long axis of the implant.

Figure 1-22 shows ideal buccolingual positioning of an anterior implant with a cement-retained restoration. Figure 1-23 shows ideal buccolingual positioning of a screw-retained prosthesis. A case of incorrect positioning toward the buccal aspect, which led to gingival recession and compromised esthetics, is shown in Fig 1-24.

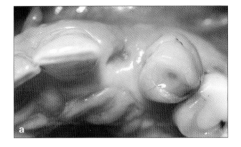
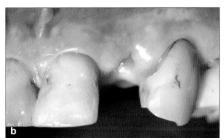
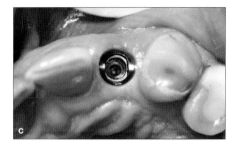
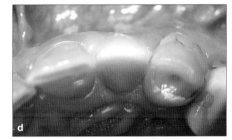
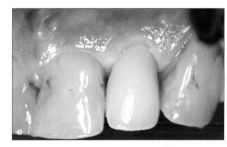

Fig 1-22 *(a to e)* Ideal buccolingual position of an anterior implant with a cement-retained prosthesis. The center of the implant is under the incisal edge of the implant crown.

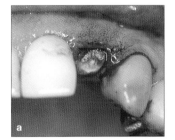
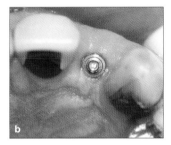
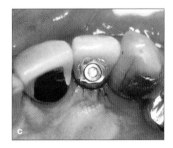
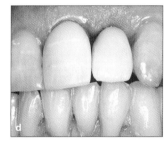

Fig 1-23 *(a to d)* Ideal buccolingual position of an anterior implant with a screw-retained prosthesis. The center of the implant is under the cingulum of the implant crown.

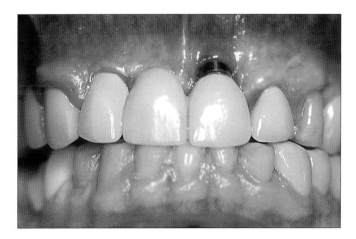

Fig 1-24 Excessive buccal positioning of an implant led to gingival recession and compromised esthetics.

Treatment of alveolar ridge width deficiency

Bone grafting procedures can be used for augmentation of the width of a deficient alveolar ridge. Some of the most common procedures are:

- Guided bone regeneration with simultaneous or delayed implant placement (Fig 1-25)

- Alveolar ridge expansion with simultaneous or delayed implant placement (Fig 1-26)
- Block grafting with delayed implant placement (Fig 1-27)

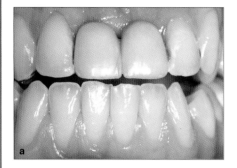
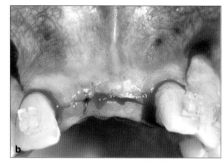
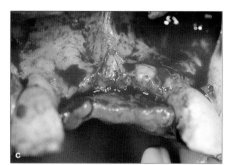
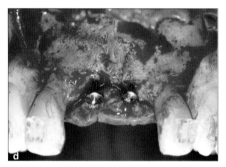
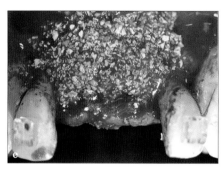
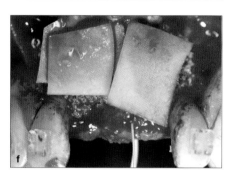
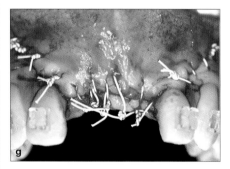

Fig 1-25 *(a to g)* A guided bone regeneration procedure is performed using particulate bone graft material and resorbable membrane to increase the width of the alveolar ridge for proper buccolingual implant positioning.

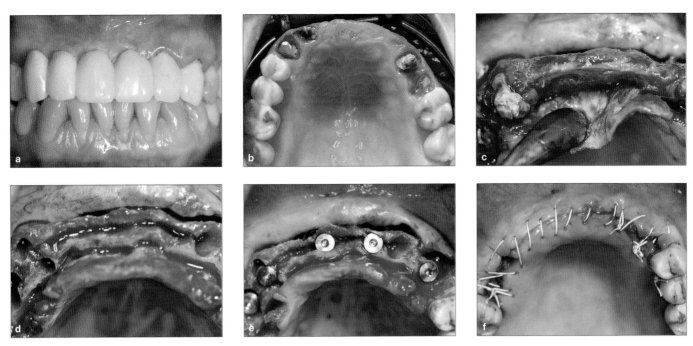

Fig 1-26 *(a to f)* Alveolar ridge expansion using the split-ridge technique is performed simultaneously with implant placement to increase the width of the alveolar ridge.

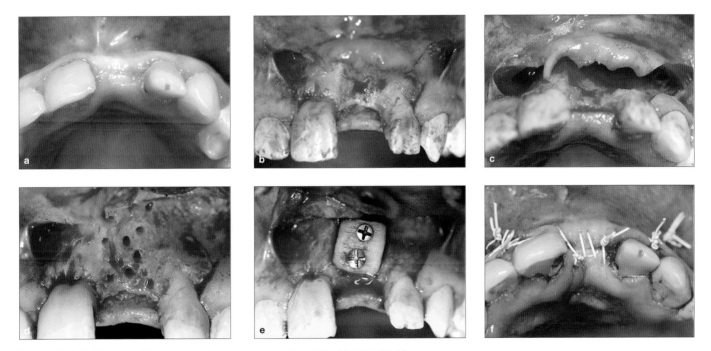

Fig 1-27 *(a to f)* A block grafting technique is used to increase the width of the alveolar ridge.

COMPLICATION 5 | Maxillary and Mandibular Tori

Maxillary tori

A maxillary torus is a mass of dense cortical bone that is typically located at the midline of the palate. Indications for removal include (1) interference with a conventional or implant-supported denture, (2) speech impediment, (3) repeated trauma to the overlying mucosa during mastication, and (4) malignancy phobia of the patient.[19] Before removal, the maxillary torus should be examined by computed tomography scan to rule out the possibility of pneumatization, in which the nasal cavity extends into the torus itself.[20]

Technique for removal

- For dentate patients, an impression is taken prior to surgery and a cast poured. The torus is removed from the cast, and a clear acrylic stent is made. Use of the stent postoperatively will assist in preventing hematoma formation and protecting the wound from irritation by food. However, if the patient wears a full or partial denture, the prosthesis can be relined with soft tissue conditioner after surgery and used as the stent (Fig 1-28).
- Anesthesia can be accomplished with bilateral greater palatine and incisive nerve blocks.
- A Y or double-Y incision is made, and a full-thickness flap is reflected to expose the torus[21] (see Figs 1-28b and 1-28c).
- After the entire torus is fully exposed, a large round diamond bur with copious irrigation is the suggested method for removal (see Fig 1-28d).
- Once the torus has been completely removed (see Fig 1-28e), the area is irrigated, and the flap is trimmed and loosely sutured using interrupted Vicryl (Ethicon) or polytetrafluoroethylene (PTFE) suture material (see Fig 1-28f).
- The stent or the relined denture (see Fig 1-28g) should be worn for 2 weeks and must be removed at least twice a day for cleaning.

Complications and solutions

- The torus is usually covered by thin mucoperiosteal tissue. Care should be taken during flap elevation not to tear this thin and friable mucosa.
- Creation of an oronasal fistula is possible because of the thin nature of the palatal bone. It is better to leave some bony elevation rather than risk perforation into the nasal cavity.
- Sloughing of the mucosal flap is common and not a cause for concern because granulation tissue will eventually cover the defect. To minimize sloughing, trim away any friable or macerated tissues during closure.

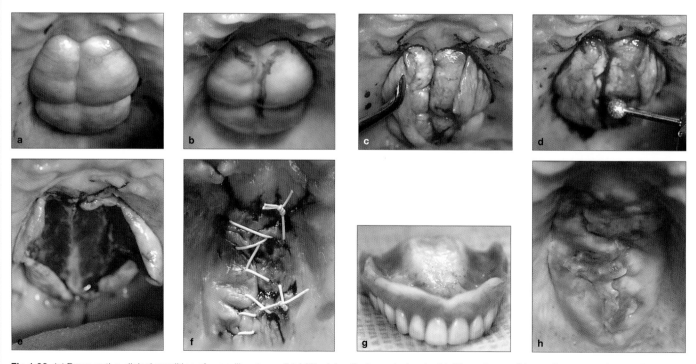

Fig 1-28 (a) Preoperative clinical condition of a maxillary torus. (b) A Y incision (for larger tori, a double Y may be used) is used to expose the maxillary torus. (c) A Molt 2/4 elevator is used to reflect a full-thickness mucoperiosteal flap. This step is done very gently to avoid tearing the friable mucosa of the flap. (d) A large, round diamond bur is used under copious irrigation to remove the torus. Care should be taken in this step not to perforate the nasal cavity. (e) The torus is completely removed. (f) The excessive tissue is removed, and the flap is sutured using PTFE suture material. (g) The denture is relined immediately after surgery using Coe Comfort (CC) tissue conditioning material. (h) Clinical condition 2 weeks after surgery.

Mandibular tori

Mandibular tori are typically located on the lingual surface of the mandible and can be bilateral, unilateral, or multiple. Indications for removal are the same as for maxillary tori.

Technique for removal

- Anesthesia is achieved with inferior alveolar block, lingual nerve block, and local infiltration.
- In an edentulous patient, a midcrestal incision of appropriate length is made to expose the entire torus (Fig 1-29a). If teeth remain, a lingual intrasulcular incision should be made.
- An envelope flap is reflected. With the use of a no. 557 fissure bur, the bone is scored at the intersection of the torus and the lingual body of the mandible (Fig 1-29b).
- The torus is removed with a bone file or large, round diamond bur. A Seldin retractor is placed under the torus to protect the floor of the mouth during the removal procedure (Fig 1-29c).
- The area is irrigated, excess soft tissue is trimmed (Fig 1-29d), and the flap is closed using interrupted Vicryl or PTFE suture material (Fig 1-29e).

Complications and solutions

- A postoperative hematoma is a potential threat to the airway. Protecting the floor of the mouth from sharp or rotating instruments is necessary for the prevention of this potential complication.
- Displacement of bony chips and debris can lead to postoperative infection in the sublingual space. Limiting the depth of the flap and performing thorough irrigation can minimize the possibility of infection.
- It is important to use an electric or surgical handpiece to prevent the possibility of inducing tissue emphysema.

Fig 1-29 *(a)* Placement of midcrestal incision for the purpose of lingual mandibular torus removal. In dentate patients, the incision is placed in the lingual gingival sulcus. *(b)* Full-thickness flap is reflected and a 1- to 2-mm groove is created using a no. 557 fissure bur at the superior buccal border of the torus. *(c)* The envelope flap is reflected further to expose the entire torus, and then a Seldin retractor is placed under the torus to prevent any damage to the floor of the mouth as the torus is removed using a round diamond bur. *(d)* Excision of the extra soft tissue of the flap is performed, and then the area is irrigated. *(e)* The flap is closed with a continuous or interrupted suturing technique.

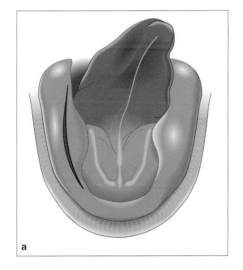
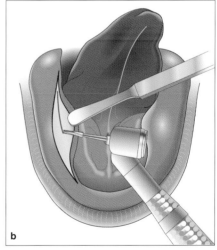
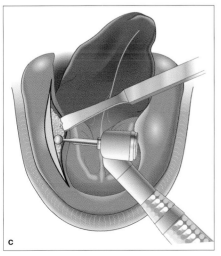
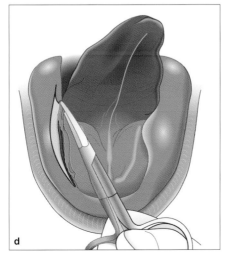
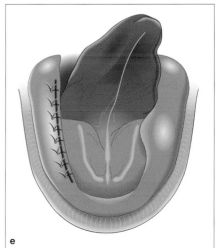

References

1. Sadowsky SJ. The implant-supported prosthesis for the edentulous arch: Design considerations. J Prosthet Dent 1997;78:28–33.
2. Sadowsky SJ. Mandibular implant-retained overdenture: A literature review. J Prosthet Dent 2001;86:468–473.
3. Chaimattayompol N, Arbree NS. Assessing the space limitation inside a complete denture for implant attachments. J Prosthet Dent 2003;89:82–85.
4. Engelman M. Clinical Decision Making and Treatment Planning in Osseointegration. Chicago: Quintessence, 1996:83.
5. Watson RM, Davis DM, Forman GH, et al. Considerations in design and fabrication of maxillary implant-supported prostheses. Int J Prosthodont 1991;4:232–239.
6. Phillips K, Wong KM. Space requirements for implant-retained bar-and-clip overdentures. Compend Contin Educ Dent 2001;22:516–518,520,522.
7. Phillips K, Wong KM. Vertical space requirement for the fixed-detachable, implant-supported prosthesis. Compend Contin Educ Dent 2002;23:750–752,754,756.
8. Gittelson GL. Vertical dimension of occlusion in implant dentistry: Significance and approach. Implant Dent 2002;1:33–40.
9. Berglundh T, Lindh J. Dimension of the peri-implant mucosa. Biologic width revisited. J Clin Periodontol 1996;23:971–973.
10. Alsiyabi AS, Felton DA, Cooper LF. The role of abutment-attachment selection in resolving inadequate interarch distance: A clinical report. J Prosthodont 2005;14:184–190.
11. Tarnow DP, Cho SC, Wallace SS. The effect of inter-implant distance on the height of inter-implant bone crest. J Periodontol 2000;71:546–549.
12. Kourkouta S, Dedi KD, Paquette DW, Mol A. Interproximal tissue dimensions in relation to adjacent implants in the anterior maxilla: Clinical observations and patient aesthetic evaluation. Clin Oral Implants Res 2009;20:1375–1385.
13. Teughels W, Merheb J, Quirynen M. Critical horizontal dimensions of interproximal and buccal bone around implants for optimal aesthetic outcomes: A systematic review. Clin Oral Implants Res 2009;20(suppl 4):134–145.
14. Salama H, Salama M, Garber D, Adar P. Developing optimal peri-implant papillae within the esthetic zone: Guided soft tissue augmentation. J Esthet Dent 1995;7:125–129.
15. Reddy MS, O'Neal SJ, Haigh S, Aponte-Wesson R, Geurs NC. Initial clinical efficacy of 3-mm implants immediately placed into function in conditions of limited spacing. Int J Oral Maxillofac Implants 2008;23:281–288.
16. Davarpanah M, Martinez H, Tecucianu JF, Celletti R, Lazzara R. Small-diameter implants: Indications and contraindications. J Esthet Dent 2000;12:186–194.
17. Petrungaro P. Management of the compromised intertooth space with small-diameter one-piece implants in the esthetic zone. Functional Esthet Restorative Dent 2007;1:70–75.
18. Renouard F, Rangert B. Risk Factors in Implant Dentistry. Chicago: Quintessence, 1990:18–24.
19. Dym H, Ogle O. Atlas of Minor Oral Surgery. Philadelphia: Saunders, 2001:196–197.
20. Goodsell J, Morin GE. Abnormalities of the mouth. In: Kruger GO (ed). Textbook of Oral Surgery, ed 4. St Louis: Mosby, 1974:chapter 6.
21. Peterson LJ (ed). Contemporary Oral and Maxillofacial Surgery, ed 3. St Louis: Mosby, 1998:300–302.

PART 2 Intraoperative Complications in Implant Placement

Complications

Incorrect Implant Angulation

The implant must be angulated correctly in the buccolingual and mesiodistal planes for optimum function and esthetics.

Buccolingual angulation

Endosseous root-form implants distribute occlusal loads most effectively when forces are applied in an axial direction. An angulation of 15 degrees or less is considered acceptable. Even natural teeth are not straight, but rather perpendicular to the *curve of Wilson,* the lateral curve of the occlusal table formed by the inclination of the posterior teeth (Fig 2-1). However, as implant angulation approaches or exceeds 25 degrees, the supporting bone is severely compromised through transmission of occlusal forces (Fig 2-2a). Moreover, if an implant is inclined buccolingually and the prosthetic reconstruction is offset relative to the implant head for improved occlusion and/or esthetics, the inclination will introduce a bending moment on the implant and will lead to a few potential problems.

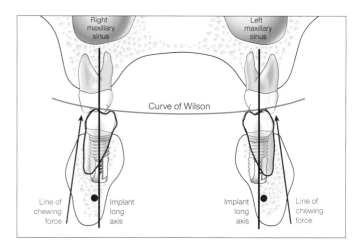

Fig 2-1 Natural posterior teeth are perpendicular to the curve of Wilson. In order for posterior implants to be aligned with the direction of chewing forces, they should also be positioned perpendicular to the curve of Wilson; however, vertical placement is acceptable because it is a minimal deviation from the direction of chewing forces.

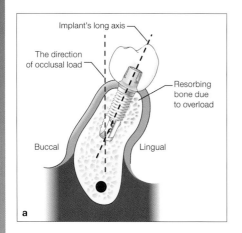 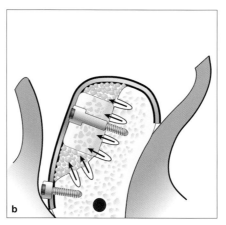 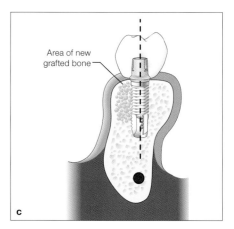

Fig 2-2 *(a)* Buccal bone resorption does not justify implant placement with severe lingual angulation (ie, greater than 15 degrees), which potentially leads to many problems. *(b and c)* The appropriate solution is ridge augmentation using a bone grafting procedure to allow proper implant placement.

Off-axis loading

Potential biomechanical problems of an excessive lingual trajectory (see Fig 2-2a) include:

- Restoration fracture
- Retaining screw fracture
- Abutment fracture
- Implant body fracture
- Osseous destruction because of unfavorable loading
- Plaque accumulation under ridge lap pontics

Placement of an overly inclined implant is not an acceptable practice, especially for single-unit restorations. If it is not possible to place an implant with an angulation of 15 degrees or less, the treatment plan should be aborted and the implant placed in a different location, or implant placement should be delayed and the area grafted using techniques such as guided bone regeneration (GBR), block grafting (Fig 2-2b), or ridge splitting, to allow optimum buccolingual angulation (Fig 2-2c).

Mesiodistal angulation

Natural teeth are perpendicular to the *curve of Spee,* the anteroposterior curve formed by the cusp tips of the posterior teeth (Fig 2-3).

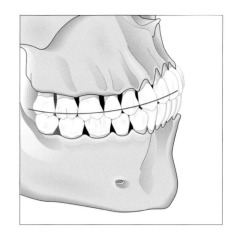

Fig 2-3 Curve of Spee.

Single implant cases

In single implant cases, excessive mesiodistal angulation should be avoided. The use of an angled abutment can compensate for slight inclinations (Fig 2-4); however, if the inclination is too severe, the implant should be removed and reinserted in a more upright position, either immediately or after a period of osseous healing.

To prevent excessive angulation, the surgeon should evaluate the position of the osteotomy after use of the pilot drill by placing a parallel pin in the pilot hole and taking a radiograph. If the angulation is not satisfactory, a Lindemann side-cutting drill can be used to adjust the angulation before continuing preparation of the implant site (Fig 2-5).

Fig 2-4 *(a to i)* The implant to replace the missing right lateral incisor was placed with imperfect angulation. However, the mesial inclination is mild, and the use of an angled abutment compensated for the inclination.

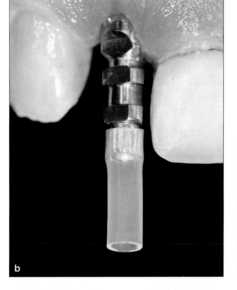

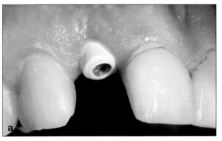
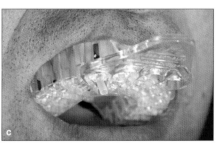

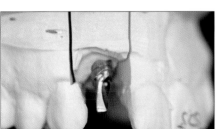
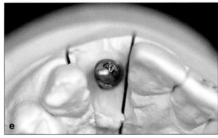
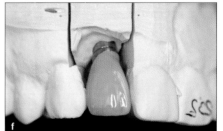

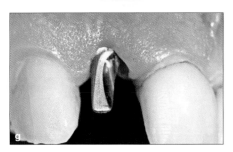
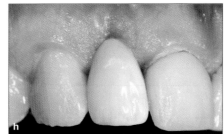
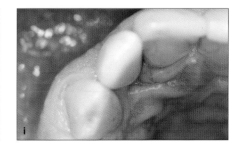

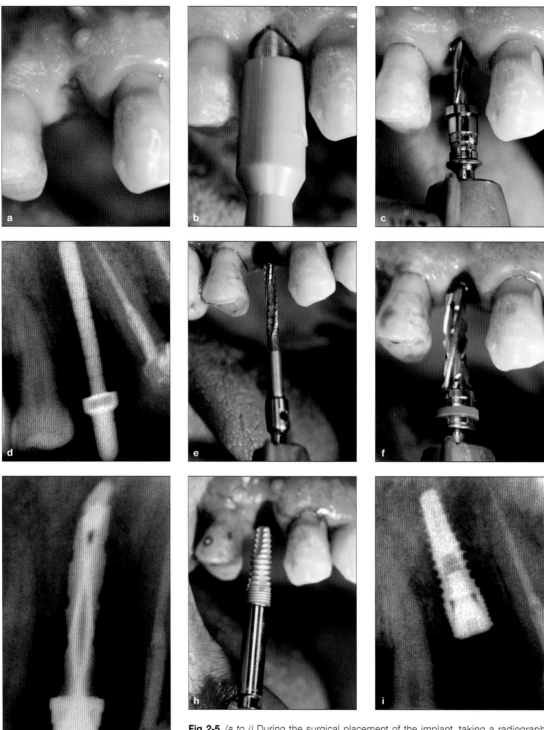

Fig 2-5 *(a to i)* During the surgical placement of the implant, taking a radiograph after the use of the pilot drill is highly recommended to check the angulation. If the angulation is incorrect, then at this point a Lindemann drill can easily be used to correct the osteotomy location and/or angulation. However, if the osteotomy has been enlarged to 3.5 mm or more in diameter, then changing its location and/or angulation will be more challenging and often mandates aborting the procedure. In such cases, bone grafting material should be placed, and implant placement can be attempted again in 2 to 4 months.

Multiple implant cases

In multiple implant cases, mesiodistal inclination has a lesser influence on occlusal load transfer to the implant and does not increase destructive forces because the prosthetic superstructure redirects occlusal forces. In fact, implant anchorage can sometimes be improved by intentional placement of an implant at a mesiodistal angulation that locates it in dense bone structure remote from the intended implant position. Survival of mesiodistally angulated implants in multiple im-

plant cases has been reported in the literature with success rates of 93% to 97.5%.[1-8]

In some cases, mesiodistally angulated implants can be an alternative to vertical ridge augmentation or sinus elevation surgery in patients with general or local contraindications to those procedures, such as medical issues, maxillary sinus pathology, or advanced age (Figs 2-6 and 2-7).

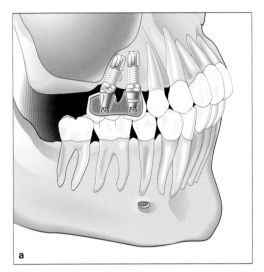 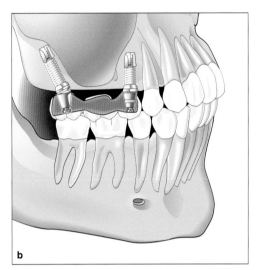

Fig 2-6 *(a and b)* Inclining the distal implant avoided the need for sinus elevation surgery, extended the prosthesis distally without the need for a cantilever, and prevented the hypereruption of the mandibular teeth opposing the maxillary edentulous area. However, it is important to note that in both scenarios it is a multi-unit, not single, implant prosthesis.

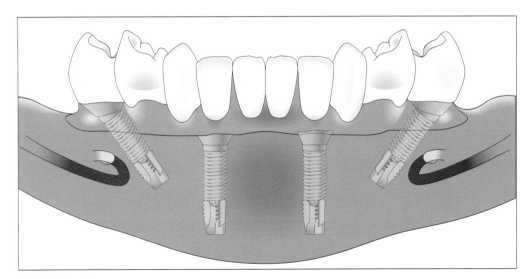

Fig 2-7 Inclining the distal implants avoided the need for vertical ridge augmentation in the posterior mandible and extended the prosthesis distally without a cantilevered section. This is a valid concept if the superstructure connects an adequate number of implants.

Malalignment

To help prevent malalignment, parallel pins can be used intraoperatively to confirm the orientation of the osteotomy, align implants to each other, and align implants to natural teeth. Pins can be placed into pilot holes or screwed onto the implants.

When multiple implants are to be placed, a pin can be placed in the first pilot hole and a radiograph taken to verify its position and angulation. If satisfactory, the pilot drill can be aligned parallel to the pin and the next pilot hole drilled. This procedure can be repeated as necessary (Fig 2-8). When the edentulous area has an adjacent natural tooth, the first pilot hole can be aligned to the long axis of its root (Fig 2-9).

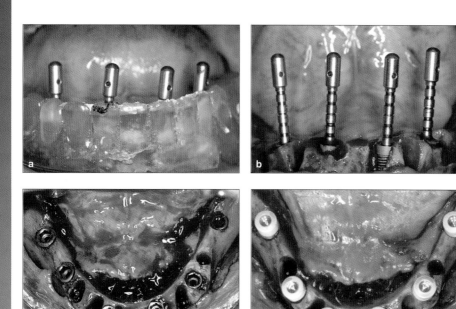

Fig 2-8 *(a to d)* Parallel pins are used to evaluate the implant osteotomy angulations, to parallel the implants to each other and to the natural teeth (if any), and to visualize the direction of the forces of occlusion.

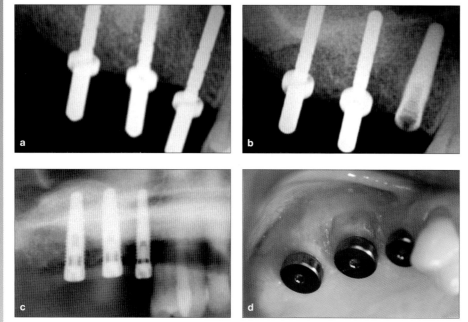

Fig 2-9 *(a to d)* The use of parallel pins in this clinical case enabled the placement of implants that are perfectly aligned to the adjacent natural tooth and to each other.

COMPLICATION 8 | Nerve Injury

Nerve injury can occur at any stage of implant surgery. Nerves can be penetrated by the local anesthetic needle, lacerated by the scalpel during incision, stretched during flap reflection, damaged by osteotomy drills, or compressed during implant insertion.

Classification of nerve injury

In 1994, Day[9] described three degrees of nerve injury:

- *Neuropraxia*: Mild injury caused by compression or prolonged traction of the nerve that results in loss of sensation. Axons remain intact, and sensation typically returns within 4 weeks after surgery.
- *Axonotmesis*: Severe compression or traction that damages the axon by edema, ischemia, or demyelination. There is a certain amount of damage to some axons, but the nerve structure itself remains intact. Partial sensation returns in 5 to 11 weeks, and sensation continues to improve over the following 10 months.
- *Neurotmesis*: Loss of continuity of the axon and its encapsulating structures. Repair requires microsurgery, and typically the prognosis for full recovery is poor.

Symptoms of nerve injury

Symptoms of nerve injury fall into the following classifications:

- *Paresthesia*: abnormal sensation
- *Hypoesthesia*: reduced feeling
- *Hyperesthesia*: increased sensitivity
- *Dysesthesia*: unpleasant (painful) sensation
- *Anesthesia*: complete loss of sensation

Spontaneous return of normal sensation after nerve injury depends on both the severity of the injury and the nerve involved. For example, a partial injury or transection involving the inferior alveolar nerve, with its bony canal to contain and direct regenerative fibers, is more likely to result in a spontaneous resolution of symptoms than a partial transection of the lingual nerve.

Prevention of nerve injury

Detailed knowledge of anatomy, careful treatment planning using computed tomography (CT) scan images and diagnostic wax-ups, surgical aids such as drill stoppers and computer-generated surgical guides, and careful manipulation of soft tissue can minimize the incidence of nerve injury. Dental specialists and general practitioners who place implants must discuss potential nerve injuries with patients and include this possibility on the consent form (see Appendix B). Specific recommendations for avoiding injury to the inferior alveolar, mental, mandibular incisive, lingual, and infraorbital nerves are provided in the following sections; in general, the implant surgeon should use common sense and avoid implant placement in areas with a high potential for injury.

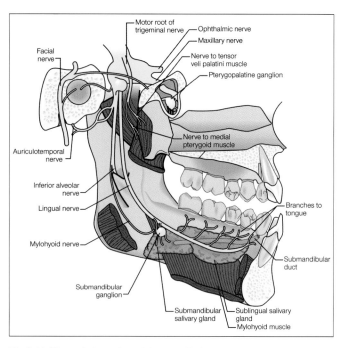

Fig 2-10 The main branches of the mandibular nerve.

Inferior alveolar nerve

The *inferior alveolar nerve* is a branch of the mandibular nerve, which is the third branch of the trigeminal nerve arising from the trigeminal ganglion. Unlike the other two branches (the maxillary and ophthalmic nerves), which are completely sensory, the mandibular nerve has both sensory and motor divisions.[10]

After passing through the foramen ovale and after giving off a meningeal branch, the mandibular nerve divides within the infratemporal fossa into sensory branches (auriculotemporal, lingual, inferior alveolar, and buccal nerves) and motor branches that innervate the muscles of mastication (masseteric, deep temporal, and pterygoid nerves) (Fig 2-10).

The inferior alveolar nerve carries motor fibers for the mylohyoid muscle and the anterior belly of the digastric muscle and sensory fibers that enter the mandibular canal through the mandibular foramen. There, it supplies the mandibular teeth with sensory branches called the *inferior dental nerves*. Anteriorly, the inferior alveolar nerve exits the canal through the mental foramen as the mental nerve. Damage to the inferior alveolar nerve will also alter sensation to areas supplied by the mental nerve.

Injury prevention

The following steps should be taken to minimize the possibility of injury to the inferior alveolar nerve:

- Use of CT scan images to determine the exact distance between the superior border of the inferior alveolar canal and the crestal bone at the planned implant site
- Maintenance of a 2-mm margin of safety between the apical end of the implant and the superior border of the inferior alveolar canal[11]

- Use of drill stoppers when possible to prevent overpenetration of the drill (Fig 2-11)
- Use of a computer-generated surgical guide such as a SurgiGuide (Materialise) to place implants in the safest and most accurate manner possible
- Compensation for the slight additional length of the drill (the drills for most implant systems are approximately 0.5 to 1.0 mm longer than the implant being placed), especially when drilling near vital anatomical structures (Fig 2-12)

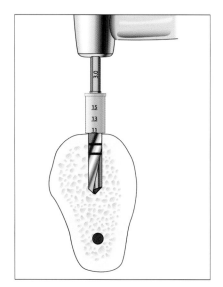

Fig 2-11 Drill stoppers prevent overpenetration of the drill.

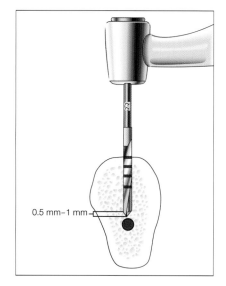

Fig 2-12 The drills for most implant systems are approximately 0.5 to 1.0 mm longer than the implant being placed. The operator should take this into consideration when drilling in close proximity to vital anatomical landmarks.

Mental nerve

The *mental nerve* exits the body of the mandible through the mental foramen, usually between the apices of the first and second mandibular premolars. It provides sensation to the chin, lower lip, labial gingiva of the mandibular anterior teeth, and skin over the mandibular body.

The position of the mental foramen can safely be used as an indicator of available bone height because the inferior alveolar nerve generally rises prior to approaching the mental foramen from the molar region. An implant placed level with the superior border of the mental foramen as it appears on a panoramic radiograph would be in reality lingual to the nerve (Fig 2-13).

It is important for clinicians to be aware of the anterior loop of the mental nerve, which traverses inferiorly and anteriorly to the mental foramen before turning back to exit the foramen.[12] The nerve may be found anterior to the mental foramen by as much as 3 mm.[13] If an implant is planned mesial and inferior to the foramen, its most posterior extent should be at least 5 mm anterior to the mesial aspect of the foramen (ie, 3 mm to allow for the mental loop plus 2 mm as a safety margin).

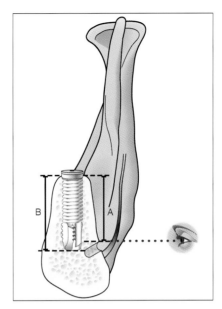

Fig 2-13 Distance A is the height of the available bone as seen on a panoramic radiograph. However, in reality (and as can be seen on a cross-sectional CT view), the actual distance (B) is greater because the inferior alveolar nerve rises as it approaches the mental foramen (compared with its height in the molar region).

Injury prevention

Several important surgical considerations will prevent damage to the mental nerve:

- The pilot drill should penetrate crestal bone 7 to 8 mm anterior to the most mesial aspect of the mental foramen to avoid drill penetration though the anterior loop (3-mm anterior loop + 2-mm safety zone + the implant radius) (Fig 2-14).
- Flap-releasing incisions mesial to the mental nerve should terminate just superior to the mucogingival junction.

- In a mandible with extensive resorption, the mental foramen may be located on the crest of the ridge. When that happens, the crestal incision should be placed toward the lingual (Fig 2-15) and the full-thickness flap carefully reflected until the foramen is identified. In some situations, a *flapless insertion protocol* should be followed to avoid damaging the mental nerve and its branches (see complication 10).

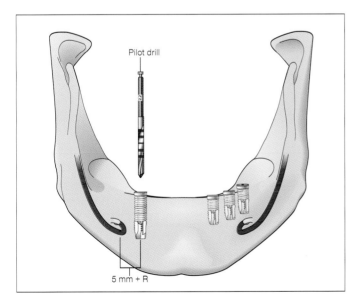

Fig 2-14 Implants can be placed anywhere mesial to the mental foramen as long as they are placed above its level. However, if implants are placed mesial to the mental foramen and below its level, then the pilot hole (ie, the center of the implant) should be located no less than 7 mm from the most mesial border of the mental foramen (3-mm anterior loop of the mental nerve + 2-mm safety margin + the radius of the implant (R) = 7 mm or more).

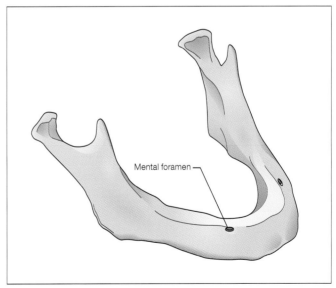

Fig 2-15 In a severely resorbed mandible, the mental foramen may be located on the crestal ridge. This should be taken into consideration if a midcrestal incision is to be made.

Mandibular incisive canal and nerve

The inferior alveolar nerve splits,[14] typically in the vicinity of the molars, into the mental nerve (to supply the skin of the mental foraminal region, the lower lip, the mucous membrane, and the gingiva) and the *incisive nerves* (to supply the mandibular anterior teeth). However, in some cases, the incisive nerve might present as a true canal with large lumen (0.48 to 2.90 mm),[15] extending anteriorly and inferiorly from the mental foramen, usually 8 to 10 mm from the lower border of the mandible. The incisive canal cannot be detected clearly on conventional radiographs; therefore, CT scans are recommended for proper assessment (Fig 2-16).

The existence of this canal can be problematic for the implant surgeon because, as an extension of the inferior alveolar nerve, it should be considered to contain the same neurovascular elements.[16] Osteotomies that would traverse this canal therefore must be avoided. Note that the position of the incisive canal, if present, will be closer to the alveolar crest in a resorbed mandible.

Injury prevention

The incisive canal must be taken into consideration when treatment planning implants in the intraforaminal zone.[17]

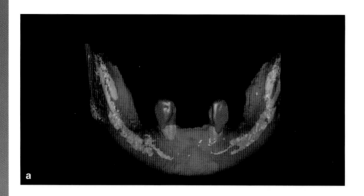

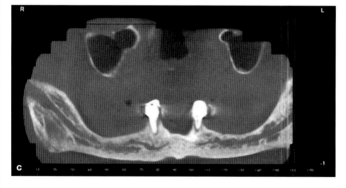

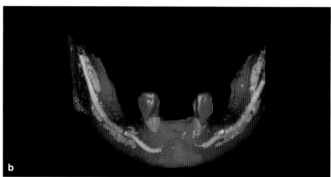

Fig 2-16 Three-dimensional *(a and b)* and panoramic *(c)* CT images of the mandibular incisive canal. Note the continuation of the inferior alveolar canal into the anterior mandible.

Lingual nerve

The *lingual nerve*, a branch of the mandibular nerve, descends to the base of the tongue just anterior and slightly medial to the inferior alveolar nerve[18] (see Fig 2-10) and supplies sensory innervation to the anterior two-thirds of the tongue. The lingual nerve receives taste fibers from the *chorda tympani*, a branch of the facial nerve.[19] It is anesthetized during the inferior alveolar nerve block.

The lingual nerve is typically located immediately medial to the lingual cortical plate of the mandible, below the crest of the ridge and posterior to the third molar roots. It is covered in this area by a thin layer of oral mucosa and may be visible clinically. Dental procedures in this region risk damage to this nerve. In a magnetic resonance study, Miloro and colleagues[20] found that the nerve crosses over the retromolar pad in 10% of patients, leading to a higher risk of traumatization during flap elevation, retraction, and suturing.

Injury prevention

Transecting the lingual nerve will anesthetize the tongue, decrease saliva flow from the submandibular gland, and affect taste. This can be avoided by:

- Placement of the distal releasing incision at 30 degrees toward the buccal in the retromolar pad area to avoid transecting the lingual nerve in case it crosses the retromolar pad
- Careful and gentle reflection of the lingual flap in the posterior mandibular region
- Avoidance of lingual releasing incisions[21]

Infraorbital nerve

The *infraorbital nerve* is a branch of the maxillary nerve, which is the second branch of the trigeminal nerve arising from the trigeminal ganglion. After giving off a meningeal branch, the maxillary nerve passes through the foramen rotundum into the pterygopalatine fossa, where it divides into the zygomatic nerve, the pterygopalatine nerves, and the infraorbital nerve.

The infraorbital nerve passes through the infraorbital fissure into the orbit and through the infraorbital canal to the cheek, where it innervates the skin between the lower eyelid and the upper lip. It gives off the posterior superior alveolar nerves to the maxillary molars, the medial superior alveolar nerves to the maxillary premolars, and the anterior superior alveolar nerve to the maxillary canines and incisors.[22]

Injury prevention

This nerve can be damaged during flap reflection for a lateral window sinus elevation procedure or for implant placement in the anterior area of a highly resorbed maxilla. Chances of damaging the infraorbital nerve can be minimized by the following:

- A three-dimensional CT scan of the infraorbital foramen prior to surgery
- Flap reflection that remains inferior to the infraorbital foramen
- Gentle management of soft tissue
- Careful use of retractors to avoid encroaching on the nerve

Management of nerve injuries

If there is a concern that nerve damage has occurred during implant placement, the situation should be assessed soon after the injury. First, a CT scan should be obtained to determine if the altered sensation is due to impingement by the implant or is the sequela of soft tissue manipulation and edema. If the implant itself appears to be the cause of altered sensation, it should be removed. If, however, the problem is pressure on the nerve because of bony compression by the implant, it may be relieved by withdrawing the implant 1 to 2 mm. Because altered sensation can be caused by an inflammatory reaction, a 3-week course of a steroidal or nonsteroidal anti-inflammatory drug such as 800-mg ibuprofen may be merited.[23] If improvement is noted, the clinician can prescribe an additional 3 weeks of anti-inflammatory treatment.

Medicolegally, it is important to document the patient's level of dysfunction postinjury, preferably the day after surgery when the effects of the anesthetic have worn off. The area of decreased or altered sensation should be outlined and described in detail, including its type and duration and suspected factors (eg, anesthesia, flap reflection, compression from implant placement). If a lingual nerve injury is suspected, taste sensation can be tested with salt and sugar. In suspected inferior alveolar and mental nerve injuries, sensitivity of the lip and gingiva can be tested with a cotton swab, thermal sensitivity with ice and a warmed mirror handle, and ability to distinguish direction of movement with a soft brush on the lip and chin with eyes closed. The examination should be repeated after 1 month. At this time, complete loss of sensation, diminishing sensation, or spontaneous pain are signs that normal sensation is unlikely to return spontaneously. Prompt referral to a microneurosurgeon is indicated. If improvement is noted at follow-up appointments, more time for spontaneous resolution—up to 4 months—can be allowed prior to surgical intervention.

The goal of early referral is to allow the patient to undergo nerve repair within 4 months of the injury, thereby minimizing distal degeneration of the nerve.[24] Robinson and colleagues[25] studied 53 patients who underwent lingual nerve repair. They reported that patients generally considered the procedure to be worthwhile, as indicated by a mean score of 7 on a scale from 0 (no change) to 10 (normal nerve function).

In all cases of suspected nerve injury, the malpractice insurance provider should be notified for guidance.

| COMPLICATION 9 | Irregular or Narrow Alveolar Crest |

After flap reflection, the clinician may discover that the alveolar crest form is irregular, sharp, or overly narrow. Alveoloplasty is recommended prior to the placement of implants to create a smoother ridge with a wider plateau that will better accommodate the planned implants.

However, in some cases, alveoloplasty does not achieve the desired ridge form because the entire residual ridge, not just the crest, is narrow (Fig 2-17a). A ridge with a pyramidal configuration on the cross-section CT image will gain crestal width with alveoloplasty (Fig 2-17b).

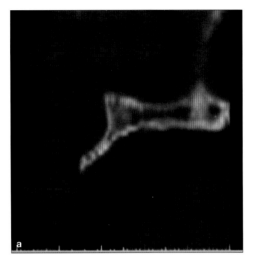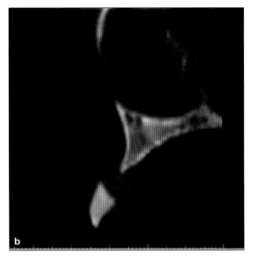

Fig 2-17 *(a)* Cross-sectional CT scan of an anterior maxilla with advanced resorption in which alveoloplasty would not be beneficial in gaining more crestal bone width for implant insertion. *(b)* A pyramid-shaped ridge in which alveoloplasty will create more crestal width for implant insertion.

Procedure

- CT scans should be taken before alveoloplasty *(1)* to determine whether the procedure is indicated and likely to be beneficial for a particular case and *(2)* to confirm that following the alveoloplasty there will be good clearance for the implants (based on anatomical landmarks).
- The flap should be adequately reflected both buccally and lingually to appreciate the full width of the ridge crest (Fig 2-18a).

- Bone removal should be kept to a minimum because loss of ridge height may present problems, including limitations on implant length and proximity of implants to anatomical structures such as the sinus floor, nasal floor, or inferior alveolar canal; it also may lead to excessive height of the restoration (Fig 2-18b).

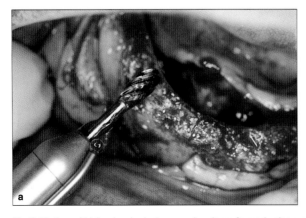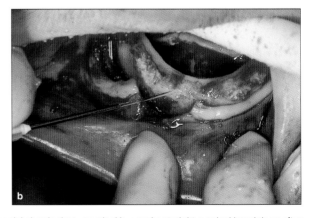

Fig 2-18 *(a and b)* An alveoloplasty procedure is performed using a special alveoloplasty surgical bur and a straight surgical handpiece after an adequate full-thickness flap has been reflected.

Tools and technique

The use of oval or round alveoloplasty burs on a straight surgical handpiece at 40,000 rpm with copious irrigation is recommended (Figs 2-19 and 2-20). Figure 2-21 shows an alveoloplasty procedure after full-arch extractions prior to immediate implant placement.

When osseous recontouring of the alveolar ridge is undesirable because the ridge is uniformly narrow or remaining bone height is crucial, the implant platform should be placed at the highest point of the ridge (Fig 2-22). If implant threads are exposed as a result of this technique, they may be addressed with GBR or covered with soft tissue if it is sufficiently thick. Positioning the implant platform lower than any part of the crestal bone will create challenges with the placement of the healing abutment, impression coping, and definitive prosthesis and may result in the formation of deep pockets, which will complicate hygiene.

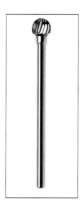

Fig 2-19 Alveoloplasty surgical bur.

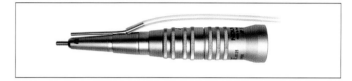

Fig 2-20 Straight surgical handpiece.

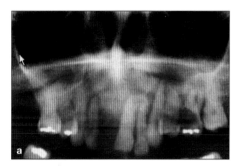
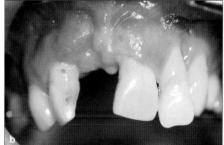
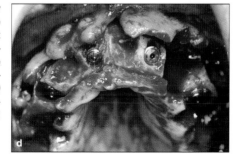
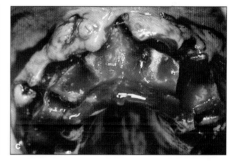
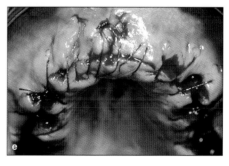

Fig 2-21 Alveoloplasty is performed immediately following full-arch tooth extraction to smooth the crestal bone and reduce the alveolar ridge height for bar overdenture implant placement. (a) Preoperative panoramic radiograph. (b) Preoperative clinical view. (c) Extraction and alveoloplasty is performed to reduce and smooth the alveolar ridge. (d) Implants are placed for the bar overdenture prosthesis. (e) A continuous suturing technique is used to close the flap.

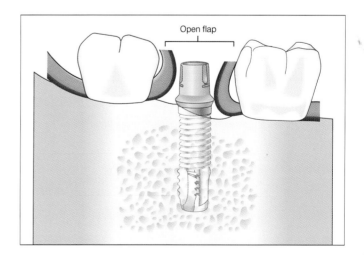

Fig 2-22 In single implant placement, if ridge recontouring is not desired (to avoid creating a deep pocket), then the implant platform should be placed at the highest crestal bone level.

Extensive Resorption of the Mandible

As noted in complication 8, the mental foramen may be positioned on the crest of the ridge in a severely resorbed mandible. Care should be taken to protect the mental nerve by placing the crestal incision lingually; however, if the resorption is extensive and the mental foramina cannot be clearly identified on the panoramic radiograph or CT scan, a flapless implant insertion protocol is recommended to avoid damage to the mental nerve or any of its branches. This technique is shown in Fig 2-23.

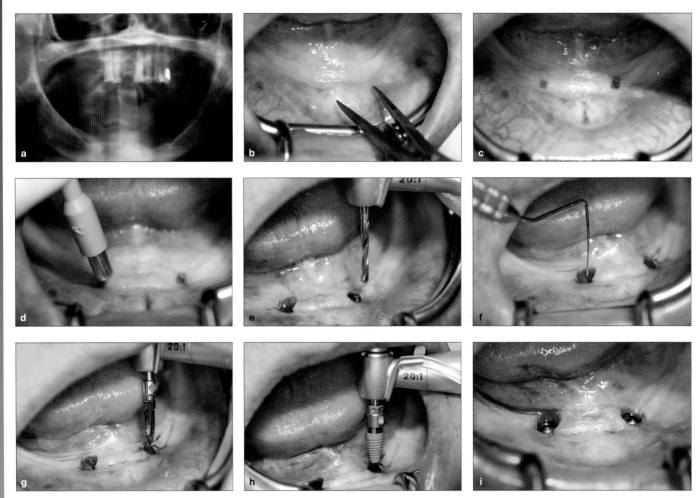

Fig 2-23 *(a)* The panoramic radiograph did not reveal the exact location of the mental foramina in this case. A decision was made to place the implants using a flapless insertion protocol to avoid transecting the mental nerve during incision. *(b and c)* The alveolar bone within 12 mm on each side of the midline was established as a low-risk area for implant placement. *(d)* A disposable tissue punch was used to access the crestal bone. *(e)* A 2.0-mm pilot drill is used to initiate the implant osteotomies. *(f)* After the use of each drill, a periodontal probe was used to verify that the osteotomy was completely within the alveolar ridge. *(g)* The implant osteotomy was enlarged as needed. *(h)* The implants were placed. *(i)* Healing screws are placed for the two-stage insertion protocol. The patient was treatment planned for a ball-retained overdenture after excessive vertical restorative space was identified. O-ring caps were incorporated into the denture to disengage the ball attachments before vertical cantilever forces became excessive.

Curved Extraction Socket

It is challenging to place an immediate implant in an ideal position into a socket after extracting a tooth with significant root curvature (Fig 2-24a). The thick palatal or lingual wall of the socket tends to direct the rotating drill toward the thinner buccal plate, placing the osteotomy and, subsequently, the implant in an unfavorable and unesthetic location. Perforation of the buccal wall of the socket may also result.

This difficulty can be overcome using a Lindemann side-cutting drill (Fig 2-24b). The drill should be placed in the socket first, then the motor activated, and a groove cut in the lingual socket wall (Figs 2-24c), facilitating movement of the subsequent implant drills in the appropriate direction for correct osteotomy positioning (Fig 2-24d). This technique is often necessary when placing immediate implants in maxillary anterior and mandibular premolar and anterior sites. Figure 2-25 shows a case of immediate implant surgery in a curved socket.

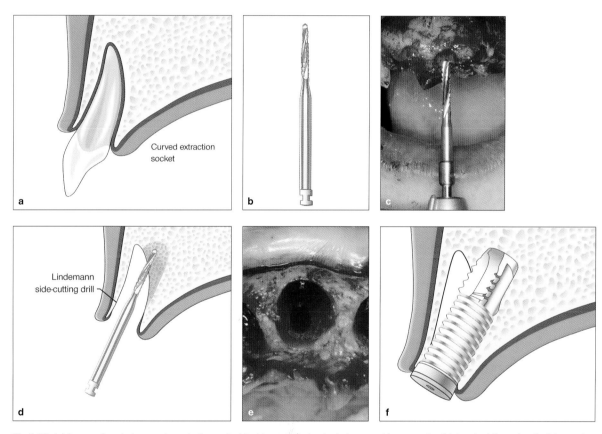

Fig 2-24 *(a)* A curved socket presents a challenge for ideal immediate implant placement because the thick palatal/lingual wall of the socket tends to redirect the drill toward the thin buccal plate. *(b and c)* The use of a Lindemann side-cutting drill enables the creation of a depression or groove in the palatal/lingual side. *(d)* Cross-sectional view of the redirection of the socket using the Lindemann drill. *(e)* Clinical view of the groove created by the Lindemann drill. *(f)* Placement of the implant in the proper direction in a curved socket.

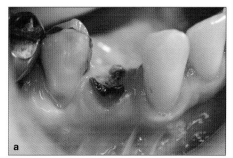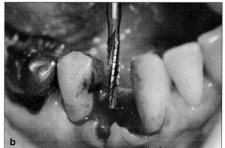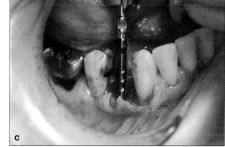

Figs 2-25a to 2-25c *(a)* Immediate implant surgery in a curved mandibular premolar socket. *(b)* A Lindemann drill was used to create a groove in the lingual surface of the alveolus. *(c)* Subsequent drills are used to further redirect the osteotomy from its natural path down the curved lingual wall of the socket, thus avoiding perforation of the buccal plate and misalignment of the implant.

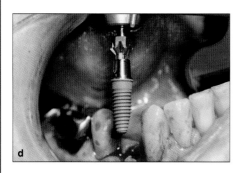
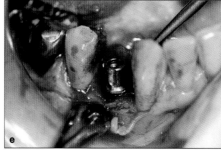
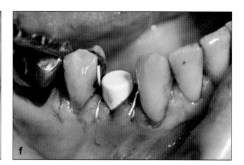

Figs 2-25d to 2-25f The implant is placed at the proper position and angulation.

Another way to manage a curved socket is to drill the pilot hole at a sharp angle into the lingual wall of the socket (Fig 2-26a). As site preparation proceeds apically and bur diameter increases, the severity of the entry angle into the lingual axial wall lessens and a straight osteotomy is created using apical and lateral pressure on the handpiece (Figs 2-26b to 2-26d). This technique is possible only in shallow sockets or those with a damaged buccal plate because a high, intact buccal plate will prohibit drilling at the required angle.

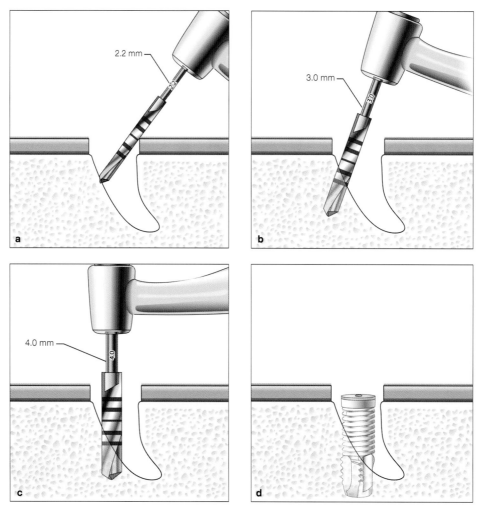

Fig 2-26 (a) In short sockets, an alternative to the use of a Lindemann drill is to start the osteotomy using a pilot drill at a sharp angle relative to the curvature of the palatal/lingual wall of the socket. (b) As the diameter of the drill increases, the severity of the drilling angle decreases. (c and d) The final drill and the implant are at the proper position and angulation in the curved socket.

COMPLICATION 12 | Injury to Adjacent Teeth During Implant Placement

Teeth adjacent to an implant site are at risk of intraoperative and postoperative damage. Placement of an implant too close to a tooth can impinge on its blood supply or overheat its surrounding bone during osteotomy preparation. In some cases, an adjacent tooth may become nonvital secondary to irreversible pulpal damage.[26-28] Endodontic therapy, apicoectomy, or extraction of the tooth and/or the implant may be necessary.

Symptoms

Patients may complain of severe pain, swelling, and thermal sensitivity after the implant is placed. Symptoms might be immediate or delayed. Once a tooth becomes nonvital, it will react to percussion tests, but thermal and electric pulp testing will not elicit a response. The radiograph will reveal a radiolucency at the apex within a short period of time after the injury occurs.

Prevention

There are a few measures that can be taken to help prevent damage to adjacent teeth during placement of implants:

- Careful space assessment of the edentulous area should be done before surgery using CT scan images. These images provide the implant surgeon with life-size, distortion-free images that allow precise measurements. The minimum recommended amount of bone between an implant and an adjacent tooth is 1 mm.
- If the space for the implant is too narrow mesiodistally, the patient should be referred for orthodontic treatment before attempting implant placement.

- It is also highly advisable to take a periapical radiograph with a parallel pin in the osteotomy immediately after drilling the pilot hole (Fig 2-27). At this point the diameter of the osteotomy is still small, ie, 2 mm or less, and adjusting its angulation will not present a challenge.
- Finally, computer-generated surgical guides should be used to direct the osteotomies when teeth are in close proximity to the planned implants.

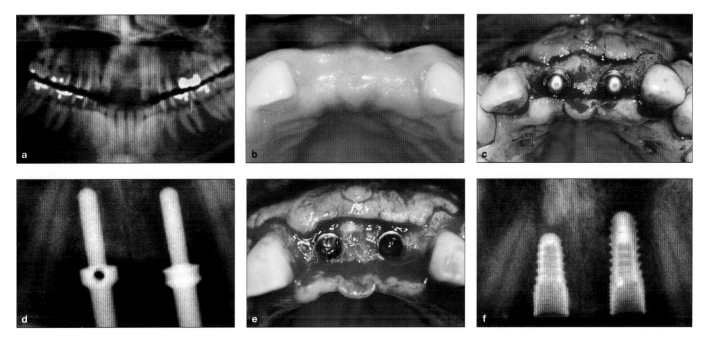

Fig 2-27 *(a)* A panoramic radiograph revealing the inclined root of the maxillary right lateral incisor. *(b)* Occlusal view of the maxillary central incisor area before surgery. *(c)* Occlusal view after drilling of pilot holes with parallel pins in place. *(d)* Periapical radiograph with parallel pins in the pilot holes shows the proximity of the pin to the root. *(e and f)* A shorter implant was placed in the right central incisor site to avoid any damage to the adjacent lateral incisor.

Management

Intraoperative

After assessing the position of the parallel pin in the pilot hole, if injury to an adjacent tooth appears imminent, the osteotomy can be redirected without difficulty using a side-cutting drill such as the Lindemann drill. If the osteotomy is enlarged well beyond the pilot hole and its direction is not satisfactory, implant placement must be delayed and bone grafting in the osteotomy site carried out instead.

Postoperative

If pulpal damage is suspected after implant placement, administration of systemic antibiotics along with endodontic therapy should be initiated immediately. Also, the implant should be removed if it appears to have penetrated the root of the affected tooth because serious injury to adjacent teeth may be critical to the fate of the implant as well. Development of an abscess can affect the osseointegration of an implant placed in close proximity to natural teeth.

| COMPLICATION 13 |

Preoperative Acute and Chronic Infections at the Implant Site

Acute infection

Any acute infection at or in close proximity to the planned implant site must be treated and implant placement delayed for 2 to 4 months (Fig 2-28). Symptoms of acute infection include tenderness, redness, swelling, suppuration, and the possibility of the presence of a fistula (see Fig 2-28b).

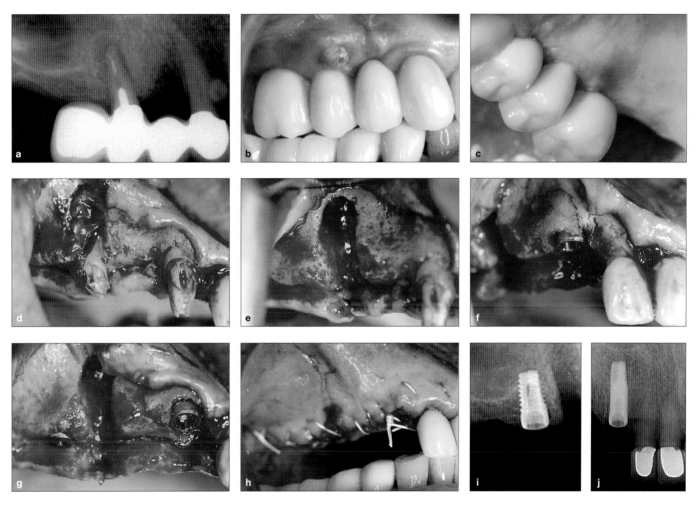

Fig 2-28 Radiograph *(a)* and clinical views *(b and c)* reveal the existence of an acute infection at the first premolar site. After tooth extraction and the debridement of the lesion *(d and e)*, collagen dressing was placed in the acute infection site and two implants were placed in the first molar and canine sites *(f and g)* for an implant-supported three-unit fixed prosthesis. The incision was sutured using polytetrafluoroethylene (PTFE) suture material *(h)*. Postoperative radiographs show the location of the implants in the first molar *(i)* and canine *(j)* sites.

Chronic infection

Chronic dentoalveolar infections include combined periodontal-endodontic lesions, chronic periodontal disease, periodontal cysts, and chronic periapical lesions, among others. Placement of implants to replace teeth with chronic asymptomatic periapical lesions presents a risk of contamination of the implant site by the bacteria of the periapical pathosis, providing an environment for a delayed *implant periapical lesion* (IPL), also referred to as *retrograde peri-implantitis* (see complication 38, part 3). Nevertheless, implant therapy is a viable treatment option if complete removal of the lesion and infected tissues is achieved (Fig 2-29).

Currently, the literature supports the successful placement of implants at the time of extraction in periapical lesion sites if the infection is removed and primary stability of the implant is achieved. Note, however, that after debridement of the infected tissues from the socket, placement of an implant in ideal position with an optimal amount of torque may be difficult. In this case, the socket should be grafted and implant placement delayed by 2 to 4 months. Lindeboom et al[29] reported a survival rate of 92% for implants immediately placed in sites with chronic periapical lesions. Novaes et al[30,31] concluded that periapical pathosis is not a contraindication to immediate implant placement if the socket is debrided and disinfected effectively. Following a strict pre- and postoperative protocol of antibiotic administration, meticulous cleaning and complete alveolar debridement before implant insertion will ensure the best chance of successful osseointegration.

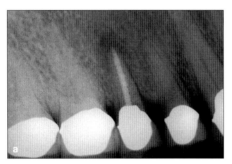 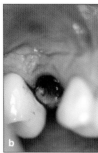 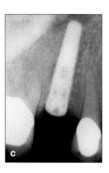

Fig 2-29 *(a and b)* A case of immediate implant placement after extraction of a tooth with a chronic periapical lesion. Debridement of the surgical area was done without the need for flap reflection and secondary surgical access. *(c)* The 6-month postoperative radiograph shows a satisfactory result.

Technique

After extraction of the hopeless teeth, the infected socket should be debrided with small surgical curettes that can reach the apex of the socket and copious irrigation. If necessary, secondary surgical access can be created at the socket apical level for meticulous debridement of the periapical lesion (Fig 2-30). This step has the added benefit of allowing better visualization during placement of the implant and/or bone grafting material. GBR is often necessary to augment the bone at the surgical access site (using bone graft material and a resorbable membrane).[32] Pre- and postsurgical systemic antibiotic therapy is recommended.

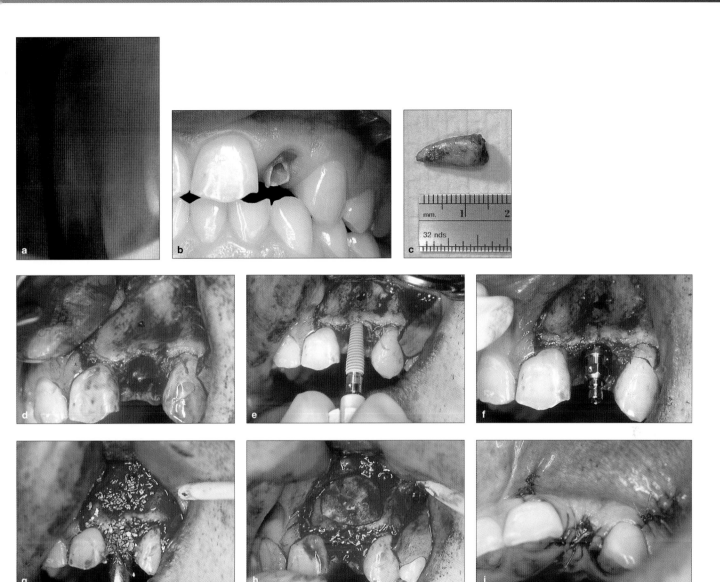

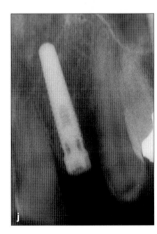

Fig 2-30 *(a to c)* A case of immediate implant placement after extraction of a tooth with a chronic periapical lesion. *(d)* The fenestration in the buccal plate was created to assure meticulous debridement. *(e and f)* The implant was placed with satisfactory angulation, depth, and torque. *(g to i)* GBR was performed with Bio-Oss bone grafting material (Geistlich) and a Bio-Gide membrane (Geistlich). *(j)* The 8-month postoperative radiograph shows an absence of lesions at the apex of the implant.

| COMPLICATION 14 | Retained Root Tips in the Implant Site |

A retained root tip at the implant site may serve as a source of infection, which may lead to an IPL or retrograde peri-implantitis.[33] Unintentional placement of dental implants in contact with retained root fragments can lead to inflammation and the subsequent need for the removal of the root fragment along with the affected implant due to peri-implantitis.[34]

However, some studies have reported an absence of inflammation, presence of cementum on the retained root surface, and functionally oriented periodontal ligament extending from the root to the implant in such cases. For example, in an animal study by Gray and Vernino,[35] several implants were unintentionally placed into root fragments. Some implants were in direct contact with the root fragments; others were in close proximity but not in direct contact. Histologic examination did not reveal inflammation at any site. Where the implant was in direct contact with a periodontal ligament, fibrous encapsulation of the implant was not observed. However, it appeared that calcified material was deposited on the implants in some areas (Fig 2-31). In a study by Buser et al,[36,37] titanium implants were placed in the mandibles of monkeys with retained apical root fragments. Histologic examination of implants in close relationship to root fragments revealed a cementum layer on the implant surface and collagen fibers inserted into the cementum and opposing bone.

These studies should not be taken as a recommendation for root tip–implant contact. Implants should never intentionally be placed in contact with retained root tips. It is important to distinguish between the placement of implants in contact with nonvital root fragments and with the root of a vital tooth (see complication 12). The unfavorable consequences of the latter include endodontic therapy, apicoectomy, or the extraction of the involved teeth.

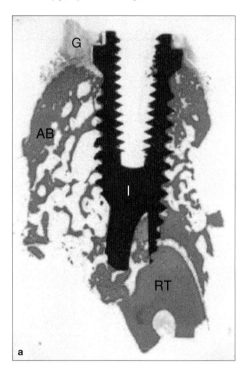
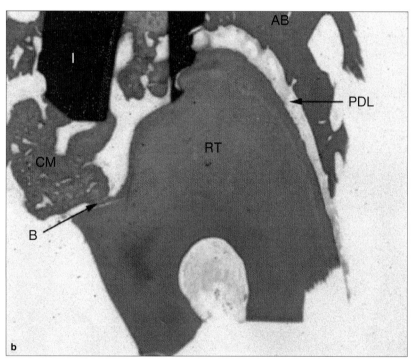

Fig 2-31 *(a)* Low-power view of an implant (I) placed into retained root fragments. G, gingiva; RT, root tip; AB, alveolar bone. *(b)* Higher-magnification view showing the periodontal ligament (PDL), a cementum-like material (CM), and a bridge (B) connecting the cementum-like material and the cementum on the root tip.

Prevention

If a retained root in the planned site is suspected prior to implant placement, a CT scan should be obtained to identify its exact location and size, and root tip removal followed by GBR should be performed. Implant placement can proceed 2 to 4 months after the removal of the retained root tip. In some cases, simultaneous implant placement with the removal of the retained root fragments can be achieved (Fig 2-32).

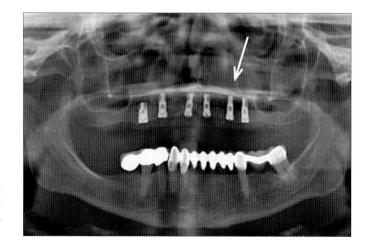

Fig 2-32 A 1-year postoperative panoramic CT image of six implants placed in the maxilla. The fixture replacing the left first premolar *(arrow)* was placed simultaneously with the removal of a root fragment. The area was asymptomatic 1 year postsurgery.

Management

If a root tip adjacent to an implant is discovered postoperatively, the implant should be observed for possible inflammatory reactions (IPL or peri-implantitis), and one or more of the treatment protocols below should be followed:

- Systemic antibiotic therapy to eliminate inflammation and infection
- Surgical retrieval of the root fragment together with the implant

- Surgical retrieval of the retained root fragment, excision of infected tissues, and GBR in the bony defect (Fig 2-33)
- Surgical retrieval of the retained root fragment and the implant followed by placement of a wide-body implant with demineralized freeze-dried bone allograft mixed with tetracycline

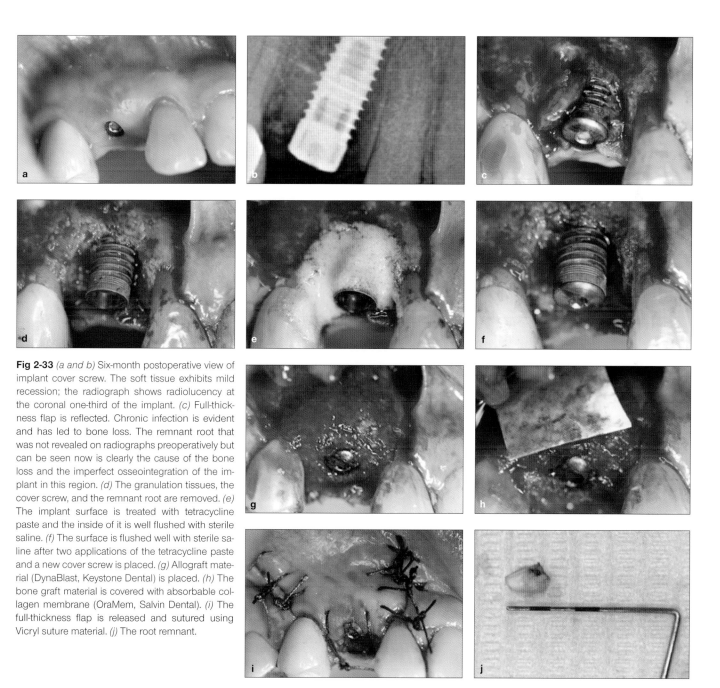

Fig 2-33 *(a and b)* Six-month postoperative view of implant cover screw. The soft tissue exhibits mild recession; the radiograph shows radiolucency at the coronal one-third of the implant. *(c)* Full-thickness flap is reflected. Chronic infection is evident and has led to bone loss. The remnant root that was not revealed on radiographs preoperatively but can be seen now is clearly the cause of the bone loss and the imperfect osseointegration of the implant in this region. *(d)* The granulation tissues, the cover screw, and the remnant root are removed. *(e)* The implant surface is treated with tetracycline paste and the inside of it is well flushed with sterile saline. *(f)* The surface is flushed well with sterile saline after two applications of the tetracycline paste and a new cover screw is placed. *(g)* Allograft material (DynaBlast, Keystone Dental) is placed. *(h)* The bone graft material is covered with absorbable collagen membrane (OraMem, Salvin Dental). *(i)* The full-thickness flap is released and sutured using Vicryl suture material. *(j)* The root remnant.

COMPLICATION 15 | Bleeding

Prevention

Medical history

When planning an implant surgical procedure, the first task should always be a thorough review of the patient's medical history. This crucial step will almost always reveal the presence of any medical complications and contraindications to surgery. It is the best prevention for bleeding problems. Key questions to ask the patient are:

- Have you had any bleeding problems in the past?
- Is there a history of bleeding problems in your family?
- Do you have hypertension and, if so, are you taking medications for it?
- Do you have a history of nonalcoholic liver disease?
- Do you consume alcohol or take any medication that could interfere with normal coagulation, such as aspirin, anticoagulants, broad spectrum antibiotics, or anticancer drugs?

If the patient gives an affirmative response to any of the above questions, one or more of the following steps should be taken:

- Consult the patient's primary physician.
- Direct the patient to stop consuming alcohol and/or taking medications that may interfere with coagulation 1 to 2 days before surgery because these substances predispose the patient to development of serious bleeding from minimal trauma.
- Request a *prothrombin time (PT)*. The PT is reported in two numbers: control time (usually 12 seconds) and patient test time. To have reasonably good hemostasis, the ratio of the patient's PT to the control PT should be 1.5 or less. Therefore, if the control is 12 seconds, the patient's PT should be no more than 18 seconds. If longer, consult with the patient's physician before performing any surgical procedures.

Radiographs

Careful review of adequate radiographs is another important factor in the prevention of bleeding complications. The radiographs must include the entire area of surgery, including the apices of the teeth to be extracted and all related anatomical structures, such as the inferior alveolar nerve, the mental foramina, and the maxillary sinuses. Intraoral and panoramic radiographs are adequate for the initial consultation; however, a CT scan is highly recommended before the implant surgery.

Management

The clinician must be aware of and prepared to address bleeding from soft tissue, bone, and arteries.

Soft tissue bleeding

The most common sign of bleeding into the soft tissues is a *contusion*, or bruise. Bruising appears as a result of intraoperative or postoperative bleeding into the soft tissue spaces, especially subcutaneous tissue spaces, adjacent to the surgical site. The likelihood and severity of bleeding are influenced by the patient's systemic health, the size of the flap, and the anatomy of the site. Bruises are named according to their diameter: *petechiae* (< 2 mm), *purpura* (2 to 10 mm), and *ecchymoses* (> 10 mm).[38]

Bruising may be limited to the site of the injury or extend to the inferior border of the mandible. Gravity may cause blood to travel under the skin along fascial planes to other locations, such as the chest (Fig 2-34). Such ecchymoses are often seen postsurgery in patients aged 50 and older when soft tissue flaps have been extensive. The patient should be informed that this sequela is not of concern and that it should resolve in 2 to 3 weeks. While bruises do not require therapy, the application of moist heat may hasten their resolution.

The following surgical techniques will minimize bleeding from soft tissue:

- Maintain clear visualization and access to the operative field with adequate lighting and suction.
- Avoid vertical releasing incisions when possible in favor of the envelope flap.
- Incise cleanly.
- Avoid crushing or tearing soft tissue.
- Smooth sharp bony areas.
- Eliminate granulation tissue.
- Identify and manage small bleeding soft tissue arteries.
- Place sufficient sutures.

To control soft tissue bleeding, the following techniques are effective:

- Ask the patient to bite on 2-inch gauze for 30 minutes.
- Control bleeding points with electrocautery.
- Apply direct pressure to bleeding vessels. If this is unsuccessful, clamp the vessel with a hemostat and ligate it with a resorbable suture soaked in hemostatic liquid such as Hemodent (Premier), ViscoStat (Ultradent), or Astringedent (Ultradent).

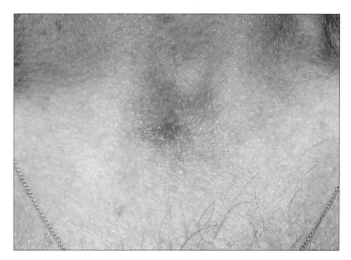

Fig 2-34 Ecchymosis extending to the chest area after extensive implant placement and bone grafting procedures.

Bony bleeding

Bleeding from an extraction socket
Bleeding from an extraction socket can be controlled by placing one of the following into the socket:

- Gelfoam absorbable gelatin (Pfizer)
- Surgicel oxidized regenerated cellulose (Ethicon)
- Topical bovine thrombin
- Avitene microfibrillar collagen (Davol)
- HeliPlug cross-linked collagen (Integra LifeSciences)

Bleeding from a bony artery
If the source of bleeding is a bony artery, or *nutrient canal*, there are three management options:

1. The adjacent bone can be crushed into the bleeding orifice with a ball burnisher or periosteal elevator.
2. Bone wax can be applied over the nutrient canal.
3. Electrocautery can be used.

Bleeding during osteotomy preparation
Bleeding during osteotomy preparation may be caused by injury to an artery within the bone. Usually placement of the implant will stop the bleeding. If the cause is an injury to the inferior alveolar artery, implant placement should be discontinued and iodoform gauze placed into the socket; pressure can be applied over it with a gauze pad. When bleeding is controlled, the soft tissue can be sutured over the iodoform gauze; the flaps will apply pressure. The patient should bite on gauze to place additional pressure on the site. The iodoform gauze can be removed after 5 to 7 days.

Arterial bleeding

The major arteries at risk for injury during implant placement are the greater palatine, incisive/nasopalatine (see complication 21), facial, lingual, sublingual, and submental arteries. Knowledge of their anatomy helps to avoid injury during surgery.

Arterial bleeding in the maxilla

Greater palatine artery

The maxillary artery enters the pterygopalatine fossa via the pterygomaxillary fissure approximately 16.6 mm above the nasal floor. The posterior superior alveolar artery, the infraorbital artery, and the descending palatine artery branch off from the portion of the maxillary artery that is in the fossa. The infraorbital artery gives off the anterior superior alveolar arteries after exiting the infraorbital foramen.

The descending palatine artery travels a short distance within the pterygopalatine fossa before entering the greater palatine canal, where it travels approximately 10 mm in an inferior, anterior, and slightly medial direction. Within the greater palatine canal, the lesser palatine arteries branch off to supply the soft palate and tonsils. The descending palatine artery exits the greater palatine foramen in the region of the second and third molars and runs across the hard palate to the incisive foramen, through which it enters the nasal cavity. The sphenopalatine artery, the terminal branch of the maxillary artery, passes through the sphenopalatine foramen to supply the lateral wall of the nose as the posterior lateral nasal artery. After crossing over the roof of the nasal cavity, its septal branches anastomose with branches of the greater palatine artery on the septum (Fig 2-35).

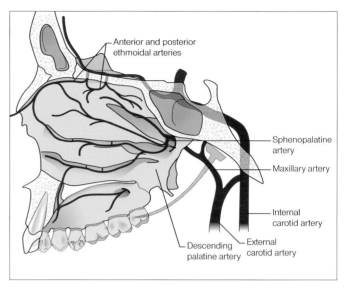

Fig 2-35 The sphenopalatine artery anastomoses with the greater palatine and the ethmoidal arteries.

When incising and reflecting a palatal flap in close proximity to the greater palatine artery, the tip of the periosteal elevator should be kept on bone at all times to prevent injury to this vessel. A study by Reiser et al[39] showed that, in patients with a high palatal vault, the greater palatine neurovascular bundle is located 17 mm from the palatal gingival margin; with a medium palatal vault, 12 mm; and with a low palatal vault, 7 mm.

Nasopalatine artery

Bleeding from the nasopalatine artery is included in the discussion of displacement of implants into the incisive canal (see complication 21).

Arterial bleeding in the mandible

Caution must be exercised when placing implants in the mandible because the floor of the mouth is highly vascularized. Perforation of the lingual cortical plate during osteotomy preparation can cause hemorrhaging that begins immediately following the vascular insult or some time after. Progressively expanding lingual, sublingual, submandibular, and submental hematomas can displace the tongue and the floor of the mouth and obstruct the airway.

Airway obstruction is a rare but potentially fatal complication of implant surgery. Detailed knowledge of regional arterial anatomy is imperative for the implant surgeon.

Anterior region of the mandible

Anatomical structures of the anterior floor of the mouth receive their blood supply from the *sublingual artery*, a branch of the lingual artery, and the *submental artery*, a branch of the facial artery (Fig 2-36).

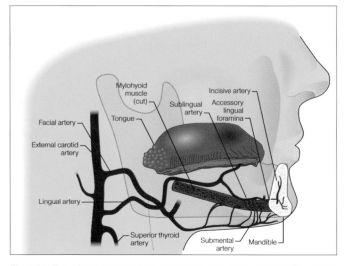

Fig 2-36 The blood supply of the anterior region of the floor of the mouth. Note the communication (anastomoses) between the submental arteries and the sublingual arteries through the mylohyoid muscle.

Lingual artery The lingual artery is one of the eight branches of the external carotid artery and arises at the level of the hyoid bone. It supplies the body and the apex of the tongue through the posterior lingual branches and its terminal branch, the *deep lingual artery*. The lingual artery gives rise to the sublingual artery at the anterior border of the hyoglossus muscle (Fig 2-37).

Sublingual artery The sublingual artery, with a mean diameter of 2 mm, supplies the sublingual salivary glands; the mylohyoid, geniohyoid, and genioglossus muscles; the mucous membranes of the floor of the mouth; and the lingual gingiva. Alveolar branches of the sublingual artery provide a complementary blood supply to the lingual anterior cortical plate of the mandible at the midline. These branches enter the cortical plate through various accessory lingual foramina. The incisive branches of the inferior alveolar artery are the primary blood supply of the mandibular symphysis.

Rosano et al[38] found that 95% of mandibles, upon dissection, had lingual foramina containing a clear vascular branch from the sublingual artery and established the proximity of these foramina to the lingual cortical plate of the mandibular midline in most cases. Their position in relation to the genial tubercles may vary and can be described as interspinal, superspinal, and subspinal.[40] Liang et al[41,42] classified lingual foramina into two groups: superior genial spinal foramina containing a vascular supply from the lingual artery and inferior genial spinal foramina containing branches from the sublingual and submental arteries. Other studies describe the existence of accessory foramina on the lingual side of the mandible in the premolar region near the inferior mandibular border[43] and near the crest of the alveolar ridge between the lateral incisors and the canines.[44]

The complementary blood supply provided by branches of the sublingual artery via the lingual foramina is especially important in edentulous mandibles. Arteriosclerotic changes of the inferior alveolar artery after tooth loss cause the blood circulation in the mandible to be increasingly dependent on the external blood supply provided by the periosteum and the accessory lingual canals. This should be taken into consideration when extensive reflection of lingual mucoperiosteal flaps is performed.[45,46]

Placing implants at the mandibular midline calls for careful planning because perforation of the lingual cortical plate presents a bleeding risk as a consequence of the close proximity of these vessels. The arteries associated with mandibular lingual foramina are of sufficient size to be implicated in severe hemorrhaging episodes after even a minor perforation during implant placement in this region.[47]

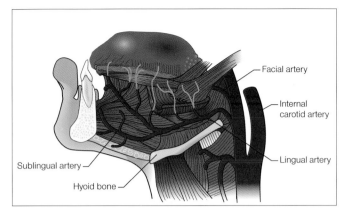

Fig 2-37 The lingual artery and its main branches. Note the proximity of the lingual artery to the hyoid bone.

Facial artery The facial artery arises from the external carotid artery superior to the lingual artery. It passes deep to the posterior belly of the digastric muscle and the stylohyoid muscle and enters a groove on the surface of the submandibular gland, which it supplies, before curving upward over the mandible at the anterior border of the masseter muscle. Its branches are the tonsillar and the lateral nasal branches and the ascending palatine, submandibular, submental, inferior labial, superior labial, and angular arteries.

Submental artery Before the facial artery crosses the border of the mandible, it gives rise to the submental artery, which courses anteriorly along the inferior border of the mylohyoid muscle together with the mylohyoid nerve. It supplies the submandibular lymph nodes, the submandibular salivary gland, and the mylohyoid and digastric muscles.

It is important to note that the sublingual and the submental arteries anastomose[48] through their respective mylohyoid branches. The sublingual artery is found on the superior aspect and the submental artery on the inferior aspect of the mylohyoid muscle (see Fig 2-36). Thus, it is a challenge to identify the source of bleeding from the floor of the mouth as the lingual artery or the facial artery. *Endovascular angiography* is a diagnostic tool that can help to define and isolate the source of bleeding.[49]

Posterior region of the mandible

In the posterior region of the mandible, the anatomy of the submandibular fossa (Fig 2-38), located below the mylohyoid muscle, should be assessed prior to implant surgery because a pronounced concavity of the fossa may lead to a perforation of the lingual plate during osteotomy preparation and the possibility of injuring a blood vessel located at the floor of the mouth.

The anatomy of the lingual aspect of the mandible cannot be observed on a panoramic radiograph (Fig 2-39); a CT scan is required for a thorough evaluation. Palpation is another valuable diagnostic tool.

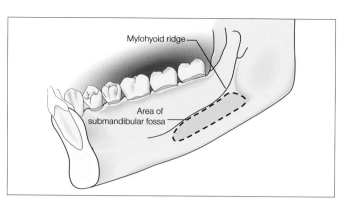

Fig 2-38 The size and depression severity of the submandibular fossa vary. It usually extends from distal of the first molar to distal of the third molar.

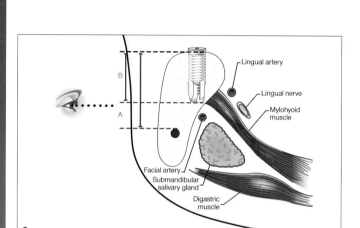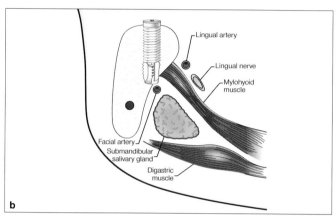

Fig 2-39 *(a)* The mylohyoid muscle will maintain the level of bone along its attachment on the medial aspect of the mandibular body. Frequently, the submandibular fossa below the mylohyoid muscle is a significant depression, and if implant size, position, and angulation are not modified, lingual perforation may result. A, apparent height of available bone on radiograph; B, actual available bone height. *(b)* If the length of the implant exceeds the height of the available bone, perforation of the lingual plate of the mandible may occur.

Hemorrhage of the floor of the mouth

As discussed previously, arterial injury of the floor of the mouth is often induced by perforation of the lingual plate with rotary instruments; however, other causes described in literature include elevation of the lingual periosteum, flap manipulation, and surgical manipulation of the deeper muscle layers. The onset of the hemorrhage is usually intraoperative but may not be detected until 4 to 6 hours postoperative.

Moreover, the anatomy of the lingual aspect of the mandible can contribute to an increased risk of intraoperative hemorrhage. The pattern of anterior mandibular alveolar ridge resorption, which occurs principally on the labial aspect of the crest, leads to a lingual trajectory of the anterior mandible. It presents a challenge for the placement of implants with a favorable prosthetic angulation and can lead to lingual perforations and hemorrhage during surgery (Fig 2-40).

Signs of hemorrhage into the floor of the mouth include swelling; elevation of the floor of the mouth; protrusion of the tongue; respiratory distress; extensive sublingual, submandibular, or submental hematomas; inability to swallow; and profuse or pulsating intraoral bleeding.

Because airway obstruction secondary to severe bleeding in the floor of the mouth is a potentially fatal complication, securing and maintaining an adequate airway should be given the highest priority. Persistent intraoral bleeding can lead to mechanical pressure on the pharyngeal lumen and consequent airway obstruction, which poses a serious threat. The clinical signs of airway obstruction—tachypnea, dyspnea,

hoarseness, cyanosis, and drooling—may be absent until significant airway occlusion has occurred. Therefore, the implant surgeon should be prepared to deal with airway obstruction quickly and efficiently.

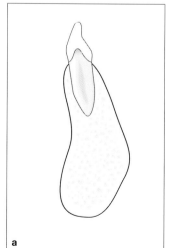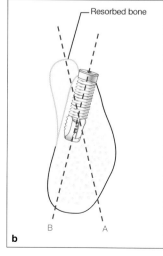

Fig 2-40 *(a)* Alveolar ridge anatomy prior to tooth loss. *(b)* Following tooth loss, resorption of the alveolar ridge mandates a change in the implant angulation from a labial inclination (A) to a lingual inclination (B) to prevent perforation of the lingual cortical plate. This will lead to an incorrect biomechanical position of the implant. The proper course of action is to augment the ridge before implant placement so the implant will be positioned correctly for prosthetic restoration.

Airway management

The airway can be secured by nasal or oral intubation, emergency tracheotomy, or cricothyroidotomy if an extensive hematoma prevents intubation. Manual tongue decompression and tactile nasal intubation have been reported as successful in airway maintenance during hemorrhagic swelling of the tongue.[50]

Bleeding management

Many bleeding control measures have been described in the literature and include the use of hemostatic agents, digital compression, and cauterization. It is important to note that bleeding may stop when the pressure of the extravasated blood exceeds the vascular pressure of the feeding bleeding vessel. Therefore, hematoma drainage may not be indicated because such intervention could potentially reverse this effect, lowering the pressure of the adjacent soft tissues and hence promoting further bleeding. This cessation of bleeding allows time for location and resolution of the source of the bleeding; meanwhile, the hematoma can be monitored and subsequently drained if it does not resolve on its own. Patient monitoring in anticipation of hemorrhage self-resolution has been successful in some cases. When conservative measures are ineffective, intraoral or extraoral surgical evacuation and ligation of the bleeding artery are necessary.

Protocol for management of hemorrhage of the floor of the mouth

It is important for the clinician to follow a protocol to effectively manage hemorrhaging in the floor of the mouth:

- At the first sign of swelling in the floor of the mouth, call 911.
- Using one hand, apply pressure to the suspected perforation site intraorally with the thumb and extraorally with the index finger (Fig 2-41).

- Calmly explain the nature of the complication to the patient.
- For buried bleeding vessels, use the technique shown in Fig 2-42 to attempt to ligate the vessel by applying pressure on the source of bleeding.
- If the bleeding vessel can be identified and isolated, close its lumen by securing it with the tips of a small hemostat and placing a knot using suture material (Fig 2-43).

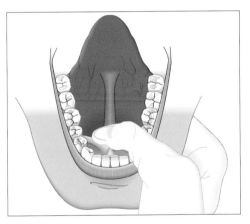

Fig 2-41 Applying pressure on a bleeding vessel will aid in stopping the bleeding.

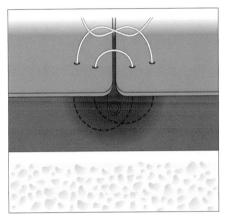

Fig 2-42 If the location of the buried bleeding vessel is identified, it can be ligated. The needle should enter the tissue about 6 mm away from the vessel on one side, exit 3 mm from it on the other side, enter the tissue 3 mm from the vessel on the original side, and exit 6 mm away from it on the other side; then a knot should be tied.

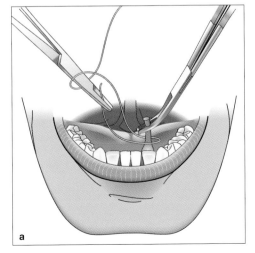

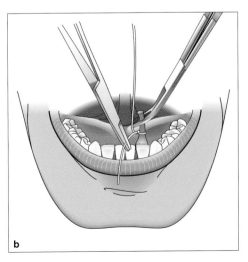

Fig 2-43 If the bleeding vessel is not buried, a hemostat can be used to isolate the vessel (a), and then it can be closed with a suture (b).

- Pull the tongue forward against the hyoid bone to reduce bleeding from the lingual artery or its branches.
- If injury is to the facial artery, press the common carotid artery against the fourth cervical vertebra to reduce bleeding.
- Do not make an incision in the floor of the mouth to relieve the hematoma.
- If the implant has already been placed, do not remove it.
- If other measures are ineffective and the patient develops signs of respiratory distress, insert a flexible nasal airway. An emergency tracheotomy or cricothyroidotomy may be necessary.
- Transfer the patient to a nearby hospital for monitoring.
- Once the rate of bleeding has slowed, use surgical ligation or electrocautery on damaged vessels if possible.

Prevention of arterial injury of the floor of the mouth is aided by:

- Detailed review of the patient's medical history.
- Knowledge of the regional arterial anatomy.
- Adequate training in surgical implant dentistry, including a thorough review of anatomy and basic sciences.
- Adequate training of the implant surgeon and staff in medical emergencies.
- Emergency equipment available in the implant surgical suite, including flexible nasal airways.

- Adherence to the appropriate surgical protocols.
- Careful positioning of implants at the mandibular midline to avoid the risk of surgical trauma or perforation of the lingual cortical plate. An even number of implants in the interforaminal region may be preferable to avoid drilling in the midline.
- Thorough examination of the anterior mandible using CT scans to detect and avoid injury to the accessory lingual foramina and canals.
- Consideration of anatomical features such as resorption patterns or sublingual and submandibular fossae when treatment planning.
- Digital palpation of the lingual mandibular surface to aid in detecting pronounced concavities in the anterior or posterior areas of the mandible.
- Monitoring of patients for a sufficient postoperative period of time, especially after surgery in the anterior mandible. There may be a latency period after arterial trauma, and hemorrhage can begin several hours later.[51]
- Adequate patient education. Patients should be advised of the warning signs of a hematoma and how it will be managed should this complication occur.[52]
- Avoidance of sites with a high potential for nerve or arterial injury given that implant therapy is an elective procedure.

Overheating of the Bone During Drilling

Production of excessively high temperatures during osseous drilling is known to impair bony regeneration.[53] Overheating of the bone during the osteotomy preparation will cause bone cell death and resorption around the implant, impairing successful osseointegration. Evidence of bony overheating will usually appear on a radiograph as a radiolucency soon after surgery. Therefore, it is essential to minimize the heat production during drilling.

In a study by Eriksson et al,[54,55] bone tissue was reported to be sensitive to heat at 47°C, irreversible bone injury occurred after a 1-minute exposure to a temperature of 53°C, and obvious bone tissue necrosis occurred at temperatures higher than 60°C. When proper technique and irrigation are used in preparation of the implant osteotomies, temperature never exceeds 33.8°C during a maximum of 5 seconds of drilling.[56]

The microscopic profile of failed implants due to overheating of the surgical site consists of the following features[57]: *(1)* bone sequestra, *(2)* lack of regeneration of the peri-implant bone, *(3)* inflammatory infiltrate in the space between bone and implant, *(4)* lack of organization of the peri-implant bone clot, *(5)* compact and mature bone around the implant, and *(6)* bacteria around the implant and the necrotic bone.

Solutions for common causes of overheating

Dull drills

Use sharp drills. Care should be taken to replace drills in a timely manner as they get dull. The number of osteotomies that can safely be made by a drill depends on the bone density. In type 1 bone, a drill can prepare 1 to 3 osteotomies; in type 2 bone, around 10; in type 3 bone, around 40; and in type 4 bone, 100 or more (Lekholm and Zarb[58] classification of bone density; Fig 2-44).

Nonsequential drilling technique

Use the correct drilling sequence as recommended by the manufacturer of the implant being placed. Enlargement of the osteotomy diameter a small fraction at a time will avoid unnecessary overheating of the osteotomy site. Large diameter drills generate more heat by friction than small diameter drills because of their large drill-bone contact zone.

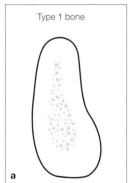 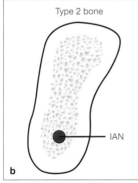 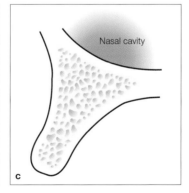 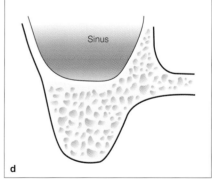

Fig 2-44 *(a)* Type 1 bone is made almost completely of cortical bone. *(b)* Type 2 bone is made of thick cortical bone and coarse trabecular bone. IAN—inferior alveolar nerve. *(c)* Type 3 bone is made of thin cortical bone and fine trabecular bone. *(d)* Type 4 bone is made of very thin cortical bone and very fine trabecular bone.

Insufficient coolant

Use an adequate amount of coolant, either sterile saline or sterile water. The coolant can be placed in the refrigerator prior to surgery. Irrigation has the greatest effect on bone temperature level during drilling; the absence of a coolant can result in temperatures in excess of 70°C.

When using implant drills on an extension shaft in the maxilla (Fig 2-45), a second source of external irrigation is necessary to compensate for the coolant loss due to gravity. The surgical assistant can use either an irrigation syringe with a catheter (Fig 2-46) or an irrigation system mounted on a stand (Fig 2-47).

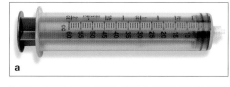

Fig 2-45 During the use of the implant drill on an extension shaft in the maxilla, the coolant will not reach the intended area due to gravity.

Improper drilling technique

Use an in-and-out motion during the osteotomy preparation to keep contact between the bone and the drill to a minimum (1 to 3 seconds). Longer periods of contact between the drill and the bone will lead to overheating of the bone.

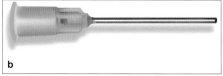

Fig 2-46 A 60-mL syringe *(a)* or blunt irrigation catheter *(b)* can be used as an additional source of external irrigation when needed.

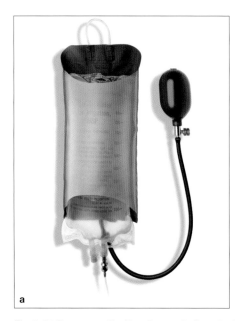

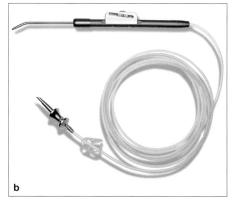

Fig 2-47 Pressure cuff with saline or sterile water bag *(a)* or fingertip irrigation control *(b)* system can be mounted on a stand and used as a source of secondary external irrigation.

Drill speed

In the presence of an adequate amount of coolant, sharp drills, and proper drilling techniques, the speed of the drill does not influence the heat generated at the osteotomy site. In a study by Iyer et al,[59] osteotomies were prepared in rabbit tibias at different speeds (2,000, 30,000, and 400,000 rpm) with appropriate irrigation. In no instance did the temperature of the bone reach 47°C, the temperature reported to lead to bone damage after 1 minute of drilling.

Treatment of failed implants due to bone overheating

The implant should be removed and any necrotic bone debrided. The patient should be prescribed antibiotic, anti-inflammatory, and pain medications, and the area should be monitored for proper healing. Bone grafting and implant placement can be reattempted after 3 to 4 months of osseous healing.

COMPLICATION 17 | # Stripping of the Implant Site

Site stripping can occur in dense bone when the clinician attempts to seat the implant deeper than the prepared osteotomy site. During insertion of the implant, torque reaches high levels and then suddenly becomes very low, indicating that stripping has occurred and the implant should be removed.

There are three options for management of a stripped osteotomy:

1. Abandon the osteotomy and prepare a new site (the original site can be grafted).
2. Remove the loose implant and drill a deeper osteotomy for a longer implant if the available bone will allow.
3. Remove the implant and place a wider implant without enlarging the osteotomy (Fig 2-48).

Technique for implant removal from a stripped site

To remove the implant, connect an impression coping and unscrew the implant using the body of the impression coping. Alternatively, if an insertion assembly is provided with the implant, it can be placed back on the implant and used for removal.

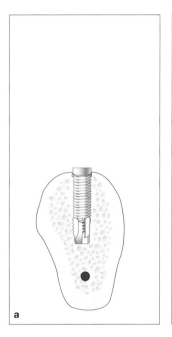
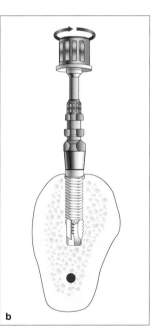

Fig 2-48 Removing an implant from a stripped osteotomy *(a)* can be accomplished by connecting the transfer assembly or an impression post to it *(b)* and unscrewing the implant using the body of one of these two components *(c and d)*. If the alveolar bone width allows, another implant with a wider diameter can be placed in the stripped site *(e)*.

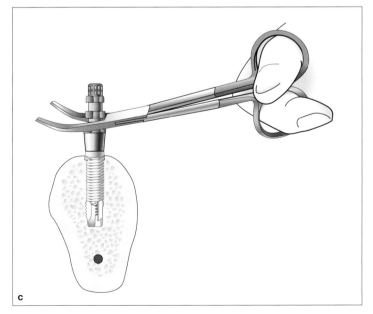
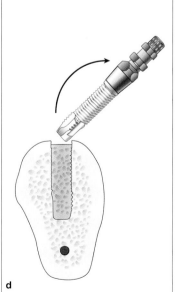
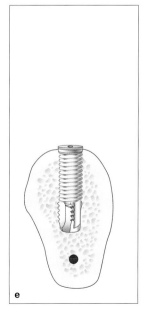

Sinus Floor Perforation

Perforation of the maxillary sinus with implant drills is usually related to inadequate surgical planning or poor surgical technique.

It is very important to take a radiograph with a parallel pin or the pilot drill in place after drilling the pilot hole. If the radiograph reveals a perforation of the sinus floor by the pilot drill, this is only a minor complication because its diameter is generally 2 mm or less. The implant placement procedure can proceed if the remaining drills and the implant do not contact the sinus floor (Figs 2-49a and 2-49b).

If a larger-diameter drill has penetrated the sinus floor, then it is recommended to abort the procedure, obtain primary soft tissue closure, and reattempt placement of the implant in this location in 3 to 4 months. A collagen dressing such as HeliPlug can be placed in the osteotomy site before closure (Fig 2-49c).

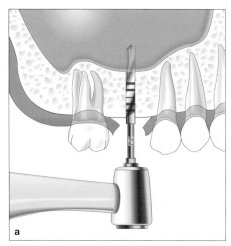

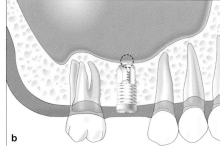

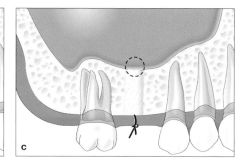

Fig 2-49 Penetrating the sinus floor with only the pilot drill (a) is usually not a concern if the rest of the drills needed to complete the osteotomy and the implant to be used remain short of the sinus floor (b). However, penetrating the sinus floor with more than the pilot drill mandates aborting the procedure for placement at a later date. The osteotomy should be filled with collagen dressing before primary closure is performed (c).

Prevention

Sinus floor perforation can be avoided by:

- Careful assessment of the presurgical CT scan
- Use of stoppers on all drills to ensure that they do not intrude into the sinus or drill deeper than what is required for placement (Fig 2-50)
- Planning sinus elevation through the osteotomy site or through a lateral window (see part 4) when the height of bone under the sinus is insufficient

The judgment of the clinician during treatment planning is paramount because each case is unique; however, guidelines can help to keep practitioners on a path that will most likely be successful. To that end, the author has developed a classification system for the available bone in the maxillary posterior quadrant to aid in treatment planning in this region.

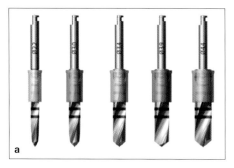

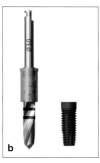

Fig 2-50 (a) Drills with removable stoppers. (b) The stopper will allow the drill to penetrate only the distance equal to the implant's length.

Al-Faraje classification of available bone for treatment planning in the maxillary posterior quadrant

- Class I: 8 mm or greater bone height between the bone crest and sinus floor with adequate width for implant placement (Fig 2-51a). Treatment plan: Placement of a 7-mm or longer implant, maintaining 1 mm of bone or more between the apex of the implant and the sinus floor.
- Class II: 5 to 7 mm bone height with adequate width for implant placement (Fig 2-51b). Treatment plan: Implant placement with simultaneous sinus elevation using a crestal approach (outlined in the next section).

- Class III: 1 to 4 mm bone height with adequate width for implant placement (Fig 2-51c). Treatment plan: Lateral window sinus elevation with delayed implant placement.
- Class IV: 1 to 4 mm bone height with inadequate width for implant placement (Fig 2-51d). Treatment plan: Lateral window sinus elevation with either delayed implant placement in a crossbite position or delayed ridge augmentation using a veneer block graft or GBR technique followed by delayed implant placement as a third stage.

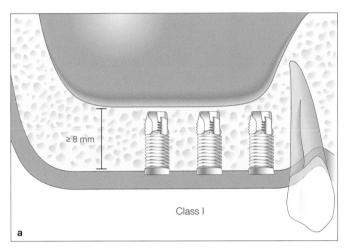

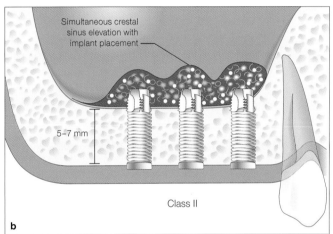

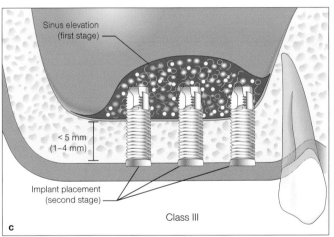

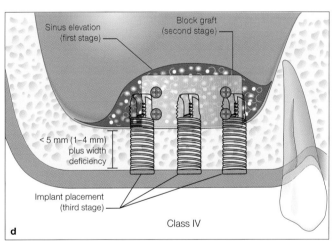

Fig 2-51 Al-Faraje classification of available bone in the posterior maxilla. *(a)* Class I: 8 mm of available bone height. Implants can be placed without a sinus bone grafting procedure. *(b)* Class II: 5 to 7 mm of available bone height. Implants can be placed with simultaneous sinus elevation using a crestal approach. *(c)* Class III: 1 to 4 mm of available bone height with sufficient alveolar ridge for implant placement. Lateral window sinus elevation procedure with delayed implant placement is the recommended treatment. *(d)* Class IV: 1 to 4 mm of available bone height with alveolar bone width deficiency. Recommended treatment is lateral window sinus elevation with either delayed implant placement in a crossbite position or delayed ridge augmentation using a veneer block graft or GBR technique followed by delayed implant placement as a third stage.

Al-Faraje technique for sinus elevation using a crestal approach

A sinus elevation procedure with surgical access through the crestal bone was first described by Tatum in 1986.[60] The technique was later modified by various authors.[61-64] This procedure and its variations are highly predictable, particularly when the height of residual alveolar bone measures 5 mm or more (Al-Faraje Class II). Its advantages and disadvantages are summarized in Box 2-1.

A modification of the original protocol has been developed by the author:

1. Flap elevation: A full-thickness flap is elevated to expose the crestal bone (Fig 2-52a).
2. Implant osteotomy: The osteotomy is completely prepared to the width of the implant but short of the sinus floor by 0.5 to 1.0 mm (Figs 2-52b and 2-52c).
3. Sinus floor elevation: A concave-tipped sinus osteotome of the same diameter as the final implant drill is gently malleted to compress the remaining 0.5 to 1.0 mm of bone against the sinus floor cortex and to infracture the sinus floor (Figs 2-52d and 2-52e). The osteotome tip should intrude into the maxillary sinus by no more than 1 to 2 mm. To avoid perforation of the sinus membrane, stoppers can be mounted on the osteotomes for depth control.
4. Bone grafting: A 15-mm resorbable collagen sponge such as HeliCote (Integra LifeSciences) is inserted into the osteotomy followed by a small amount (0.25 mL) of Bio-Oss grafting material. The collagen membrane protects the si-

Box 2-1	Advantages and disadvantages of sinus elevation using the crestal approach
Advantages	**Disadvantages**
• Small mucoperiosteal flap (limited to the crestal area and thus less disruption to the sinus lateral wall blood supply) • Limited incidence of membrane perforation • Limited incidence of membrane bleeding • Limited incidence of introducing bone graft material into the sinus cavity	• The use of the mallet can be traumatic for the patient • Unless the procedure is performed under sinuscopic control, it is hard to detect membrane perforation • Limited elevation (3 to 5 mm[65-67] compared with 10 mm or more for the lateral window technique) • A minimum of 5 mm of available alveolar bone required

nus membrane from perforation by sharp bone fragments (Fig 2-52f).

5. Implant placement: The implant selected should not exceed the original available bone height by more than 3 mm to avoid exceeding the stretching limit of the sinus membrane. The apical portion of the implant will compress the bone graft material and the collagen membrane, providing further elevation of the sinus membrane. The implant should be inserted at a speed of 30 rpm or less (Fig 2-52g).
6. Flap closure: Primary closure is recommended but not required.

A case completed with the above technique is shown in Fig 2-53.

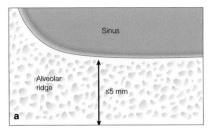

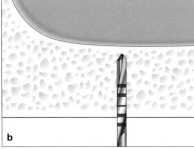

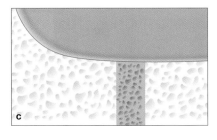

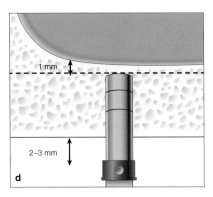

Fig 2-52 *(a)* Simultaneous crestal bone sinus graft procedure with implant placement in an insufficient alveolar ridge. *(b and c)* A complete osteotomy that stops short of the sinus floor is created using all drills recommended for a particular implant diameter. *(d and e)* The next step is to infracture the floor of the sinus using sinus osteotomes (preferably with stoppers to avoid penetrating the sinus cavity by more than 3 mm). *(f)* Collagen dressing and bone grafting material are inserted and pushed gently toward the superior part of the osteotomy. *(g)* The implant is placed, using a slow speed to gently push the bone grafting material as needed.

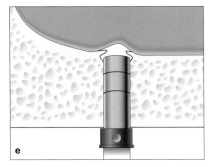

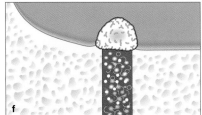

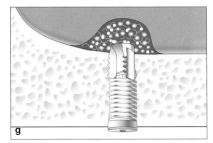

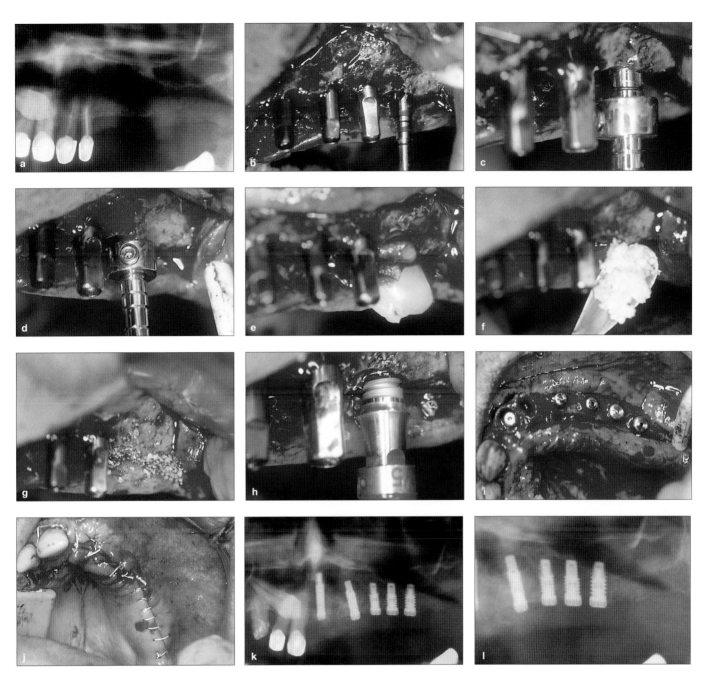

Fig 2-53 *(a to l)* Clinical case in which the procedure described in Fig 2-52 was carried out.

| Nasal Floor Perforation

Inadequate treatment planning for implant placement in the maxillary anterior region can lead to perforation of the nasal floor if the alveolar bone is deficient in height or if, in a case of immediate implant placement, there is insufficient bone apical to the sockets of the extracted teeth. A study by Brånemark et al[68] found no complications secondary to incidental penetration of implants into the nasal cavity, so long as the implant was sufficiently stabilized in bone.

Symptoms

Minimal perforation of the nasal floor might not be accompanied by any symptoms (Fig 2-54). Bleeding is a rare but possible sequela of perforation of the nasal floor with a rotary instrument. The arterial blood supply to the nasal cavity is derived from both the external and internal carotid arteries[69] (Fig 2-55). Other signs of perforation are postoperative swelling and pain.

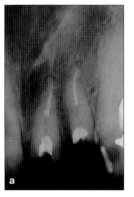 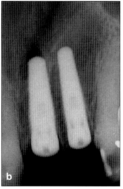 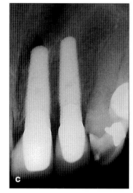

Fig 2-54 *(a and b)* Placement of two immediate implants in the maxillary anterior region. The implant that replaced the right central incisor has penetrated the nasal floor. A clinical decision was made to let the implant osseointegrate and observe the area for any possible adverse reactions. *(c)* One year after placement, the radiograph shows no adverse reaction. This unnecessary complication could have been avoided by selection of a shorter implant.

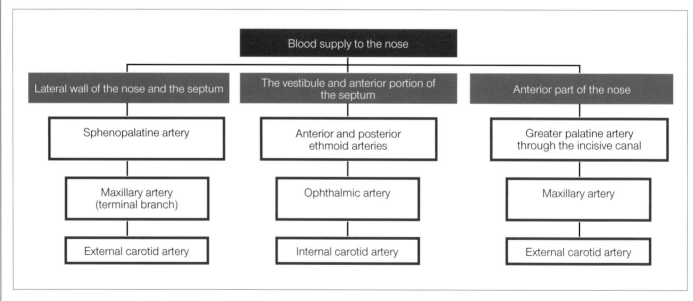

Fig 2-55 Flow chart describing how blood is supplied to the nose.

Prevention and management

When the anterior maxillary alveolar ridge is less than 10 mm in height, nasal floor elevation with bone augmentation is indicated to provide adequate bone for implant placement (Fig 2-56). The thick nasal mucosa is resistant to injury and can be predictably elevated 3 to 5 mm.[70]

Antibiotics, anti-inflammatory medications, and a chlorhexidine mouthrinse should be prescribed to reduce the incidence of infection. The patient should be advised to avoid blowing the nose, smoking, or coughing with the mouth closed.

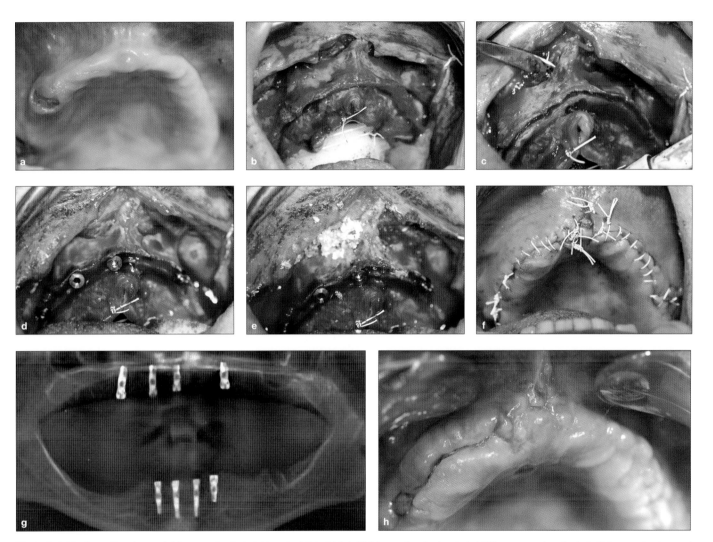

Fig 2-56 *(a)* Patient with advanced ridge atrophy (in height and width). *(b)* A full-thickness flap is elevated. *(c)* The mucosa is reflected off the nasal spine and the anterior part of the nasal floor. *(d)* Implants are placed. *(e)* Bone graft material (a combination of autogenous bone and Bio-Oss) is placed. *(f)* Primary incision line closure is obtained using PTFE suture material. *(g)* Immediate postoperative radiograph. *(h)* Clinical situation 2 weeks postoperative.

<table>
<tr><td>COMPLICATION 20</td><td>

Accidental Partial or Complete Displacement of Dental Implants into the Maxillary Sinus

</td></tr>
</table>

Implant placement for reconstruction of an atrophic maxillary posterior quadrant always presents a risk for introduction of the implants into the sinus cavity, even if a sinus elevation procedure has been done preoperatively or is being performed simultaneously with implant placement.

Partial displacement

Partial intrusion of an implant into the sinus cavity (Fig 2-57) can occur if the implant placed is longer than the available alveolar ridge height.

Prevention

Careful assessment of the preoperative CT scan should reveal the exact height, quality, and density of available bone inferior to the sinus cavity. Additional caution should be taken not to introduce the implant into the sinus cavity in cases where there is a dehiscence in the sinus floor apical to the root that is being extracted for immediate implant placement.

Management

If the alveolar bone height is not at least approximately 2 mm longer than the planned implant, a shorter implant should be substituted or a sinus elevation performed through the osteotomy or extraction site (Fig 2-58).

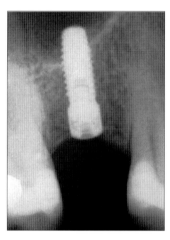

Fig 2-57 Partial displacement of the implant into the maxillary sinus due to poor preoperative assessment of the available bone.

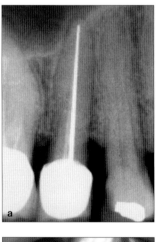
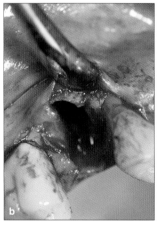
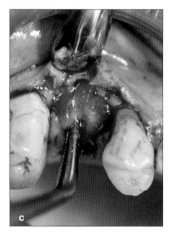

Fig 2-58 Sinus augmentation through a fresh extraction site. *(a)* The socket displays dehiscence between its apex and the sinus floor; therefore, drilling is not necessary. *(b)* The tooth is extracted. *(c)* Collagen dressing (HeliCote) is inserted. *(d)* Bone graft is placed. *(e)* The implant is placed. *(f)* The cover screw is placed for a two-stage protocol, and the flap is sutured. *(g)* Postoperative radiograph.

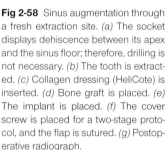

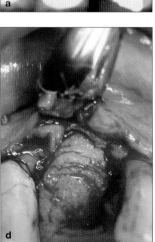
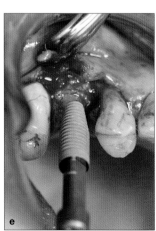
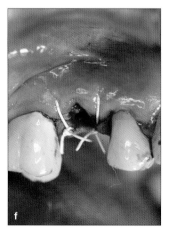
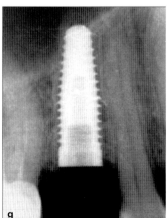

Complete displacement

Complete displacement of dental implants into the maxillary sinus can occur during implant placement[71] (Fig 2-59) or later as a postoperative complication.[72] Guler and Delilbasi[73] reported a case in which an implant migrated into the sinus cavity 8 years after placement. This risk of complete displacement is higher when implants are placed simultaneously with lateral window sinus elevation because the bone below the sinus usually is of poor quality and lacks sufficient bone volume for proper implant stability.

Prevention

Because of the anatomy and physiology of the maxillary posterior quadrant, primary stability of the implant is essential to avoid this complication. To ensure acceptable primary stability with the single-stage approach (ie, simultaneous sinus elevation and implant placement), there must be at least 5 mm of bone with good density between the floor of the sinus and the crest of the ridge; otherwise, the clinician should treatment plan a two-stage surgical approach. In a two-stage approach, the implants are placed 4 to 12 months after the sinus elevation is performed, depending on the graft material used.

Management

If an implant migrates into the maxillary sinus, it should be removed in order to avoid sinus pathology.[74] Various methods of removal have been reported in literature, several of which are detailed below.

Chiapasco et al[75] reported on the progress of 27 patients seen for postoperative complications involving the paranasal sinuses following displacement of implants in the maxillary sinuses. Complications included asymptomatic implant displacement, reactive sinusitis, and/or associated oroantral communication. Patients were treated with functional endoscopic sinus surgery (FESS), an intraoral approach, or a combination of both procedures according to the type of complication. Twenty-six patients recovered completely within 1 year, showing that the choice of an appropriate surgical protocol for a specific complication following displacement of implants in the maxillary sinuses is important for reliable results.

Ramotar et al[76] described a technique for the removal of migrated implants from the maxillary sinus via image-guided transnasal endoscopy. In this technique, reconstructed CT images were used to guide the endoscopy procedure in two patients. Removal was successful with no complications in both cases.

A modified transantral endoscopic approach for the removal of displaced implants has been successfully combined with simultaneous grafting of the sinus cavity.[77]

Other surgical techniques available for the removal of displaced implants are the Caldwell-Luc procedure and extraction through the tooth socket; both procedures have higher rates of conversion to open procedures, more damage to the nasal sinuses, and higher postoperative complication rates compared with endoscopic approaches.

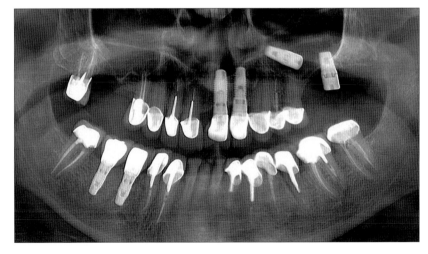

Fig 2-59 Delayed complete displacement of a dental implant into the maxillary sinus occurred during stage-two surgery (placement of the healing abutment).

Accidental Displacement of Dental Implants into the Maxillary Incisive Canal

When planning the placement of implants into the maxillary anterior region, it is essential to consider the size and position of the incisive canal. Penetrating the incisive canal will compromise osseointegration because of the epithelial tissue found in the canal. Replacement of the maxillary central incisors or placement of an implant at the maxillary midline for an implant-supported overdenture are two situations in which the incisive canal is at risk.

Anatomy and morphology

The incisive canal is located at the midline of the anterior hard palate. Its position is posterior to the focal trough of routine panoramic radiographs and therefore is poorly visualized on these films.[78] Moreover, on periapical radiographs, a pathology such as an incisive canal cyst may be misdiagnosed as an endodontic lesion.[79] Preoperative study of cross-sectional CT images is invaluable in determining canal morphology and dimensions and assessing anterior bone width for placement of implants buccal to the canal.

The incisive canal contains the nasopalatine nerve and the anterior branch of the greater palatine artery. There are at least two neurovascular bundles in the canal (Fig 2-60a) because the nerves and the arteries originate bilaterally.[80]

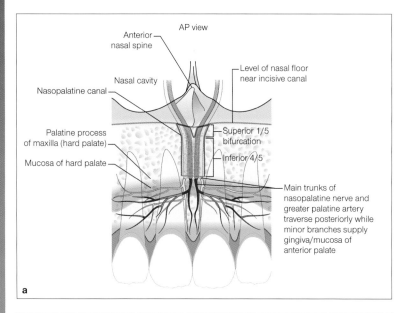

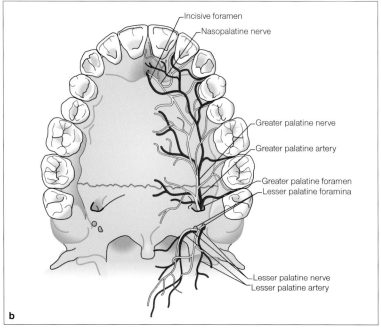

Fig 2-60 *(a)* Bilateral source of the contents of the nasopalatine canal (ie, the nasopalatine nerve and the anterior branch of the greater palatine artery) and the area supplied by them. *(b)* Communication between the nasopalatine nerve and the greater palatine nerve.

The nasopalatine nerve is a branch of the posterior superior nasal nerve that arises from the pterygopalatine ganglionic branches of the maxillary nerve. It runs downward and forward on the nasal septum to the incisive foramen, through which it passes to supply the anterior part of the palate; it communicates in this area with the corresponding nerve of the opposite side and with the greater palatine nerve (Fig 2-60b). Therefore, anesthesia for surgery involving the maxillary anterior region, the maxillary central incisors, the nasal septum, or the nasal floor can be achieved by injection into the incisive foramen.

The greater palatine artery emerges from the pterygopalatine fossa through the greater palatine foramen and runs across the hard palate to the incisive foramen (Fig 2-60c), through which it enters the nasal cavity to anastomose with the sphenopalatine artery on the nasal septum. This anastomosis may also occur within the incisive canal.

A study of two- and three-dimensional CT images[81] found that the nasopalatine canal has a mean length of 8.1 mm. Its palatal opening, the incisive foramen, has a mean inner diameter of 4.6 mm. At the level of the nasal floor, the foramen contains typically two, but possibly three or four, openings (Fig 2-60d). The average maximum width of the nasopalatine canal structure at the level of the nasal floor is 4.9 mm. The buccopalatal width of the bone anterior to the canal is 7.4 mm. However, the anatomy of the nasopalatine canal may vary greatly with regard to morphology and dimensions.

Iordanishvili[82] found that the distance between the incisive foramen and the central incisor roots is approximately 3.5 mm in adults. In individuals with a resorbed maxillary anterior region, the distance between the anterior portion of the canal and the buccal plate of the anterior maxilla is compromised. Bone resorption together with an enlarged incisive foramen can challenge proper implant placement.

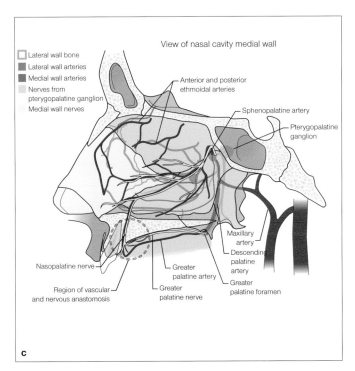

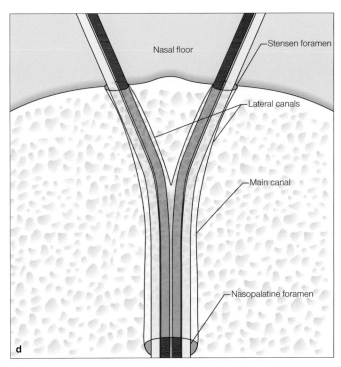

Fig 2-60 *(cont)* *(c)* The origin and the path of the contents of the incisive/nasopalatine canal. *(d)* The anatomy of the incisive/nasopalatine canal.

Grafting of the incisive canal

In some cases, the location of the incisive canal may prevent the replacement of maxillary central incisors with dental implants. However, if ideal prosthetic planning dictates use of this site, excision of the nerves and the blood vessels of the incisive canal, placement of bone graft material, and immediate or delayed implant placement is a viable technique that can be accomplished without detriment to the patient.[83–85]

The nerve and the artery of the incisive canal anastomose with the greater palatine artery and nerve, permitting immediate revascularization and a gradual reinnervation of the region within 3 to 6 months. Loss of sensation in the anterior palate is a possibility about which the patient must be informed; however, it is rarely a cause of patient complaint.

This procedure can be performed under local anesthesia. After reflection of a full-thickness flap, curettes and a round bur are used with copious irrigation to remove the contents of the canal. The bone inside the canal is scored to ensure sufficient bleeding, and bone grafting material (autogenous bone or a mixture of xenograft and allograft materials) is placed for simultaneous or delayed implant placement.

Deep Implant Placement

Osseointegration, the proper anchorage of an implant in bone, is a prerequisite for implant stability, but long-term retention of an implant depends on many factors, including a proper epithelial and connective tissue attachment to the titanium surface, which serves as a complete soft tissue seal protecting the bone from the oral environment.[86]

In general, the ideal implant position for the creation of an esthetic emergence profile is 3 mm apical to the ideal buccal free gingival margin.[87] In a healthy periodontium, there is a soft tissue seal measuring approximately 3 mm around natural teeth extending from the crestal bone to the free gingiva: 2 mm free gingiva, including the junctional epithelium, and 1 mm supracrestal connective tissue with a 2-mm biologic width.[88] Collagen fibers are perpendicular to the root and insert into its cementum. Studies by Berglundh et al[89] and Listgarten et al[90] revealed that healthy peri-implant mucosa has a tissue structure similar to that surrounding natural teeth, although the collagen fibers in the connective tissue zone are parallel to the implant surface because of the lack of cementum on the implant surface (Fig 2-61).

If the 2-mm biologic width is encroached upon by a restoration placed on a natural tooth (in case of general dentistry) or by the deeper-than-ideal positioning of the implant-abutment microgap relative to the ridge crest (in implant dentistry), the result is either bone resorption and the consequent soft tissue recession due to remodeling of both buccal and proximal marginal bone (in cases of thin bone and thin soft tissue biotype) or an increased risk of deep pocket formation and chronic inflammation (in cases of thick bony walls and thick soft tissue biotype). Bone loss in reaction to the microgap at the implant-abutment interface is discussed below in the "Implant design" section.

Placement of the implant platform at the bone level in the esthetic zone provides at least 3 mm of buccal soft tissue for an esthetic emergence profile of the implant crown without creating a deep pocket. In some cases, the position of the most apical point of the free gingival margin cannot be assessed during implant placement because a soft tissue flap has been reflected. When that happens, the clinician can use the level of the crestal bone or the position of the cementoenamel junction (CEJ) on an adjacent tooth. The crestal bone level (in the absence of bone loss) is generally equivalent to 3 mm below the most apical point of the free gingival margin and to a point 1 to 2 mm below the CEJ of adjacent teeth. However, in some scenarios, such as severe hard tissue scalloping, compliance with this guideline can lead to an implant that is positioned too deep mesially and distally. Therefore, although crestal bone morphology is the most important factor to consider when planning the depth of an implant, there are other important factors that must be carefully examined and assessed before insertion of the implant, including:

- Soft tissue quality, or *biotype*
- Implant platform design: conventional or platform switching
- Buccolingual position of the planned implant
- Implant location: esthetic or nonesthetic zone
- Susceptibility of the patient to periodontal disease
- History of orthodontic treatment
- Presence of implant or natural tooth adjacent to the implant
- Patient age and genetics

Each of these factors is discussed in greater detail in the following sections.

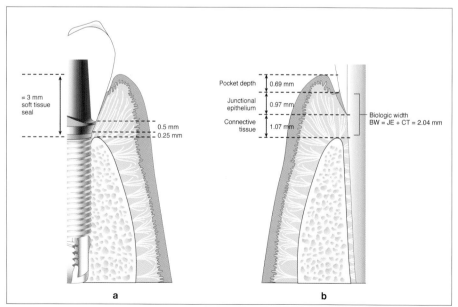

a   b

Fig 2-61 Anatomy of healthy soft and hard tissue surrounding an implant *(a)* and a tooth *(b)*. The biologic width (BW) is an average number that is subject to patient variability but usually is around 2 mm. It represents a combination of the connective tissue layer and the junctional epithelium (part of the free gingiva). In general dentistry, crown margins should not invade the BW. The same is true in implant dentistry; however, most often the implant-abutment margin is within the BW, and thus about 1 mm of bone loss is noticed around most implants because of the reestablishment of the BW by the body for the purpose of its own protection from the oral environment.

Crestal bone morphology/Soft tissue biotype: Al-Faraje classification system for coronoapical implant placement

The author has developed a system for the classification of crestal bone morphology and the soft tissue biotype to simplify the coronoapical positioning of dental implants.

Class I: Straight alveolar crestal bone

Class IA: Straight alveolar crestal bone in a nonesthetic zone

The implant platform should never be positioned below the crestal bone level, but rather at least 0.25 mm above the alveolar crest, as dictated by the thickness of the soft tissue: If the thickness of the soft tissue is 2 mm, the implant platform should be placed 0.5 mm above the crestal bone level. If the thickness of the soft tissue is 3 to 4 mm, the implant platform can be placed 0.5 to 1.0 mm above the crestal bone level (Fig 2-62). If the thickness of the soft tissue is greater than 4 mm, soft tissue reduction should be performed using electrosurgery, a soft tissue laser, or a scalpel to create the optimal soft tissue height and decrease the risk of deep pocket formation around the implant restoration. Otherwise, the implant would have to be placed above the bone to keep the platform from being any deeper than 3 to 4 mm below the most apical point of the free gingival margin. If the soft tissue thickness is less than 2 mm, then the implant would have to be placed at the

crestal bone level or alveoloplasty (if possible) could be performed to place the implant more apically and have a greater amount of soft tissue above the platform.

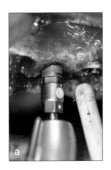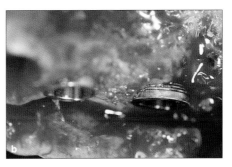

Fig 2-62 *(a and b)* Placement of implants slightly above the crestal bone in Class IA crestal bone morphology (flat alveolar crest in nonesthetic zone with no loss of alveolar height).

Class IB: Straight alveolar crestal bone in an esthetic zone

The crestal bone can be scalloped with a round or oval bur to re-create the interdental bony papillae, after which the soft tissue is modified accordingly (Fig 2-63).

Fig 2-63 Placement of an implant in a straight crestal alveolar ridge *(a)* in the esthetic zone (Class IB). The recommended protocol is to create a mildly scalloped crest using a round or football-shaped bur *(b and c)*, place the implant *(d to f)*, contour the soft tissues *(g)*, and then close the flap *(h)*.

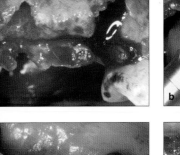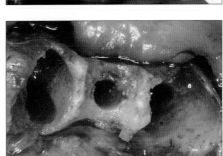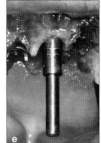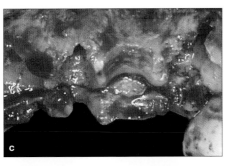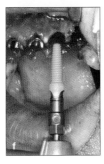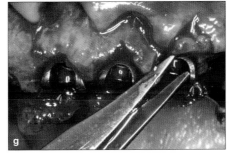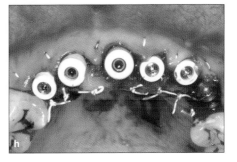

Figure 2-64 summarizes implant placement in Class IA and Class IB bone.

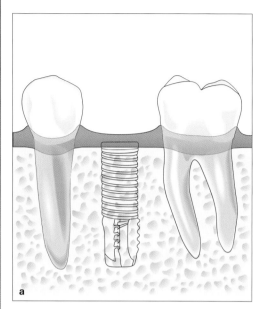
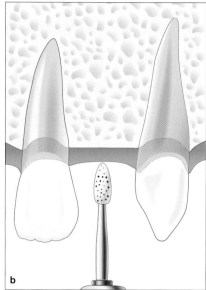
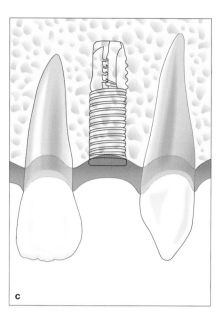

Fig 2-64 Recommended depth placement for Al-Faraje Class IA and IB crestal bone morphology. *(a)* Placement of the implant's platform slightly above the crestal bone in Class IA (nonesthetic zone). *(b and c)* Implant placement slightly above the crestal bone in Class IB (esthetic zone) after creation of a scalloped ridge using a bur.

Class II: Irregular alveolar crestal bone

Class IIA: Irregular alveolar crestal bone in single-unit edentulous areas

If the crestal bone is irregular, the implant platform should be placed at the greatest height of crestal bone (Fig 2-65). Otherwise, any bone coronal to the implant platform will cause difficulty in seating the healing abutment, placing the impression coping, and delivering the prosthesis. Moreover, the bone coronal to the implant platform will eventually resorb.

Note that any suprabony part of the implant body must be well covered by soft tissue. If placement of the implant platform at the greatest height of bone will lead to implant exposure in the oral cavity, recontouring of the crestal bone level is indicated so that the implant can be placed in a more apical position. GBR and/or soft tissue regeneration can also be performed before or simultaneously with the implant placement. Figure 2-66 summarizes implant placement in Class IIA bone.

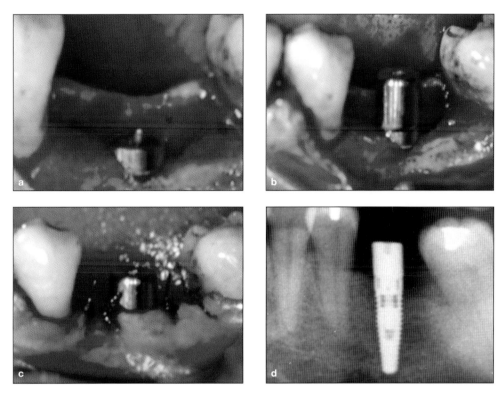

Fig 2-65 Placement of an implant in Class IIA bone (irregular alveolar crest level in a single-unit edentulous span). (a) The implant's platform is placed at the highest crestal bone level. (b) A healing abutment is placed for stage-one protocol. (c) The flap is sutured back. (d) Six-month postoperative radiograph.

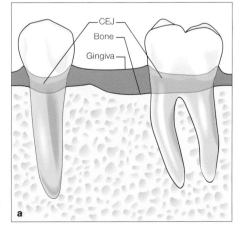
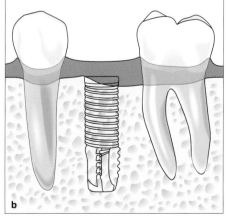

Fig 2-66 (a) Class IIA crestal bone morphology. (b) The implant platform is placed at the highest crestal bone level. Soft tissue covers the areas of the implant that are supracrestal.

Class IIB: Irregular alveolar crestal bone in a fully or partially edentulous arch

Using an oval or round alveoloplasty bur, the crestal bone can be leveled before implant placement if a removable or a fixed-detachable prosthesis such as a bar-retained overdenture is planned, or the bone can be scalloped if a fixed implant-supported prosthesis is planned (Fig 2-67). Figure 2-68 summarizes implant placement in Class IIB bone.

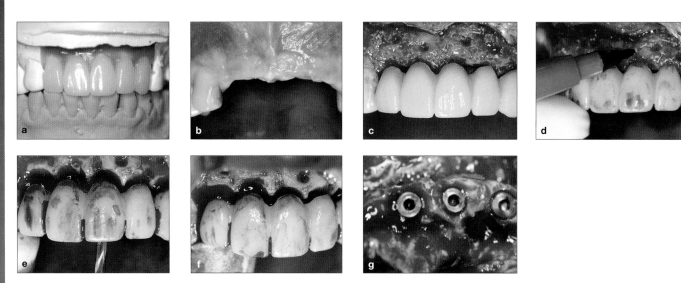

Fig 2-67 This clinical case demonstrates placement of implants in a Class IIB ridge. A diagnostic wax-up *(a)* is fabricated for a partially edentulous anterior maxillary ridge *(b)*. After flap elevation, the surgical stent is placed *(c)*, and the center of the teeth is marked on the bony ridge *(d)*. A round diamond bur is used to scallop the ridge and create bony papillae *(e)*, and then implants are placed in the center of the scalloped areas *(f and g)*.

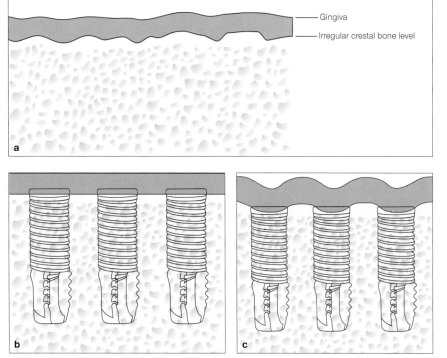

Fig 2-68 Class IIB crestal bone morphology *(a)* is managed by flattening *(b)* or scalloping *(c)*.

Class III: Scalloped alveolar crestal bone

Scalloped alveolar crestal bone is commonly encountered after extractions for immediate implant placement and is an esthetic risk factor. Despite scalloping, the surgical goals do not change: placement of the implant platform 3 mm below the most apical point of the free gingival margin and avoidance of deep pocket formation mesial and distal to the implant crown.

Tissue biotype must be considered when treatment planning to achieve an esthetic result. Current literature classifies the gingiva–crestal bone complex into two biotypes: thick and thin. The author prefers a more accurate subdivision of the complex into thin, medium, and thick biotypes.

The crestal bone morphology of Class III fresh extraction sites can be subclassified into four groups.

Class IIIA: Mildly scalloped crestal bone with thick soft tissue (thick biotype)

If the scalloping of the bone is minimal, the implant platform can be placed at the lowest crestal bone height. Two cases are shown in Figs 2-69 and 2-70.

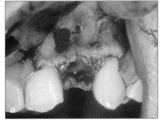
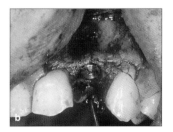

Fig 2-69 *(a)* Clinical view of Class IIIA crestal bone morphology. *(b)* Note the placement of the implant's platform flush with the level of the mildly scalloped crestal bone in a fresh extraction socket.

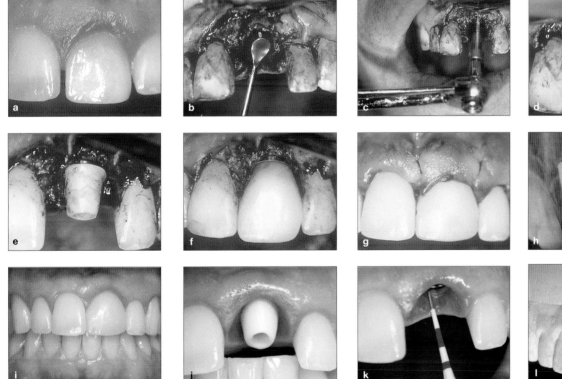

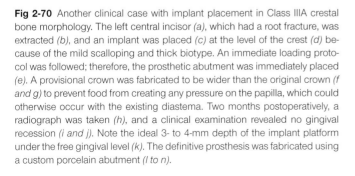

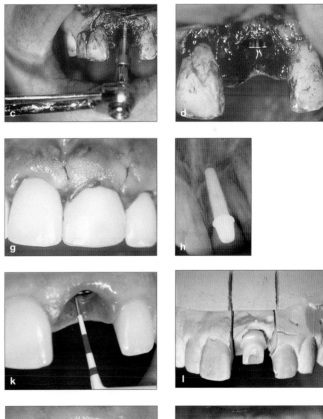

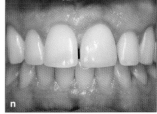

Fig 2-70 Another clinical case with implant placement in Class IIIA crestal bone morphology. The left central incisor *(a)*, which had a root fracture, was extracted *(b)*, and an implant was placed *(c)* at the level of the crest *(d)* because of the mild scalloping and thick biotype. An immediate loading protocol was followed; therefore, the prosthetic abutment was immediately placed *(e)*. A provisional crown was fabricated to be wider than the original crown *(f and g)* to prevent food from creating any pressure on the papilla, which could otherwise occur with the existing diastema. Two months postoperatively, a radiograph was taken *(h)*, and a clinical examination revealed no gingival recession *(i and j)*. Note the ideal 3- to 4-mm depth of the implant platform under the free gingival level *(k)*. The definitive prosthesis was fabricated using a custom porcelain abutment *(l to n)*.

Class IIIB: Moderately scalloped crestal bone with medium soft tissue (medium biotype)

The implant can be positioned above the lowest crestal bone height, but a minimum of 2 mm of soft tissue must be maintained over the implant platform. The relative thickness of the soft tissue will prevent exposure of the implant to the oral cavity (Fig 2-71).

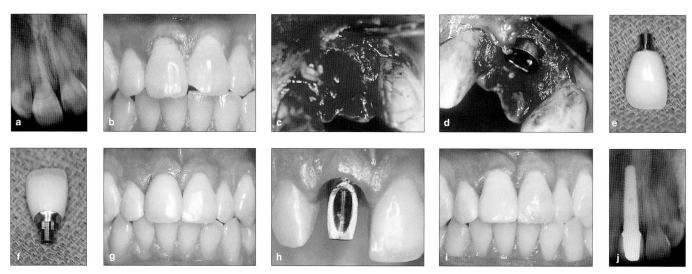

Fig 2-71 Clinical case with Class IIIB crestal bone morphology. The maxillary right central incisor exhibited root fracture due to trauma *(a and b)* and was extracted. Note the moderate scalloping *(c)*. The gingiva has a medium biotype; therefore, it was possible to place the implant platform above the crestal bone level by 1 to 2 mm without the risk of implant neck exposure into the oral cavity *(d)*. The provisional laboratory prosthesis was fabricated from composite material *(e and f)* and delivered the same day to the patient *(g)*. Two months later, the definitive crown was fabricated and delivered with excellent esthetic soft tissue results *(h and i)*. The 6-month postoperative radiograph *(j)* shows good hard tissue levels.

Class IIIC: Severely scalloped crestal bone with thin soft tissue (thin biotype)

Ideally, in this scenario, the implant platform should be positioned 1 to 2 mm above the lowest crestal bone height and at least 2 mm below the most apical point of the free gingival margin. Thick tissue is required to meet these specifications, but thin tissue often covers severely scalloped bony crests.

One-piece implants or implants with a scalloped platform are ideal for placement in severely scalloped crestal bone. The scalloped platform will support the interdental bony septa yet is short enough buccally not to risk exposure to the oral cavity (Fig 2-72). The one-piece implant can be shaped with burs, allowing the clinician to place the implant crown margin in an ideal position (Fig 2-73). When placing one-piece or scalloped-platform implants, the clinician should follow the manufacturer's guidelines for insertion to achieve an optimal result. In some cases, a fixed partial denture (FPD) should be considered as a reasonable alternative. An FPD may be the treatment of choice in cases where the biotype is very thin or the possibility of significant resorption and its impact on esthetics is high.

Figure 2-74 summarizes implant placement in Classes IIIA and IIIB. Figure 2-75 describes implant placement in severely scalloped (Class IIIC) bone.

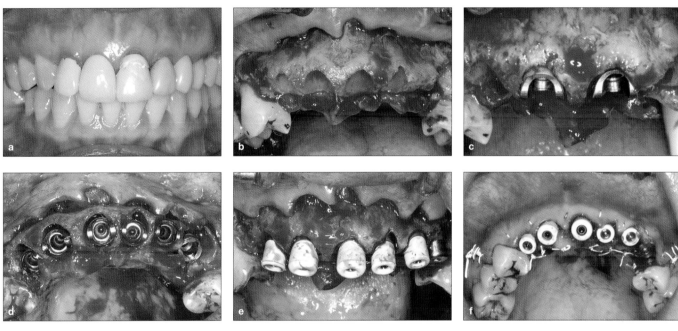

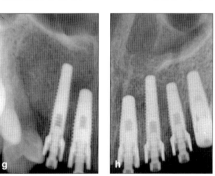

Fig 2-72 Clinical case with implant placement in Class IIIC crestal bone morphology. Note the thin biotype (a) and the severely scalloped crestal bone (b). Scalloped implants were chosen for placement in the fresh extraction sockets (c and d) following a one-stage protocol (e and f). Radiographs taken 9 months postoperatively (g and h) display no bone loss at the crestal bone level.

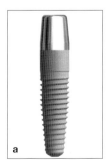
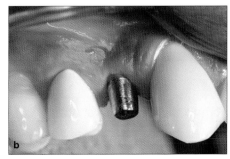
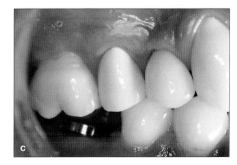
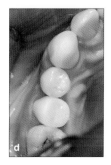

Fig 2-73 A one-piece implant (a) also can be used in Class IIIC crestal bone because the operator has control over the location of the implant crown margin, which can be created at the neck of the implant using special titanium burs (b). Implant crown 1 year after placement (c and d).

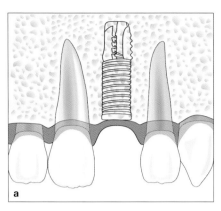 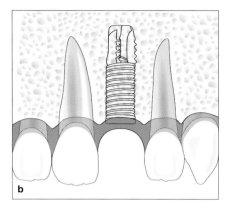

Fig 2-74 Recommended depth of implant placement for Classes IIIA and IIIB crestal bone morphology. *(a)* Class IIIA. *(b)* Class IIIB.

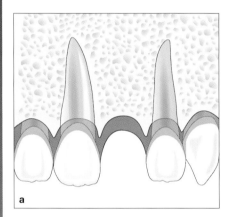 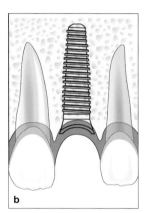 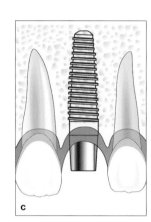 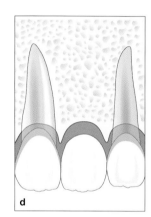

Fig 2-75 *(a)* Severely scalloped crestal bone with thin soft tissue (Class IIIC). *(b)* Placement of an implant with a scalloped platform. *(c)* Placement of a one-piece implant. *(d)* Fabrication of an FPD or performing socket grafting and/or soft tissue grafting and reevaluating the site for implant placement in 3 to 6 months.

Class IIID: Severely scalloped crestal bone due to bone resorption secondary to infection or trauma

Bone resorption at the extraction site does not justify placing the implant overly deep. In a case of severe bone resorption and concomitant soft tissue resorption following trauma or chronic infection, the implant platform should still be placed no deeper than 3 to 4 mm from where the most apical point of the free gingival margin would be without the soft tissue recession. However, to augment the bone and/or soft tissue deficiency, GBR and possibly soft tissue grafting should be performed simultaneously with implant placement. Figure 2-76 shows the treatment of a Class IIID case with GBR at the time of implant placement.

Another treatment option is bone grafting of the extraction site, with or without soft tissue grafting, followed by delayed implant insertion. Figure 2-77 summarizes the two treatment options for Class IIID bone.

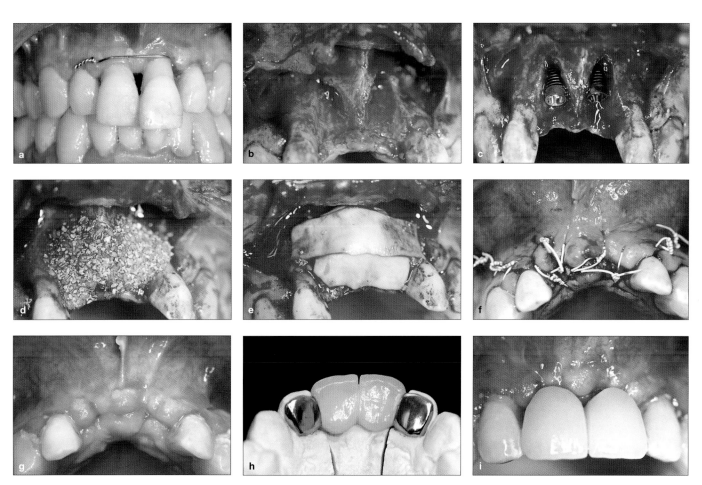

Fig 2-76 Clinical case example of implant placement in Class IIID crestal bone morphology. The patient presented for replacement of the maxillary central incisors *(a)*, which were mobile because of chronic infection and bone resorption secondary to trauma. The teeth were extracted *(b)* and the implants placed with platforms approximately 3 mm from the free gingival margin *(c)*. GBR was performed simultaneously using a particulate bone graft material mixture of Bio-Oss with demineralized allograft *(d)* and two layers of Bio-Gide membrane *(e and f)*. At the 2-week postoperative appointment *(g)*, a Maryland bridge was fabricated as the provisional restoration *(h and i)*.

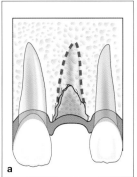
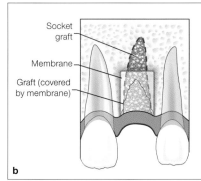
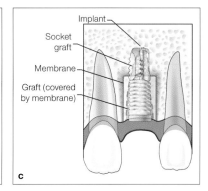

Fig 2-77 Protocols recommended for implant placement in Class IIID crestal bone morphology. *(a)* Class IIID crestal bone morphology. *(b)* Socket bone graft with or without soft tissue graft for delayed implant placement. *(c)* Placement of the implant immediately after extraction and removal of any granulation tissues with simultaneous GBR procedure.

Soft tissue biotype

The differences in gingival tissue biotype must be considered during implant treatment planning, particularly when determining the coronoapical position of the implant. The characteristics of the thick and thin biotypes and their response to surgical or restorative trauma are well established in the literature[91–95] and are summarized in Table 2-1.

Knowledge of these differences will help the implant dentist to choose the proper strategy to manage different periodontal clinical scenarios for a predictable implant treatment outcome. For example, identifying a thin tissue biotype at a planned implant site should alert the clinician to the need for a more careful extraction technique with the objective being bony ridge preservation because ridge resorption postsurgery may be unpredictable. The bone loss can be 1.5 to 2 mm over the 12 months after extraction, with most of the loss occurring during the initial 3 months.[96] Patients with thick biotypes are better candidates for immediate implant placement because there is less risk of postoperative bone resorption and soft tissue recession, and thus esthetic results are more predictable and stable. If immediate placement is performed in patients with a thin biotype, there may be a higher risk of abutment or implant thread exposure into the oral cavity because the frequency of gingival recession greater than 1 mm is higher than in thick biotype tissue. Moreover, sites with implants placed immediately after extraction reported 50% resorption of the original buccal plate width.[97] As a result, immediate implants are not often recommended in areas with thin tissue biotype.

Table 2-1	Thick vs thin tissue biotypes	
	Thick biotype	**Thin biotype**
Tissue quality	Dense, with a large zone of attached gingiva	Thin, with a minimum of attached gingiva
Periodontal probing	Probe not visible through gingiva	Probe visible through gingiva
Papilla architecture	Short	Long
Gingival topography	Flat	Scalloped
Osseous form	Thick	Thin, with dehiscence and fenestration
Course of periodontal disease	Bone loss and pocket formation	Rapid bone loss and gingival recession
Pattern of postsurgery healing	Minimal ridge atrophy with predictable soft tissue contours	Ridge resorption and unpredictable soft tissue contours

Implant design

Following implant placement, peri-implant crestal bone changes differ significantly and are dependent on many factors, including implant design. In one-piece implants, crestal bone loss depends on whether the implant-bone interface is rough or smooth; in two-piece implants, the interface (microgap) between the implant and the abutment (in cement-retained restorations) or between the implant and the restoration (in screw-retained restorations) is the key variable.[98–100] Movement between implant components and the size of the microgap are two factors among many that may influence the resulting crestal bone level. In general, placement of the microgap closer to crestal bone provides a niche for bacteria and inflammatory cells and contributes to soft tissue recession.[101,102] *Platform switching* is a design concept that moves the microgap inward, away from the bone and toward the center of the implant. Less vertical crestal bone loss has been observed around platform-switched implants, although the bone is still likely to react.[103–107]

Buccolingual position of the implant

After extraction and implant placement, the alveolar crestal bone undergoes an initial phase of remodeling. When the implant is placed in a buccally inclined position, gingival tissue and crestal bone are more likely to continue receding. Therefore, in the anterior area, the implant should be positioned under the incisal edge of the planned implant restoration or slightly lingual/palatal to it.

Implant location

As discussed earlier, some decisions regarding depth of implant placement are dictated by the location of the implant in the mouth, ie, in an esthetic or nonesthetic zone.

Susceptibility of the patient to periodontal disease

Risk factors for developing periodontal disease should be taken into consideration, such as the periodontal tissue status of adjacent teeth, large teeth, small embrasures, and crowding.

History of orthodontic treatment

Previous orthodontic treatment predisposes the patient to gingival recession and should be taken into consideration during treatment planning.

Patient age and genetics

Some patients are genetically more resistant to oral bacteria, including those bacteria that colonize the implant-abutment interface; vertical crestal bone loss will be minimal in these patients. In other patients, slow, continuous bone remodeling or a biologic complication such as peri-implantitis will be observed.

Implant vs natural tooth adjacent to implant

Interdental bony and soft tissue papillae have a higher incidence of recession between two implants. An implant between two natural teeth is a more favorable situation for the preservation of the adjacent papillae.

In conclusion, it is the operator's experience with the nine factors described above that will help predict which patient, site, or situation will have issues related to bone or gingival remodeling and to what extent.

Complications associated with deep implant placement

Bone loss around the implant neck

When the implant is placed below the height of the crestal (cortical) bone, the occlusal load is sustained less effectively by the weaker trabecular bone, which leads to bone loss and soft tissue recession. A significant difference between the bone levels at the implant site and at adjacent teeth compromises periodontal and peri-implant tissue health and esthetics (Fig 2-78). Figure 2-79 shows gingival recession subsequent to deep apicocoronal positioning of the implant.

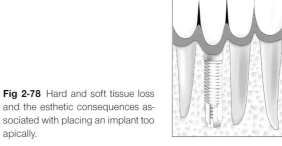

Fig 2-78 Hard and soft tissue loss and the esthetic consequences associated with placing an implant too apically.

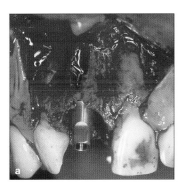 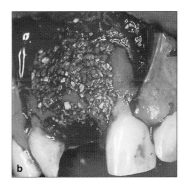 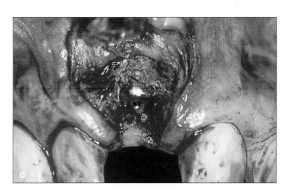

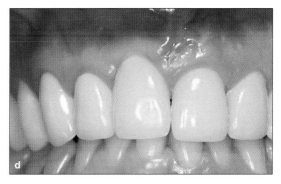

Fig 2-79 *(a to c)* Clinical case with deep implant placement. *(d)* Note the soft tissue recession secondary to hard tissue loss that was triggered by the deep apicocoronal placement of the implant.

Increased crown height

Placement of an implant below the alveolar bone crest increases the vertical restorative space and the crown-implant ratio.

Increased occlusal forces

Increased crown height leads to an increase in undesirable vertical cantilever forces.

Increased sulcus depth

The more subgingivally the implant is placed, the deeper the resulting pocket, which causes difficulty in maintaining proper hygiene.

Compromised esthetics

The most demanding and critical step in anterior implant esthetics is preservation of the papillae. The position and size of the papillae are determined by the interproximal bone level of the adjacent teeth. When an implant is placed in an excessively subcrestal position, the level of interproximal bone is not maintained, and the support of papillary tissues is compromised. According to Tarnow et al,[108] papillary fill of the embrasure between two teeth depends on the distance between the crestal bone and the interproximal contact (Table 2-2). A distance greater than 5 mm is correlated with an absence of the interproximal papilla, seen intraorally as a black triangle (Fig 2-80).

Table 2-2	Papillary fill of the embrasure as a function of distance from interproximal contact to crestal bone*	
Distance from crestal bone to interproximal contact (mm)		Probability of papillary fill in interdental embrasure
4		100%
5		98%
6		56%
7		27%

*Data from Tarnow et al.[108]

Difficulty seating prosthetic components

Complete seating of the healing abutment, the impression coping, and the definitive abutment may be prevented by bone above the implant platform.

Difficulty removing excess cement

Deep implant placement can make it difficult to remove excess cement when placing the definitive restoration (see complication 39, part 3).

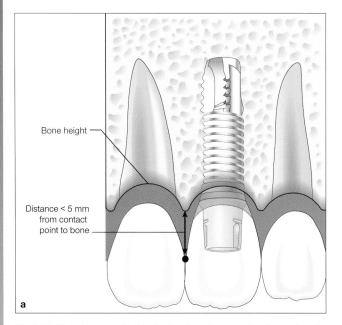
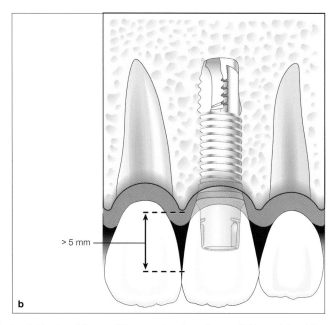

Fig 2-80 The absence of a black triangle between restorations when the contact point is at a distance of 5 mm or less from the crestal bone *(a)* and the formation of a black triangle when this distance exceeds 5 mm *(b)*.

| # Shallow Implant Placement

Complications associated with implant placement in an overly supracrestal position include:

- Exposure of the cover screw during healing (Fig 2-81).
- Poor emergence profile because of inadequate soft tissue thickness over the implant platform (Fig 2-82). Use of a ceramic abutment can resolve esthetic complications in this situation (Fig 2-83).
- Decreased crown height.
- Exposure of the abutment. A preparable ceramic abutment can be used to place the crown-abutment margin below the free gingival margin (Fig 2-84).
- Exposure of the implant body is also a possibility in shallow placement with thin soft tissue. Solutions include bone and/or soft tissue grafting or implant removal.

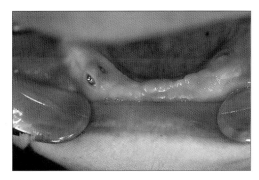

Fig 2-81 Exposure of the cover screw during the healing period due to a combination of shallow implant placement and thin mucosa.

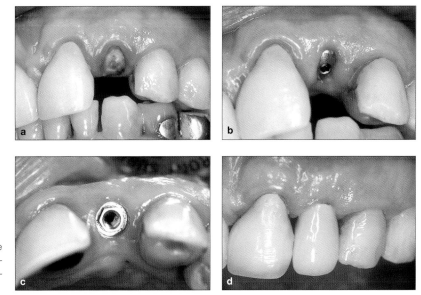

Fig 2-82 *(a to d)* An esthetically compromised emergence profile due to shallow implant placement. The shallow placement led to inadequate soft tissue thickness above the platform of the implant.

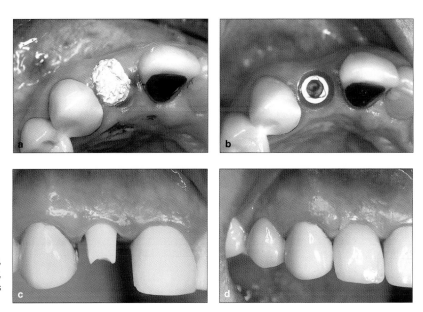

Fig 2-83 *(a and b)* A case similar to that shown in Fig 2-81 (ie, shallow implant placement after tooth extraction). However, the use of a ceramic abutment *(c)* and a metal-free prosthesis *(d)* led to better esthetic results.

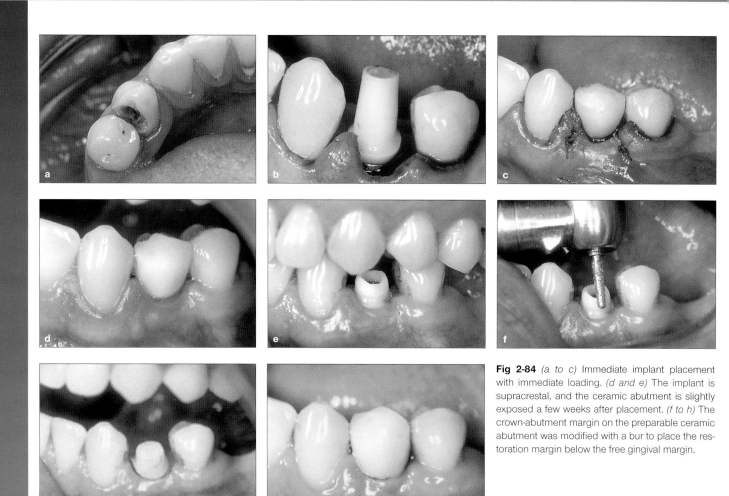

Fig 2-84 *(a to c)* Immediate implant placement with immediate loading. *(d and e)* The implant is supracrestal, and the ceramic abutment is slightly exposed a few weeks after placement. *(f to h)* The crown-abutment margin on the preparable ceramic abutment was modified with a bur to place the restoration margin below the free gingival margin.

Achieving ideal soft tissue esthetics

When indicated, immediate implant placement combined with immediate loading is the best strategy for achieving optimal soft tissue esthetics. Ideal esthetics can be achieved without the need for additional bone or soft tissue grafting provided that the following conditions are met:

- No bone resorption
- No soft tissue recession
- Presence of interdental bony papillae
- Presence of soft tissue papillae
- Healthy soft tissue (no gingivitis or periodontitis)
- Mildly scalloped crestal bone with thick tissue biotype
- No peri-implant infection

| COMPLICATION 24 | Complications in Flapless Implant Placement |

Flapless implant surgery can give predictable results if patient selection and surgical technique are appropriate.[109] Studies of this technique indicate a high overall implant survival of 95% or greater.[110] Although the flapless protocol was initially suggested for novice implant surgeons, a successful outcome often requires advanced clinical experience.

Technique

In this protocol, the gingival tissue must first be perforated at the insertion site by a rotary or hand tissue punch to access the bone before the initiation of the drilling phase (Fig 2-85).

Use of a tissue punch narrower than the implant diameter will result in better peri-implant tissue healing, a shorter junctional epithelium, and less crestal bone loss.[111]

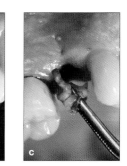
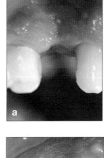
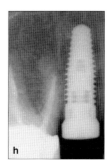

Fig 2-85 Flapless implant placement technique. *(a)* Flapless placement is planned for the missing maxillary right second premolar. The width of the alveolar ridge and the amount of the attached keratinized gingiva present the right conditions for this insertion protocol. *(b to d)* The procedure starts with access to the crestal bone by removal of a tissue plug with a rotary or hand tissue punch. *(e to g)* The osteotomy is then created, and the implant is placed (with a single-stage protocol in this case). *(h)* Four-month postoperative radiograph.

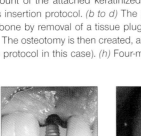
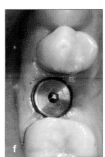
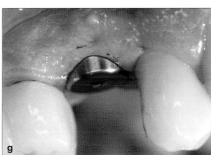

Advantages

- No need for flap reflection and suturing, thus minimizing the duration of surgery.
- Minimal intraoperative bleeding.
- Minimal patient discomfort with reduced swelling and pain. In a study by Fortin et al[112] that assessed postoperative discomfort after flapless and conventional implant surgery, patients experienced significantly less pain and used fewer analgesics for a shorter period of time when the flapless approach was used. These findings were supported in a study by Nkenke et al[113] that found less patient morbidity following flapless surgery compared with conventional surgery.
- Preservation of soft and hard tissues by maintaining vascular supply and existing soft tissue contours.[114–116]

Disadvantages

- Inability to visualize certain anatomical landmarks. Because flapless implant placement is a mostly "blind" surgical technique, the clinician must be cautious when placing implants. Perforation of the cortical bone may occur, especially in the maxillary anterior or the lingual mandibular molar regions. However, selection of appropriate patients with sufficient available bone width will reduce the incidence of buccal or lingual perforation.
- Inability to clearly visualize the crestal bone level, which may result in implants being placed too deep or too shallow.
- Potential for overheating the bone during drilling due to the limited effect of external irrigation.
- Reduction in the amount of the keratinized gingiva, which may have a negative effect on the health of the peri-implant gingiva and increase the implant failure rate.[117,118]

Recommendations

Because of the disadvantages discussed above, the author does not recommend the use of flapless insertion as a routine protocol for implant surgery; instead, this protocol should be limited to indicated cases treated by experienced implant dentists. Figure 2-86 shows a case in which flapless insertion was discontinued midsurgery because of previously unrecognized contraindications.

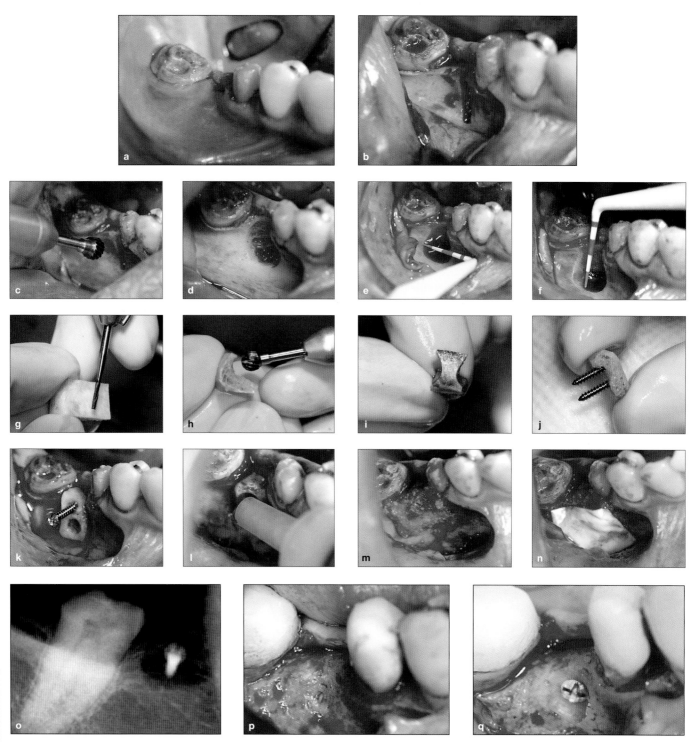

Fig 2-86 (a) A flapless insertion was attempted; however, it was an inappropriate approach for this thin ridge. The dentist aborted the procedure, and the patient was referred for ridge augmentation (a preoperative CT scan would have helped to avoid this complication). (b) A full-thickness flap is reflected. (c and d) The recipient site is prepared for the block graft. (e and f) The dimensions of the area to be grafted are measured. (g to j) The block graft is prepared. (k) Two screws are used to fix the block at the recipient site. (l to n) Bone graft material (allograft) and a resorbable membrane (Bio-Gide) are used to augment the areas around the block. (o) Postoperative radiograph. (p) The area is exposed 4 months postoperatively to remove the fixation screws and to insert the implant. Compare the bone volume with that shown in Fig 2-85b. (q) Some bone was removed to gain access to the top of the fixation screws for removal. A successful outcome was achieved.

When the flapless approach is used, the precise location of the implant must be planned in advance. In accordance with the concept of *prosthetic-driven implantology*, CT images, dedicated interactive computer software programs,[119,120] and mucosa-supported stereolithographic surgical guides[121] (Fig 2-87) for computer-guided surgery are valuable treatment-planning and surgical tools. If CT images are not available, ridge-mapping calipers (Fig 2-88) should be used to measure precisely the alveolar ridge width.

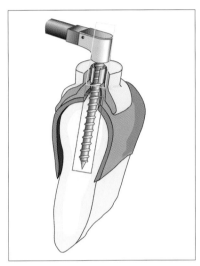

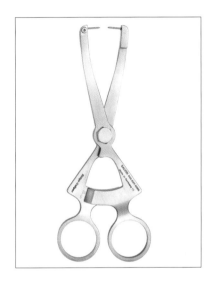

Fig 2-87 *(left)* Computer-generated surgical stent that enables the operator to place implants in the exact locations determined using virtual treatment-planning computer software and 5-mm cylindric tubes (incorporated at the drill access points) that prevent changing the angulation during drilling, leading to safer and more predictable flapless implant insertion.

Fig 2-88 *(right)* Ridge-mapping caliper, a useful tool in determining the width of the alveolar ridge (along its entire height) in the absence of a CT scan.

Aspiration or Ingestion of Foreign Objects

Aspiration or ingestion of instruments and materials can occur during any dental procedure. Accidental inhalation of dental instruments (drills, files, screwdrivers, parallel pins) can present a life-threatening complication[122] more serious than ingestion and must always be treated as an emergency situation. When this happens, patients must be referred to an emergency room immediately for evaluation and treatment. If intraoperative ingestion is suspected, the patient should be referred to a gastroenterologist.

Aspiration

Often aspiration of a foreign body will be accompanied by one or more of the following symptoms: coughing, decreased breath sounds, choking, fever, breathing noises such as wheezing or stridor, or cyanosis. However, patients may be asymptomatic initially. When in doubt, the patient must always be referred for a chest radiograph (Fig 2-89).

Plain chest radiography is the initial imaging modality for patients with suspected aspiration of a foreign body. If the plain chest radiograph is negative but suspicion of foreign-body aspiration remains, a multidetector CT scan of the chest, possibly with virtual bronchoscopy, should be considered in order to avoid unnecessary rigid bronchoscopy.[123] *CT virtual bronchoscopy* is a noninvasive technique that creates a three-dimensional reconstruction of the interior of the trachea and major bronchi. *Rigid bronchoscopy* is usually successful in removing the dental instrument under general anesthesia.[124]

Due to bronchial anatomy, the instrument or foreign body is most likely to become lodged in the right main bronchus.[125] In a study by Haliloglu et al,[126] out of seven patients with foreign-body aspiration, CT virtual bronchoscopy and conventional bronchoscopy revealed the location of the foreign body to be in either the right (four patients) or left (two patients) main bronchi or, in one patient, the lower lobe bronchus.

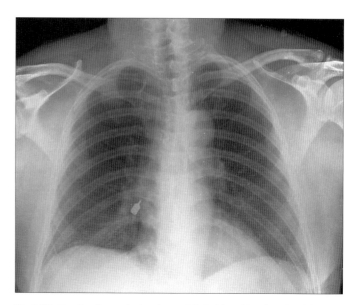

Fig 2-89 Chest radiograph showing an inhaled hex driver into the right lung.

Ingestion

Ingestion of dental instruments can potentially result in serious consequences, including infection and gastrointestinal blockage.[127] Moreover, esophageal foreign bodies, particularly sharp ones, can eventually erode through the thin esophageal wall and lead to deadly complications. Partial dentures sometimes are accidentally swallowed and become lodged in the esophagus, where the clasp arms can tear the esophageal wall upon retrieval.

Prevention

Prevention of ingestion and aspiration is the best approach.[128] Small instruments such as screwdrivers and parallel pins should be tied with floss before they are inserted in the mouth (Fig 2-90) to simplify their retrieval if necessary. In addition, a large piece of gauze or a sponge can sometimes be used to shield the airway.

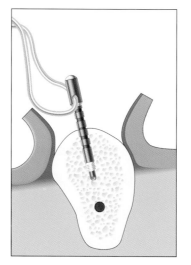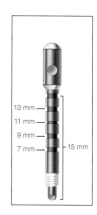

Fig 2-90 Tying components with floss before their use in the mouth prevents them from being inhaled or aspirated.

Mandibular Bone Fracture

Mandibular fracture is a rare complication and can occur with the insertion or removal of implants[129] in severely resorbed mandibular bone. This complication is most likely to occur in very atrophic edentulous mandibles with a bone height less than 10 mm. Placement of four or more implants or wide-body implants in an atrophic mandible may further weaken the bone and lead to a fracture. Patients should be warned about the possibility of this complication. Fractures can occur during or after implant surgery as a result of stress concentration in weakened areas such as an osteotomy site or the site of a removed implant, especially in an already compromised mandible. Moreover, the site of an implant that has not yet osseointegrated acts as a site of tensile stress concentration, and repeated functional forces can lead to a spontaneous fracture without trauma.[130]

Prevention

The following considerations are essential to preventing mandibular bone fracture:

- When treatment planning implant placement in a severely resorbed mandible, consideration should be given to the quantity of bone needed to maintain mandibular strength, keeping in mind that an increase in the number of implants will increase the risk of bone fracture.
- A CT scan of the mandible should be used to evaluate the height and width of the available bone and determine if the patient's anatomy will accommodate insertion of implants. A minimum of 10 mm in height and 5 mm in width should be available for implant placement.
- Clinicians should pay special attention to the bone density, especially in patients with osteoporosis and osteomalacia.
- Procedures such as inferior alveolar nerve transposition may make more bone available for implant insertion but may also lead to a fracture because they compromise the structural integrity of the atrophic mandible.[131-133]
- Bone grafting procedures such as block grafting and GBR can be used to increase the bone volume and strength before the insertion of implants.
- Implants should be placed 10 mm apart for better stress distribution.
- Using short abutments in cases with fixed prostheses can also minimize the force or stress on the implants.
- Excessive tightening of implants during placement can result in strain or microfractures in the surrounding bone; in mandibles with poor density or mineralization, this may predispose the region to fracture.
- During the healing period after placement or removal of implants, patients should limit stress to the jaw with appropriate measures such as a soft diet.

Symptoms of implant-related mandibular fracture

- Pain
- Swelling with or without fluctuation
- Presence or absence of mobility in the mandible
- Change in occlusion
- Fracture with no history of trauma

Management of mandibular fractures

The management of mandibular fractures always begins with a complete and careful clinical and radiographic examination. The basic principles in fracture treatment are anatomical reduction and immobilization of the fractured site, restoration of occlusion, application of stable fixation to neutralize negative forces on the fracture, gentle handling of soft tissues, avoidance of iatrogenic dental trauma, extraction of diseased teeth within the fracture line, and avoidance of excessive soft tissue elevation. The clinician should adhere to these principles for mandibular fractures, although fixation of the fracture is not necessary in the absence of abnormal mobility.

Removal of an implant in a fracture line is not necessary if stabilization and fixation can be achieved because implants, which do not have pulp tissue, are less likely to become a focus of infection.[134] However, it is essential to avoid movement or exposure of the implant during reduction of the fracture.

Additional healing time before stage-two surgery and abutment connection should also be provided. Other factors[135] influencing the decision to keep or remove an implant in a fracture line include:

- The importance of the implant to the overall treatment plan
- The presence or absence of infection
- The mobility or immobility of the implant

Minimally displaced stress fractures that occur during the healing phase can result from the placement of implants in a severely resorbed edentulous mandibular ridge. A nonsurgical approach is indicated in the management of this type of fracture because an open procedure requires extensive reflection of the periosteum to rigidly fixate the fracture, compromising the blood supply to the fracture site and jeopardizing healing. In a nonsurgical approach, a provisional fixed or removable denture or an acrylic resin splint on the remaining integrated implants and/or teeth serves as the external fixation device.

Other methods of treatment of a fracture include extraoral or intraoral open reduction, stainless steel reconstructive bone plates (Fig 2-91), the use of screw-retained corticocan-cellous bone block grafts to bridge nonunion fracture areas, occlusolingual splints, and maxillomandibular fixation. Choice of treatment should be based on the type and location of the fracture and the degree of atrophy.[136]

Fracture patients should be closely observed, prescribed antibiotics, and instructed to limit jaw movements and follow a soft diet.

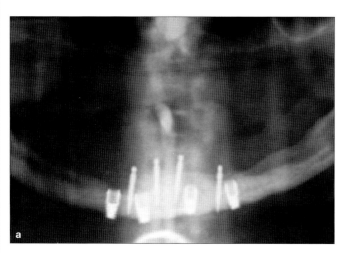 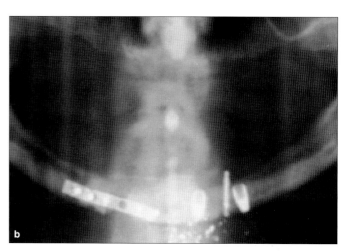

Fig 2-91 *(a)* Placement of several implants in this severely resorbed mandible led to delayed mandibular fracture due to stress concentration in the most weakened areas of the mandible. *(b)* Implants located in the fracture line or close to it were removed, and the fracture site was immobilized using a stainless steel reconstructive plate.

COMPLICATION 27   Implant Fracture

Implant fracture can happen intraoperatively or after delivery of the prosthesis.

Intraoperative implant fracture

Some implant designs are more apt to fracture at the neck than others, particularly small-diameter internal hex implants (Fig 2-92). The metal at the neck of some of these implants is thin because of their internal hex design, and it often cannot withstand the torque of being placed in dense bone. Therefore, when placing these implants in type 1 or type 2 bone, precise preparation of the osteotomy site should be performed to minimize torque on the implant neck during placement.

Because fractured implants have generally been placed under high torque, their removal requires the use of a trephine drill that is slightly longer and slightly wider than the implant (Fig 2-93). Some implant manufacturers offer tools that can be used with some degree of success to remove an implant in case of fracture during placement.

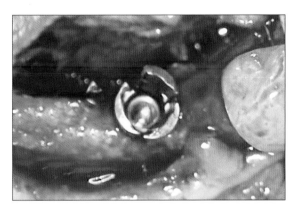

Fig 2-92 Small-diameter internal hex implant fractured at the neck level. The thin internal hex walls could not withstand the stress from the torque applied to the implant during placement.

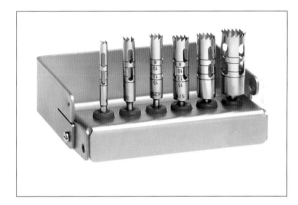

Fig 2-93 Trephine drills that can be used to remove fractured implants.

Postsurgical implant fracture

Occlusal overload can cause fracture of an implant after delivery of the provisional or definitive prosthesis. Parafunctions such as bruxism and clenching, cantilever forces, premature loading, prostheses without passive fit, and poor prosthetic design can lead to occlusal overload and fracture.

In most cases of postsurgical fracture, the implant has osseointegrated and therefore must be removed with a trephine drill (Fig 2-94). Placement of a new implant immediately after removal of a broken implant with a trephine drill is sometimes not possible (because of the high volume of bone removed or destroyed during implant removal); in such cases, the implant site should be grafted for delayed implant placement (Fig 2-95).

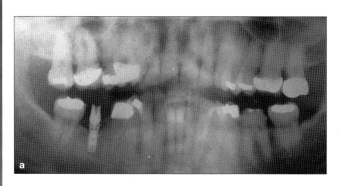

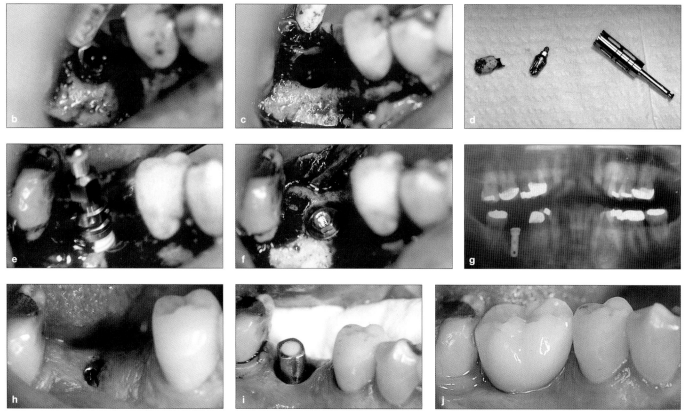

Fig 2-94 *(a)* Implant fracture. The narrow-diameter implant could not withstand the occlusal forces applied to its large restoration. *(b to d)* Removal using an appropriately sized trephine drill. *(e to g)* A wider and longer implant was placed using a two-stage insertion protocol. *(h to j)* The restoration was delivered 4 months postsurgery.

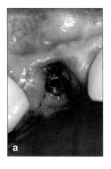
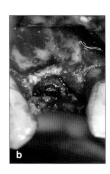
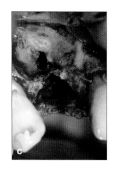

Fig 2-95 *(a)* Implant fracture. *(b)* A full-thickness flap has been reflected. *(c)* The implant has been removed using a trephine drill. Note the large osteotomy site and the buccal plate defect created by the trephine drill, which mandate delayed implant placement after bone grafting and an appropriate healing period.

COMPLICATION 28	# Excessive Torque During Insertion and Compression Necrosis

A variety of factors contribute to early bone loss around implants, and it can be difficult to determine the exact cause (see complication 37, part 3). Compression necrosis should be suspected when implants were placed in dense bone without tapping and when no other systemic or local factors are present.

Excessive insertion torque may lead to ineffective osseointegration because of bone compression beyond its physiologic tolerance, resulting in ischemia and subsequent necrosis. The crestal region around an implant is generally dense cortical bone and is the most susceptible to bone necrosis because of its minimal blood supply. Bone necrosis due to excessive compression forces during insertion will appear usually within the first month after placement. Histology of the area surrounding a failed implant because of necrotic compression will reveal nonviable bony sequestra with bacterial colonization and subacutely inflamed granulation tissue.[137]

Determining the optimum level of torque

Primary implant stability is a critical factor in achieving osseointegration and in the survival of an implant. Bone density, bone volume, and drilling and insertion techniques influence primary stability. An initial torque of approximately 20 Ncm is generally adequate to achieve osseointegration if all other healing factors are met, including an adequate healing period, a low-trauma surgical technique, an absence of micromovement during healing, precise osteotomy preparation, and an implant surface uncontaminated by organic or inorganic materials.

However, when an immediate loading protocol is followed, the initial torque must be increased to withstand the micromovement and stress applied to the implant by the immediate provisional prosthesis in the critical early stages after placement.[87,138,139] An optimum insertion torque of approximately 35 to 45 Ncm for immediately loaded implants is generally agreed upon in the literature. Even when immediate loading is not planned, an initial torque greater than 20 Ncm is recommended to reduce the healing period and increase the likelihood of osseointegration.

Methods for achieving the optimum level of torque

High-density bone

In high-density (type 1 or 2) bone, exceeding the optimum torque of 35 to 45 Ncm may cause bone necrosis and loss of implant stability. Sites consisting of dense bone seem to be at increased risk for compression necrosis.[137]

It is important to use the full series of drills recommended by the implant manufacturer when preparing the osteotomy. Also, special drills like tapping drills or threadformers are necessary in dense bone. The tapping drill should be used in an incremental fashion to form the threads in the osteotomy site.

It is worth noting that if the surgeon is not careful, he or she may overtap or perform too many in-and-out motions during drilling in high-density bone, resulting in a loose implant.

Low-density bone

In low-density (type 3 or 4) bone, the techniques available to facilitate initial stability include:

* Omitting the final one or two drills in the drilling sequence
* Not using the tapping drill
* Using osteotomes (in certain cases with poor-quality type 4 bone) to condense the bone laterally rather than removing bone from the osteotomy site

Clinical tip

Although placement of the implant with a handpiece is an acceptable and common practice, the author recommends that the clinician switch to a hand ratchet when the implant is just short of its definitive position (by 3 to 4 mm) so as to have better control over the level of torque and the apicocoronal position relative to the crestal bone level.

Predicting and measuring implant stability

Bone-quality and implant-stability parameters are correlated, allowing the clinician to predict the level of primary stability before surgery. When bone quality is poor, the treatment plan can be modified accordingly.[140]

Following are methods of measuring implant stability following implant placement:

- Subjective evaluation.[141]
- Resonance frequency analysis (RFA).[142,143] In this method, the stiffness of the bone-implant interface is calculated from a resonance frequency in reaction to oscillations applied to the implant-bone system by the SmartPeg (Osstell), which attaches to the implant (Fig 2-96). The more stable the implant, the higher the frequency.
- Insertion torque.[144,145] This method records the torque required to place the implant and provides valuable information about local bone quality.

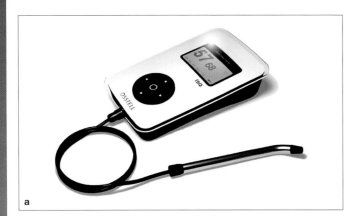

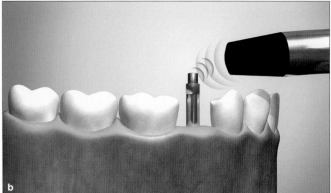

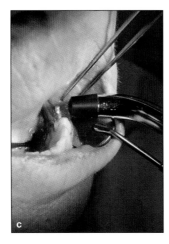

Fig 2-96 *(a)* Resonance frequency analysis machine. *(b and c)* The Smart-Peg attaches to the implant and creates oscillations; the stiffness of the implant-bone interface is determined by measuring the resulting resonance frequency.

Inadequate Initial Stability

Inadequate insertion torque

Low-torque implant placement can be a factor in implant failure. Loose implants are subject to movement during the healing period, which interferes with osseointegration. There are a few reasons why implants may lack primary stability, including:

- Overpreparation of the site with excessive in-and-out motions during drilling
- Use of dense bone drills or tapping drills in low-density bone
- Following an elliptical or imprecise pathway during drilling

Prevention

Conservative drilling of the osteotomy is essential for preventing inadequate initial stability (Fig 2-97). In type 1 bone, for example, all drills, including the tapping drill, should be used. In type 2 bone, the tapping drill is most often not needed. In type 3 bone, the osteotomy should be a little narrower than the implant diameter for good initial stability. In type 4 bone, the osteotomy should be created with osteotomes (after the use of the pilot drill) to condense bone laterally rather than removing bone using drills.

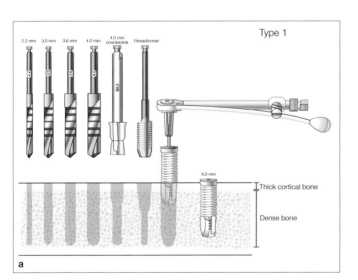

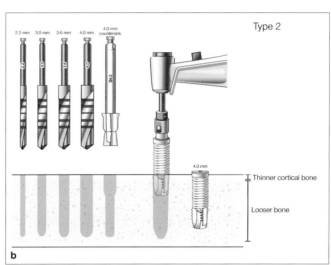

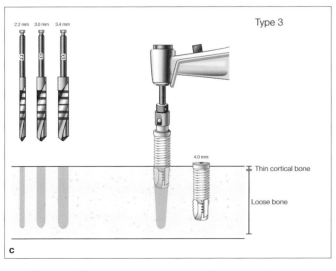

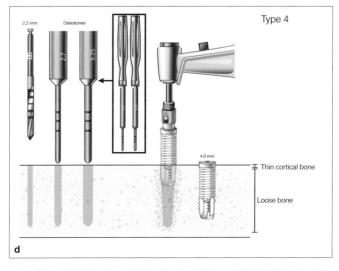

Fig 2-97 *(a to d)* The recommended sequence for enlarging the implant osteotomy in all four bone-density types to achieve optimal initial stability. More drills are required for denser bone, and minimal drilling is recommended for type 4 bone, with preference for the use of osteotomes.

Management

Loose implants should be removed and replaced by a wider or longer implant if sufficient bone and space are available (Fig 2-98). If sufficient bone is not available, the osteotomy site should be abandoned in lieu of a more suitable site. This is usu-ally possible in fully edentulous arches or in long-span edentu-lous areas. If maintaining the original site is crucial to the treat-ment plan, the osteotomy site should be grafted and an implant can be placed in the same location 3 to 4 months later.

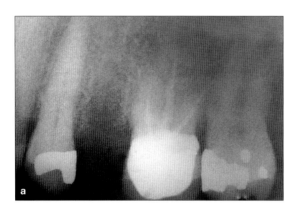

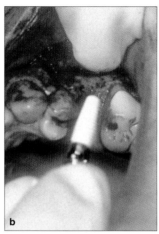

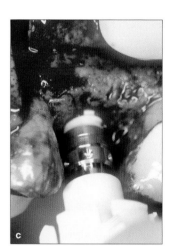

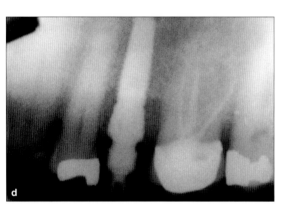

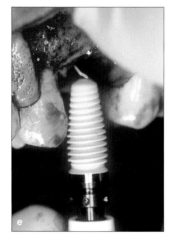

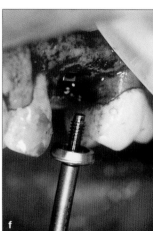

Fig 2-98 *(a to d)* The placement of a 4.3-mm implant with unsatisfactory initial torque. *(e to g)* It was removed and, without any further drilling, replaced by a 5.0-mm implant with satisfactory initial stability.

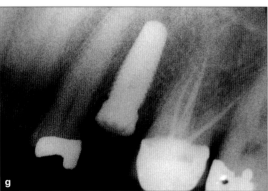

Al-Faraje torque and depth control technique

To prevent compression necrosis due to excessive initial stability in dense bone and to prevent unstable implants in low-density bone, the author has developed a technique for achieving the optimal torque for implant stability (35 to 45 Ncm) with the correct position of the implant platform relative to the crestal bone.

The first step in achieving high initial stability, especially in low-density bone, is to forgo using the full drilling sequence recommended by the manufacturer. Instead, the clinician should stop short of the tapping drill in type 2 bone and short of the final drill in type 3 bone. For example, if the drilling sequence calls for five drills to place a 4.0-mm-diameter implant in type 1 bone (2.2-, 3.0-, 3.6-, and 4.0-mm, plus the tapping drill), in lower-quality bone (ie, type 3 bone density), the clinician should forgo the last one to three drills, attempting to seat the implant after the use of the 3.6-mm drill, or even the 3.0-mm drill. In doing so, the implant will be very tight in the osteotomy upon seating, and the handpiece will not be able to seat the implant to the definitive depth.

At this point, the clinician should switch to the ratchet driver for the final seating of the implant. Using the larger handle on the ratchet, the clinician should force the implant further into the osteotomy, back it out, then use the smaller ratchet handle to torque it until the implant cannot move further or until 45 Ncm is reached. If the implant is still shallow, the above steps can be repeated until the implant is fully seated with good primary stability (Fig 2-99).

Guidelines for applying the technique

- This technique should not be used in type 1 or type 4 bone. In type 1 bone, all drills plus the tapping drill should be used to place the implant. In type 4 bone, the clinician should use mostly osteotomes to place the implant. The technique described above is for type 2 and type 3 bone in the range of 300 to 700 Hounsfield units.
- This technique should not be used with narrow-diameter internal hex implants (< 4 mm).
- This technique should not be repeated more than three to four times because the metal may reach its fatigue curve and implant neck fracture might occur. If the implant is under high torque forces and is still well above the crestal bone level, it should be removed and the osteotomy enlarged further using drills.

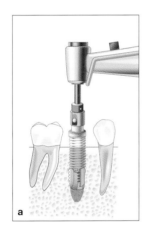
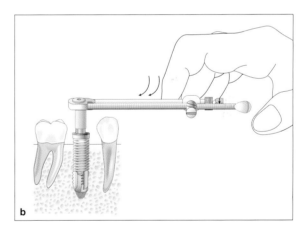
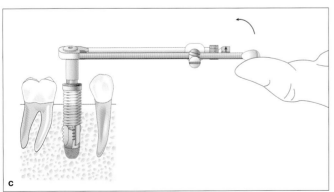
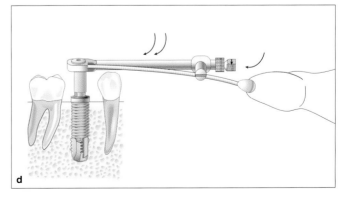

Fig 2-99 *(a)* When the final one to three drills are skipped during drilling of the osteotomy site, the implant initially will be seated above the crestal bone level, a bit higher than ideal. *(b)* The clinician should switch from the handpiece to a hand ratchet, and using the large handle of the ratchet, force the implant to a deeper level. The torque on the implant may exceed 50 to 60 Ncm. *(c)* At this point, the clinician should back the implant out slightly to relieve the pressure. *(d)* Then, using the smaller handle of the ratchet, the implant should be seated until the torque reaches 45 Ncm. This technique enables the implant to be seated a bit deeper than the handpiece initially allowed and with good torque. The steps shown in *b* and *c* can be repeated three to four times if deeper placement is desired.

References

1. Bahat O. Osseointegrated implants in the maxillary tuberosity: Report on 45 consecutive patients. Int J Oral Maxillofac Implants 1992;7:459–467.

2. Bahat O. Brånemark system implants in the posterior maxilla: Clinical study of 660 implants followed for 5-12 years. Int J Oral Maxillofac Implants 2000;15:646–653.

3. Venturelli A. A modified surgical protocol for placing implants in the maxillary tuberosity: Clinical results at 36 months after loading with fixed partial dentures. Int J Oral Maxillofac Implants 1996;11:743–749.

4. Fortin Y, Sullivan RM, Rangert BR. The Marius implant bridge: Surgical and prosthetic rehabilitation for the completely edentulous upper jaw with moderate to severe resorption: A 5-year retrospective clinical study. Clin Implant Dent Relat Res 2002;4:69–77.

5. Krekmanov L, Kahn M, Rangert B, Lindstrom H. Tilting of posterior mandibular and maxillary implants for improved prosthesis support. Int J Oral Maxillofac Implants 2000;15:405–414.

6. Krekmanov L. Placement of posterior mandibular and maxillary implants in patients with severe bone deficiency: A clinical report of procedure. Int J Oral Maxillofac Implants 2000;15:722–730.

7. Capelli M, Zuffetti F, Del Fabbro M, Testori T. Immediate rehabilitation of the completely edentulous jaw with fixed prostheses supported by either upright or tilted implants: A multicenter clinical study. Int J Oral Maxillofac Implants 2007;22:639–644.

8. Testori T, Del Fabbro M, Capelli M, Zuffetti F, Francetti L, Weinstein RL. Immediate occlusal loading and tilted implants for the rehabilitation of the atrophic edentulous maxilla. 1-year interim results of a multicenter prospective study. Clin Oral Implants Res 2008;19:227–232.

9. Day RH. Diagnosis and treatment of trigeminal nerve injury. J Calif Dent Assoc 1994;22:48–54.

10. Guyton A. Anatomy & Physiology. New York: CBS College, 1985:264–266.

11. Worthington P. Injury to the inferior alveolar nerve during implant placement: A formula for protection of the patient and clinician. Int J Oral Maxillofac Implants 2004;19:731–734.

12. Greenstein G, Tarnow D. The mental foramen and nerve: Clinical and anatomical factors related to dental implant placement. A literature review. J Periodontol 2006;77:1933–1943.

13. Peterson LJ, Ellis E, Hupp JR, Tucker MR. Contemporary Oral and Maxillofacial Surgery. St Louis: Mosby, 1998:378–379.

14. Wadu SG, Penhall B, Townsend GC. Morphological variability of the human inferior nerve. Clin Anat 1997;10:82–87.

15. Mardinger O, Chaushu G, Arensburg B, Taicher S, Kaffe I. Anatomic and radiologic course of the mandibular incisive canal. Surg Radiol Anat 2000;22:157–161.

16. Monsour PA, Dudhia R. Implant radiography and radiology. Aust Dent J 2008;53(suppl 1):S11–S25.

17. Romanos GE, Greenstein G. The incisive canal. Considerations during implant placement: Case report and literature review. Int J Oral Maxillofac Implants 2009;24:740–745.

18. Fehrenbach M, Herring S. Illustrated Anatomy of the Head and Neck. Philadelphia: Saunders, 1996:205–206.

19. Hall-Craggs ECB. Anatomy as a Basis for Clinical Medicine. Munich: Urban & Schwarzenberg, 1985:546–547.

20. Miloro M, Halkias LE, Slone HW, Chakeres DW. Assessment of the lingual nerve in the third molar region using magnetic resonance imaging. J Oral Maxillofac Surg 1997;55:134–137.

21. Greenstein G, Cavallaro J, Romanos G, Tarnow D. Clinical recommendations for avoiding and managing surgical complications associated with implant dentistry. A review. J Periodontol 2008;79:1317–1329.

22. Kahle W, Leonhardt H, Platzer W. Color Atlas and Textbook of Human Anatomy, vol 3. Stuttgart, Germany: George Thieme Verlag, 1986:118.

23. Kraut RA, Chahal O. Management of patients with trigeminal nerve injuries after mandibular implant placement. J Am Dent Assoc 2002;133:1351–1354.

24. Ruggiero S. Trigeminal nerve injury and repair. N Y State Dent J 1996;62:36–40.

25. Robinson PP, Loescher AR, Smith KG. A prospective, quantitative study on the clinical outcome of lingual nerve repair. Br J Oral Maxillofac Surg 2000;38:255–263.

26. Sussman HI. Tooth devitalization via implant placement: A case report. Periodontal Clin Investig 1998;20:22–24.

27. Kim SG. Implant-related damage to an adjacent tooth: A case report. Implant Dent 2000;9:278–280.

28. Margelos JT, Verdelis KG. Irreversible pulpal damage of teeth adjacent to recently placed osseointegrated implants. J Endod 1995;21:479–482.

29. Lindeboom JA, Tjiook Y, Kroon FH. Immediate placement of implants in periapical infected sites: A prospective randomized study in 50 patients. Oral Surg Oral Med Oral Pathol Oral Radiol Endod 2006;101:705–710.

30. Novaes AB Jr, Novaes AB. Immediate implants placed into infected sites: A clinical report. Int J Oral Maxillofac Implants 1995;10:609–613.

31. Novaes AB Jr, Vidigal GM Jr, Novaes AB, Grisi MF, Polloni S, Rosa A. Immediate implants placed into infected sites: A histomorphometric study in dogs. Int J Oral Maxillofac Implants 1998;13:422–427.

32. Naves Mde M, Horbylon BZ, Gomes Cde F, Menezes HH, Bataglion C, Magalhães D. Immediate implants placed into infected sockets: A case report with 3-year follow-up. Braz Dent J 2009;20:254–258.

33. Park SH, Sorensen WP, Wang HL. Management and prevention of retrograde peri-implant infection from retained root tips: Two case reports. Int J Periodontics Restorative Dent 2004;24:422–433.

34. Guarnieri R, Giardino L, Crespi R, Romagnoli R. Cementum formation around a titanium implant: A case report. Int J Oral Maxillofac Implants 2002;17:729–732.

35. Gray JL, Vernino AR. The interface between retained roots and dental implants: A histologic study in baboons. J Periodontol 2004;75:1102–1106.

36. Buser D, Warrer K, Karring T. Formation of a periodontal ligament around titanium implants. J Periodontol 1990;61:597–601.

37. Buser D, Warrer K, Karring T, Stich H. Titanium implants with a true periodontal ligament: An alternative to osseointegrated implants? Int J Oral Maxillofac Implants 1990;5:113–116.

38. Rosano G, Taschieri S, Gaudy JF, Testori T, Del Fabbro M. Anatomic assessment of the anterior mandible and relative hemorrhage risk in implant dentistry: A cadaveric study. Clin Oral Implants Res 2009;20:791–795.

39. Reiser GM, Bruno JF, Mahan PE, Larkin LH. The subepithelial connective tissue graft palatal donor site: Anatomic considerations for surgeons. Int J Periodontics Restorative Dent 1996;16:130–137.

40. Krenkel C, Holzner K, Poisel S. Hemoatoma of the mouth floor following oral surgery and its anatomical characteristics [in German]. Dtsch Z Mund Kiefer Gesichtschir 1985;9:448–451.

41. Liang X, Jacobs R, Lambrichts I. An assessment on spiral CT scan of the superior and inferior genial spinal foramina and canals. Surg Radiol Anat 2006;28:98–104.

42. Liang X, Jacobs R, Lambrichts I, Vandewalle G. Lingual foramina on the mandibular midline revisited: A macroanatomical study. Clin Anat 2007;20:246–251.

43. Shiller WR, Wiswell OB. Lingual foramina of the mandible. Anat Rec 1954;119:387–390.

44. McDonnell D, Reza Nouri M, Todd ME. The mandibular lingual foramen: A consistent arterial foramen in the middle of the mandible. J Anat 1994;184:363–369.

45. Bradley JC. The clinical significance of age changes in the vascular supply to the mandible. Int J Oral Surg 1981;10(suppl 1):71–76.

46. Castelli WA, Nasjleti CE, Diaz-Perez R. Interruption of the arterial inferior alveolar flow and its effects on mandibular collateral circulation and dental tissues. J Dent Res 1975;54:708–715.

47. Kalpidis CD, Setayesh RM. Hemorrhaging associated with endosseous implant placement in the anterior mandible: A review of the literature. J Periodontol 2004;75:631–645.

48. Bavitz JB, Harn SD, Homze EJ. Arterial supply to the floor of the mouth and lingual gingiva. Oral Surg Oral Med Oral Pathol 1994;77:232–235.

49. Zimmerman RA, McLean G, Freiman D, Golestaneh Z, Perez M. The diagnosis and therapeutic role of angiography in lingual arterial bleeding. Radiology 1979;133:639–643.

50. Piper SN, Maleck WH, Kumle B, Deschner E, Boldt J. Massive postoperative swelling of the tongue: Manual decompression and tactile intubation as a life-saving measure. Resuscitation 2000;43:217–220.

51. Ten Bruggenkate CM, Krekeler G, Kraaijenhagen HA, Foitzik C, Oosterbeek HS. Hemorrhage of the floor of the mouth resulting from lingual perforation during implant placement: A clinical report. Int J Oral Maxillofac Implants 1993;8:329–334.

52. Ferneini E, Gady J, Lieblich SE. Floor of the mouth hematoma after posterior mandibular implants placement: A case report. J Oral Maxillofac Surg 2009;67:1552–1554.

53. Kerawala CJ, Martin IC, Allan W, Williams ED. The effects of operator technique and bur design on temperature during osseous preparation for osteosynthesis self-tapping screws. Oral Surg Oral Med Oral Pathol Oral Radiol Endod 1999;88:145–150.

54. Eriksson AR, Albrektsson T. Temperature threshold levels for heat-induced bone tissue injury: A vital-microscopic study in the rabbit. J Prosthet Dent 1983;50:101–107.

55. Eriksson AR, Albrektsson T, Grane B, McQueen D. Thermal injury to bone. A vital-microscopic description of heat effects. Int J Oral Surg 1982;11:115–121.

56. Eriksson AR, Adell R. Temperatures during drilling for the placement of implants using the osseointegration technique. J Oral Maxillofac Surg 1986;44:4–7.

57. Piattelli A, Piattelli M, Mangano C, Scarano A. A histologic evaluation of eight cases of failed dental implants: Is bone overheating the most probable cause? Biomaterials 1998;19:683–690.

58. Lekholm U, Zarb GA. Patient selection and preparation. In: Brånemark P-I, Zarb G, Albrektsson T (eds). Tissue-Integrated Prostheses: Osseointegration in Clinical Dentistry. Chicago: Quintessence, 1985:199–210.

59. Iyer S, Weiss CM, Mehta A. Effects of drill speed on heat production and the rate and quality of bone formation in dental implant osteomies. Part I: Relationship between drill speed and heat production. Int J Prosthodont 1997;10:411–414.

60. Tatum OH Jr. Maxillary and sinus implant reconstructions. Dent Clin North Am 1986;30:207–229.

61. Summers RB. The osteotome technique. Part IV: Future site development. Compend Contin Educ Dent 1995;16:1090–1092.

62. Bruschi GB, Scipioni A, Calesini G, Bruschi E. Localized management of sinus floor with simultaneous implant placement: A clinical report. Int J Oral Maxillofac Implants 1998;13:219–226.

63. Fugazzotto PA. Immediate implant placement following a modified trephine/osteotome approach: Success rate of 116 implants to 4 years of function. Int J Oral Maxillofac Implants 2002;17:113–120.

64. Nkenke E, Schlegel A, Schultze-Mosgau S, Neukam FW, Wiltfang J. The endoscopically controlled osteotome sinus floor elevation: A preliminary prospective study. Int J Oral Maxillofac Implants 2002;17:557–566.

65. Deporter D, Todescan R, Caudry S. Simplifying management of the posterior maxilla using short, porous-surfaced dental implants and simultaneous indirect sinus elevation. Int J Periodontics Restorative Dent 2000;20:477–485.

66. Komarnyckyj OG, London RM. Osteotome single-stage dental implant placement with and without sinus elevation: A clinical report. Int J Oral Maxillofac Implants 1998;13:799–804.

67. Zitzmann NU, Scharer P. Sinus elevation procedures in the resorbed posterior maxilla. Comparison of the crestal and lateral approaches. Oral Surg Oral Med Oral Pathol 1998;85:8–17.

68. Brånemark PI, Adell R, Albrektsson T, Lekholm U, Lindström J, Rockler B. An experimental and clinical study of osseointegrated implants penetrating the nasal cavity and maxillary sinus. J Oral Maxillofac Surg 1984;42:497–505.

69. Krmpotic-Nemanic J, Draf W, Helms J. Surgical Anatomy of the Head and Neck. Berlin: Springer-Verlag, 1985:126,133.

70. Garg AK. Subnasal elevation and bone augmentation. In: Jensen OT (ed). The Sinus Bone Graft, Chicago: Quintessence, 1999:177–181.

71. Chappuis V, Suter VG, Bornstein MM. Displacement of a dental implant into the maxillary sinus: Report of an unusual complication when performing staged sinus floor elevation procedures. Int J Periodontics Restorative Dent 2009;29:81–87.

72. Ziccardi VB, Betts NJ. Complications of maxillary sinus augmentation. In: Jensen OT (ed). The Sinus Bone Graft. Chicago: Quintessence, 1999:201–208.

73. Guler N, Delilbasi C. Ectopic dental implants in the maxillary sinus. Quintessence Int 2007;38:e238–e239.

74. Ridaura-Ruiz L, Figueiredo R, Guinot-Moya R, et al. Accidental displacement of dental implants into the maxillary sinus: A report of nine cases. Clin Implant Dent Relat Res 2009;11(suppl 1):e38–e45.

75. Chiapasco M, Felisati G, Maccari A, Borloni R, Gatti F, Di Leo F. The management of complications following displacement of oral implants in the paranasal sinuses: A multicenter clinical report and proposed treatment protocols. Int J Oral Maxillofac Surg 2009;38:1273–1278.

76. Ramotar H, Jaberoo MC, Koo Ng NK, Pulido MA, Saleh HA. Image-guided, endoscopic removal of migrated titanium dental implants from maxillary sinus: Two cases. J Laryngol Otol 2010;124:433–436.

77. Ucer TC. A modified transantral endoscopic technique for the removal of a displaced dental implant from the maxillary sinus followed by simultaneous sinus grafting. Int J Oral Maxillofac Implants 2009;24:947–951.

78. Kraut RA, Boyden DK. Location of incisive canal in relation to central incisor implants. Implant Dent 1998;7:221–225.

79. Terry BR, Bolanos OR. A diagnostic case involving an incisive canal cyst. J Endod 1989;15:559–562.

80. Song WC, Jo DI, Lee JY, et al. Microanatomy of the incisive canal using three-dimensional reconstruction of microCT images: An ex vivo study. Oral Surg Oral Med Oral Pathol Oral Radiol Endod 2009;108:583–590.

81. Mraiwa N, Jacobs R, Van Cleynenbreugel J, et al. The nasopalatine canal revisited using 2D and 3D CT imaging. Dentomaxillofac Radiol 2004;33:396–402.

82. Iordanishvili AK. Age-related characteristics and sex differences in the anatomical structure of the incisive canal [in Russian]. Stomatologiia (Mosk) 1991;(4):25–27.

83. Rosenquist, JB, Nyström E. Occlusion of the incisal canal with bone chips. A procedure to facilitate insertion of implants in the anterior maxilla. Int J Oral Maxillofac Surg 1992;21:210–211.

84. Spin-Neto R, Bedran TB, de Paula WN, de Freitas RM, de Oliveira Ramalho LT, Marcantonio E Jr. Incisive canal deflation for correct implant placement: Case report. Implant Dent 2009;18:473–479.

85. Scher EL. Use of the incisive canal as a recipient site for root form implants: Preliminary clinical reports. Implant Dent 1994;3:38–41.

86. Palacci P. Esthetic Implant Dentistry. Soft and Hard Tissue Management. Chicago: Quintessence, 2001:33–45.

87. Wöhrle PS. Single-tooth replacement in the aesthetic zone with immediate provisionalization: Fourteen consecutive case reports. Pract Periodontics Aesthet Dent 1998;10:1107–1114.

88. Gargiulo AW, Wentz FM, Orban B. Dimensions and relations of the dentogingival junction in man. J Periodontol 1961;32:261–267.

89. Berglundh T, Lindhe H, Ericsson I, Marinello CP, Liljenberg B, Thomsen P. The soft tissue barrier at implants and teeth. Clin Oral Implants Res 1991;2:81–90.

90. Listgarten MA, Buser D, Steinemann SG, Donath K, Lang NP, Weber HP. Light and transmission electron microscopy of the intact interfaces between nonsubmerged titanium-coated epoxy resin implants and bone or gingiva. J Dent Res 1992;71:364–371.

91. Ochsenbein C, Ross S. A re-evaluation of osseous surgery. Dent Clin North Am 1969;13:87–102.

92. Kao RT, Pasquinelli K. Thick vs thin tissue: A key determinant in tissue response to disease and restorative treatment. J Calif Dent Assoc 2002;30: 521–526.

93. Kao RT, Fagan MC, Conte GJ. Thick vs thin gingival biotypes: A key determinant in treatment planning for dental implants. J Calif Dent Assoc 2008;36:193–198.

94. Olsson M, Lindhe J. Periodontal characteristics in individuals with varying forms of the upper central incisors. J Clin Periodontol 1991;18:78–82.

95. Kois JC. Predictable single tooth peri-implant esthetics: Five diagnostic keys. Compend Contin Educ Dent 2001;22:199–206.

96. Schropp L, Wenzel A, Kostopoulos L, Karring T. Bone healing and soft tissue contour changes following single-tooth extraction: A clinical and radiographic 12-month prospective study. Int J Periodontics Restorative Dent 2003;23:313–323.

97. Botticelli D, Berglundh T, Lindhe J. Hard-tissue alterations following immediate implant placement in extraction sites. J Clin Periodontol 2004; 31:820–828.

98. Hermann JS, Buser D, Schenk RK, Cochran DL. Crestal bone changes around titanium implants. A histometric evaluation of unloaded non-submerged and submerged implants in the canine mandible. J Periodontol 2000;71:1412–1424.

99. Hermann JS, Schoolfield JD, Schenk RK, Buser D, Cochran DL. Influence of the size of the microgap on crestal bone changes around titanium implants. A histometric evaluation of unloaded non-submerged implants in the canine mandible. J Periodontol 2001;72:1372–1383.

100. Buser D, Mericske-Stern R, Dula K, Lang NP. Clinical experience with one-stage, non-submerged dental implants. Adv Dent Res 1999;13:153–161.

101. Broggini N, McManus LM, Hermann JS, et al. Peri-implant inflammation defined by the implant-abutment interface. J Dent Res 2006;85:473–478.

102. Hermann JS, Buser D, Schenk RK, Schoolfield JD, Cochran DL. Biologic width around one- and two-piece titanium implants. Clin Oral Implants Res 2001;12:559–571.

103. Lazzara RJ, Porter SS. Platform switching: A new concept in implant dentistry for controlling postrestorative crestal bone levels. Int J Periodontics Restorative Dent 2006;26:9–17.

104. Luongo R, Traini T, Guidone PC, Bianco G, Cocchetto R, Celletti R. Hard and soft tissue responses to the platform-switching technique. Int J Periodontics Restorative Dent 2008;28:551–557.

105. Cappiello M, Luongo R, Di Iorio D, Bugea C, Cocchetto R, Celletti R. Evaluation of peri-implant bone loss around platform-switched implants. Int J Periodontics Restorative Dent 2008;28:347–355.

106. Crespi R, Capparè P, Gherlone E. Radiographic evaluation of marginal bone levels around platform-switched and non-platform-switched implants used in an immediate loading protocol. Int J Oral Maxillofac Implants 2009;24:920–926.

107. Trammell K, Geurs NC, O'Neal SJ, et al. A prospective, randomized, controlled comparison of platform-switched and matched-abutment implants in short-span partial denture situations. Int J Periodontics Restorative Dent 2009;29:599–605.

108. Tarnow DP, Magner AW, Fletcher P. The effect of the distance from the contact point to the crest of the bone on the presence or absence of the interproximal dental papilla. J Periodontol 1992;62:995–996.

109. Campelo LD, Camara JR. Flapless implant surgery: A 10-year clinical retrospective analysis. Int J Oral Maxillofac Implants 2002;17:271–276.

110. Brodala N. Flapless surgery and its effect on dental implant outcomes. Int J Oral Maxillofac Implants 2009;24(suppl):118–125.

111. Lee DH, Choi BH, Jeong SM, Xuan F, Kim HR, Mo DY. Effects of soft tissue punch size on the healing of peri-implant tissue in flapless implant surgery. Oral Surg Oral Med Oral Pathol Oral Radiol Endod 2010;109:525–530.

112. Fortin T, Bosson JL, Isidori M, Blanchet E. Effect of flapless surgery on pain experienced in implant placement using an image-guided system. Int J Oral Maxillofac Implants 2006;21:298–304.

113. Nkenke E, Eitner S, Radespiel-Troger M, Vairaktaris E, Neukam FW, Fenner M. Patient-centred outcomes comparing transmucosal implant placement with an open approach in the maxilla: A prospective, non-randomized pilot study. Clin Oral Implants Res 2007;18:197–203.

114. Wood DL, Hoag PM, Donnenfeld OW, Rosenfeld LD. Alveolar crest reduction following full and partial thickness flaps. J Periodontol 1972; 43:141–144.

115. Van der Zee E, Oosterveld P, Van Waas MA. Effect of GBR and fixture installation on gingiva and bone levels at adjacent teeth. Clin Oral Implants Res 2004;15:62–65.

116. Sclar AG. Guidelines for flapless surgery. J Oral Maxillofac Surg 2007; 65:20–32.

117. Block MS, Kent JN. Factors associated with soft- and hard-tissue compromise of endosseous implants. J Oral Maxillofac Surg 1990;48:1153–1160.

118. Buser D, Weber HP, Lang NP. Tissue integration of non-submerged implants. 1-year results of a prospective study with 100 ITI hollow-cylinder and hollow-screw implants. Clin Oral Implants Res 1990;1:33–40.

119. Azari A, Nikzad S. Flapless implant surgery: Review of the literature and report of 2 cases with computer-guided surgical approach. J Oral Maxillofac Surg 2008;66:1015–1021.

120. Azari A, Nikzad S, Kabiri A. Using computer-guided implantology in flapless implant surgery of a maxilla: A clinical report. J Oral Rehabil 2008;35:690–694.

121. D'haese J, Van De Velde T, Elaut L, De Bruyn H. A prospective study on the accuracy of mucosally supported stereolithographic surgical guides in fully edentulous maxillae [epub ahead of print 10 Nov 2009]. Clin Implant Dent Relat Res.

122. Bergermann M, Donald PJ, aWengen DF. Screwdriver aspiration. A complication of dental implant placement. Int J Oral Maxillofac Surg 1992;21:339–341.

123. Pinto A, Scaglione M, Pinto F, et al. Tracheobronchial aspiration of foreign bodies: Current indications for emergency plain chest radiography. Radiol Med 2006;111:497–506.

124. Pingarrón Martín L, Morán Soto MJ, Sánchez Burgos R, Burgueño García M. Bronchial impaction of an implant screwdriver after accidental aspiration: Report of a case and revision of the literature. Oral Maxillofac Surg 2010;14:43–47.

125. Agarwal RK, Banerjee G, Shembish N, Jamal BA, Kareemullah C, Swaleh A. Foreign bodies in the tracheobronchial tree: A review of 102 cases in Benghazi, Libya. Ann Trop Paediatr 1988;8:213–216.

126. Haliloglu M, Ciftci AO, Oto A, et al. CT virtual bronchoscopy in the evaluation of children with suspected foreign body aspiration. Eur J Radiol 2003;48:188–192.

127. Worthington P. Ingested foreign body associated with oral implant treatment: Report of a case. Int J Oral Maxillofac Implants 1996;11:679–681.

128. Barkmeier WW, Cooley RL, Abrams H. Prevention of swallowing or aspiration of foreign objects. J Am Dent Assoc 1978;97:473–476.

129. Raghoebar GM, Stellingsma K, Batenburg RH, Vissink A. Etiology and management of mandibular fractures associated with endosteal implants in the atrophic mandible. Oral Surg Oral Med Oral Pathol Oral Radiol Endod 2000;89:553–539.

130. Mason ME, Triplett RG, Van Sickels JE, Parel SM. Mandibular fractures through endosseous cylinder implants: Report of cases and review. J Oral Maxillofac Surg 1990;48:311–317.

131. Luna AH, Passeri LA, de Moraes M, Moreira RW. Endosseous implant placement in conjunction with inferior alveolar nerve transposition: A report of an unusual complication and surgical management. Int J Oral Maxillofac Implants 2008;23:133–136.

132. Karlis V, Bae RD, Glickman RS. Mandibular fracture as a complication of inferior alveolar nerve transposition and placement of endosseous implants: A case report. Implant Dent 2003;12:211–216.

133. Kan JY, Lozada JL, Boyne PJ, Goodacre CJ, Rungcharassaeng K. Mandibular fracture after endosseous implant placement in conjunction with inferior alveolar nerve transposition: A patient treatment report. Int J Oral Maxillofac Implants 1997;12:655–659.

134. Tolman DE, Keller EE. Management of mandibular fractures in patients with endosseous implants. Int J Oral Maxillofac Implants 1991;6:427–436.

135. Shonberg DC, Stith HD, Jameson LM, Chai JY. Mandibular fracture through an endosseous implant. Int J Oral Maxillofac Implants 1992; 12:401–404.

136. Eyrich GK, Grätz KW, Sailer HF. Surgical treatment of fractures of the edentulous mandible. J Oral Maxillofac Surg 1997;55:1081–1087.

137. Bashutski JD, D'Silva, NJ, Wang HL. Implant compression necrosis: Current understanding and case report. J Periodontol 2009;80:700–704.

138. Szmukler-Moncler S, Salama H, Reingewirtz Y, Dubruille JH. Timing of loading and the effect of micromotion on bone-dental implant interface: Review of experimental literature. J Biomed Mater Res 1998;43:192–203.

139. Brunski JB. In vivo bone response to biomechanical loading at the bone/dental-implant interface. Adv Dent Res 1999;13:99–119.

140. Turkyilmaz I, McGlumphy EA. Influence of bone density on implant stability parameters and implant success: A retrospective clinical study. BMC Oral Health 2008;8:32.

141. Orenstein IH, Tarnow DP, Morris HF, Ochi S. Three-year post-placement survival of implants mobile at placement. Ann Periodontol 2000;5:32–41.

142. Meredith N, Alleyne D, Cawley P. Quantitative determination of the stability of the implant-tissue interface using resonance frequency analysis. Clin Oral Implant Res 1996;7:261–267.

143. Meredith N. Assessment of implant stability as a prognostic determinant. Int J Prosthodont 1998;11:491–501.

144. Tricio J, van Steenberghe D, Rosenberg D, Duchateau L. Implant stability related to insertion torque force and bone density: An in vitro study. J Prosthet Dent 1995;74:608–612.

145. Johansson P, Strid KG. Assessment of bone quality from placement resistance during implant surgery. Int J Oral Maxillofac Implants 1994;9:279–288.

PART 3 # Postoperative Complications

Complications

COMPLICATION 30	Postoperative Pain

In general, pain and swelling experienced by patients following the surgical placement of dental implants is mild and gradually decreases over time. Generally, pain is at its maximum 1 day postsurgery and inflammation, 48 hours postsurgery. The patient should expect to limit his or her daily activities, especially for the first 3 days after surgery.[1–3]

Nonetheless, from the patient's perspective, implant placement is one of the most stressful and anxiety-provoking procedures in dentistry.[4] Therefore, minimally invasive surgical protocols should be applied whenever possible to reduce the patient's pain and anxiety and increase the rate of treatment acceptance.

Factors influencing level of pain after dental implant placement

Flap techniques

Flapless technique

A study by Fortin et al[5] compared postoperative pain experienced after implant placement using two different surgical protocols: a flapless protocol using an image-guided system with a surgical template and an open-flap procedure. The study concluded that patients experienced less intense pain for a shorter period of time after the flapless procedure. Pain after the flapless protocol is minimized by decreased postoperative edema or hematoma.

Figure 3-1 shows a case of flapless implant insertion. The postoperative photo (see Fig 3-1j) demonstrates a lack of postoperative swelling. The patient reported no discomfort postoperatively, and painkillers were not needed. Nonetheless, patients should not be promised a painless recovery from flapless surgery; instead, they can be told to expect less pain over a shorter duration of time.

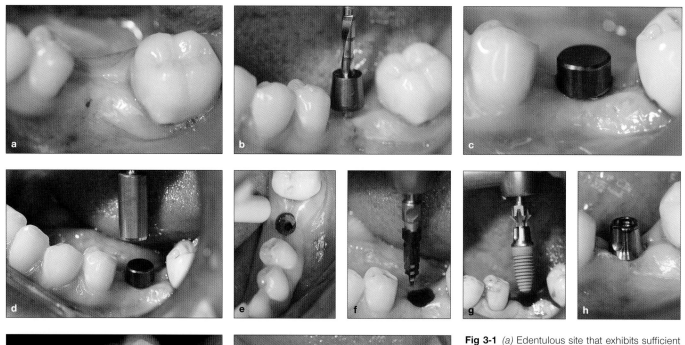

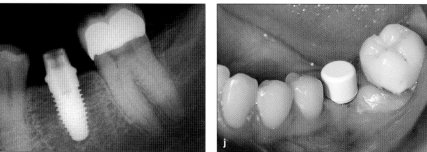

Fig 3-1 *(a)* Edentulous site that exhibits sufficient alveolar ridge width and adequate soft tissue quality and quantity. The site is a candidate for flapless insertion protocol. *(b)* A pilot hole is created. *(c)* The tissue punch guide is placed. *(d and e)* A rotary tissue punch is used to remove the soft tissue at the intended implant site. *(f)* The osteotomy is enlarged to the desired depth and diameter. *(g to i)* The implant is seated to the desired depth, as confirmed on the postoperative radiograph. *(j)* One-week postoperative photo demonstrates the lack of swelling. The patient reported no discomfort postoperatively.

Open-flap technique

The open-flap technique is necessary in some cases because it gives the clinician clearer access to and visualization of the surgical field. It also enables the clinician to manipulate the soft tissue into a desirable position after implant placement. When using this technique, precise incisions, intact reflected periosteum, atraumatic handling of soft tissues, and proper suturing technique minimize postoperative swelling and pain. Improper soft tissue manipulation can lead to incision line opening and subsequent *healing by secondary intention,* or closure of the wound by tissue granulation. This type of healing is usually accompanied by more discomfort than is *healing by primary intention.*

Manipulation of hard tissue

Pain can arise from improper handling of the bone. Overheating the bone during drilling (see complication 16, part 2), overcompression of the bone during implant placement (see complication 28, part 2), and excessive pressure while drilling are three factors that can contribute to postoperative pain. Proper handling of hard tissue can reduce postoperative pain.

Nerve damage

Perforation of the roof of the mandibular canal during osteotomy preparation or implant insertion in close proximity to the inferior alveolar canal can provoke irritation of the inferior alveolar nerve, resulting in chronic pain. The canal cannot be detected in conventional dental radiographs, but computed tomography (CT) images can reveal the close proximity of the implant apex to the mandibular canal (Fig 3-2). Leckel et al[6] used a high-resolution dental magnetic resonance imaging (MRI) technique to show the effect of surgical proximity to the inferior alveolar nerve by measuring the vascular reaction of the neurovascular bundle in the mandibular canal.

No treatment should be performed before obtaining a high-resolution CT or MRI scan to confirm the cause of the pain, especially in cases of multiple implant placements where there is a need to identify the exact implant(s) causing the pain or inflammatory reaction of the nerve. This practice will prevent unnecessarily performing interventions such as endodontic treatment, extraction of teeth in close proximity to the affected area, or the removal of an implant.

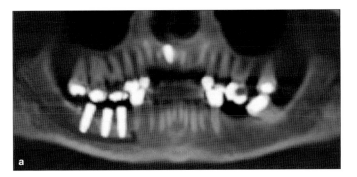
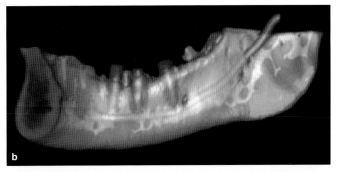
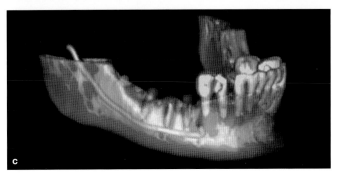

Fig 3-2 Panoramic *(a)* and three-dimensional *(b and c)* CT images reveal that the two distal implants are in contact with the inferior alveolar nerve in a patient who complained about pain and paresthesia postoperatively. Regular posteroanterior or panoramic radiographs could not confirm the exact proximity of the implants to the inferior alveolar nerve.

Delayed wound healing

Many factors play a role in delayed wound healing,[7] including late infection, flap design, incision line opening, malnutrition, aging, immune deficiency, and smoking. Prompt management of these problems with antibiotics, surgical revision, hyperbaric oxygen treatment, diet, and proper postoperative instructions can reduce postsurgical pain.

Postoperative swelling

Postoperative swelling contributes to increased pain. Proper postoperative care and adherence to a medication protocol can minimize pain and swelling.

Medications

Postoperatively, the patient should start on a protocol of antibiotics for prevention of infection and anti-inflammatory medications such as ibuprofen and dexamethasone. Analgesics of sufficient strength should be taken immediately after surgery and can play an important role in pain control. For more information on pharmacologic management of pain, see complication 73, part 5.

Home care

The patient's postoperative compliance also plays an important role in postoperative pain management. Abstaining from smoking, maintaining good oral hygiene, taking all medications as prescribed, applying ice packs, and following a soft diet are all important instructions that should be followed for quicker, uneventful healing.

Patient emotions

Patient emotions such as stress and anxiety can exacerbate the postoperative experience of pain. Antianxiety medications can help in this regard.

Skill of the surgeon

The sound judgment and hands-on expertise of an experienced surgeon is an important factor in minimizing the patient's discomfort.

Tissue Emphysema Induced by Dental Procedures

Tissue emphysema can be induced by the inadvertent introduction of air into the soft tissues (ie, skin or mucous membranes) during dental procedures, particularly during the removal of mandibular third molars.[8] High-speed air-driven handpieces, air-water syringes, air abrasive devices, and endotracheal intubation or ventilation can all force air into the soft tissues. Air introduced into a sulcus or a surgical wound can move through the fascial planes and create a unilateral enlargement of the facial and/or the submandibular region.[9]

Bergendal et al[10] reported a case of submucosal emphysema arising from an air-powder abrasive device (Prophy-Jet, Dentsply) used to remove calculus and debris from the titanium abutments during a 6-month recall visit, resulting in an acute clinical reaction with marginal bone loss around the implants.

Symptoms

Tissue emphysema is identified by swelling that is coincident with dental treatment. The onset of swelling is almost immediate, although the onset may be delayed when coughing or sneezing is the cause, resulting in the entry of air through an oral wound. Palpation of skin usually produces *crepitus*, a crackling sensation, as the air is pushed through the tissue. Pain is not a typical feature of tissue emphysema.

Differential diagnosis

Angioedema caused by the use of nonsteroidal anti-inflammatory drugs or local anesthetics, soft tissue infections, and hematomas must be ruled out.

Although many cases of tissue emphysema go unnoticed, some emphysemas can have potentially life-threatening effects[9,11–13] if the air moves into deeper fascial spaces. Serious complications include mediastinitis, airway compromise, fatal air embolism, and infections caused by the spread of microorganisms along the fascial planes dissected by the emphysematous air. Quick diagnosis and proper management will reduce the incidence of further complications.

Prevention

- Handpieces that vent air away from the surgical field should be used during surgical procedures[14] (Fig 3-3).
- Mucoperiosteal flaps should not extend onto the lingual aspect of the mandibular third molar area or onto the medial side of the vertical ramus.
- Use of the air-water syringe in areas of soft tissue and periodontal infections should be avoided.
- Preparation of the pulp chamber during endodontic therapy should be done with a slow-speed handpiece.

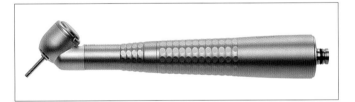

Fig 3-3 Rear-exhaust high-speed surgical handpiece.

Management

Most tissue emphysemas are mild. Treatment usually consists of broad-spectrum antibiotic therapy because of the possible introduction of bacteria along with the compressed air, mild analgesic therapy, reassurance, and observation. Patients should also be warned to avoid forceful sneezing, blowing of the nose, or restrained coughing. Symptoms usually subside in 3 to 10 days; however, consultation with a physician is necessary to rule out further complications.

If the patient reports any respiratory distress, he or she should be immediately referred to a hospital for close observation and high-dose intravenous antibiotics.

| COMPLICATION 32 | Incision Line Reopening |

The incision line can reopen soon after surgery and can compromise the final results of implant surgery by increasing the risk of infection in the surgical area and by affecting the postoperative soft tissue esthetic outcome.

Preventive techniques

Midcrestal incision lines

When the crestal incision is not made in the middle of the crestal ridge, the sutures will be located on the buccal or the lingual side of the alveolar ridge, where activity of the underlying muscles can increase the incidence of incision line reopening upon movement of the lips, cheeks, and tongue because of tension on the sutures (eg, during speaking or laughing). Placement of the midline incision in a midcrestal position will minimize this risk. Another advantage of the midcrestal midline incision is less bleeding because of the smaller blood vessels in this area.

Smoking abstinence

The association between cigarette smoking and delayed wound healing is well recognized.[15] Nicotine is a vasoconstrictor that causes tissue ischemia and impaired healing. Moreover, nicotine increases platelet adhesiveness, which contributes to thrombotic microvascular occlusion and tissue ischemia. In addition, proliferation of red blood cells, fibroblasts, and macrophages is reduced by nicotine. Carbon monoxide and cyanide, two components of tobacco smoke, have a negative effect on oxygen transport and metabolism. Compared with nonsmokers, smokers are more likely to have unsatisfactory healing after dental surgical procedures.

Smoking increases the incidence of implant postoperative complications,[16] including the extent of marginal bone loss, the incidence of peri-implantitis, and the success rate of bone

grafts. While cigarette smoking is not an absolute contraindication for implant placement, smokers should be informed that there is an increased risk of implant loss and peri-implantitis.[17]

Proper suturing technique

Proper suturing is an important aspect of implant placement. Many implants and bone grafts have become infected because the sutures did not provide a proper seal for the surgical site. Exposed membranes and gingival recession can be a result of technically deficient suturing.

Technique

Sutures should be placed every 3 to 5 mm along the entire incision line, with the needle penetrating the tissue approximately 3 mm from the incision line. In most cases, the corner of the flap at the junction of the midcrestal incision and the releasing incision(s) should be secured first (Fig 3-4a). However, the author recommends closing large flaps by first placing one suture in the middle to secure it (Fig 3-4b).

Well-sutured flaps heal more quickly and by primary intention with reduced edema, whereas open flaps heal by secondary intention, which is generally accompanied by tissue loss and scarring. Tables 3-1 and 3-2 summarize the phases of healing by primary and secondary intention, respectively. Table 3-3 summarizes the most popular oral surgery suturing techniques and their indications, including the continuous locking suture, shown in Fig 3-5.

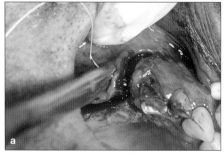 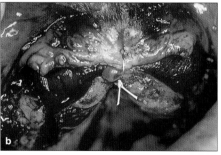 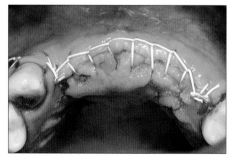

Fig 3-4 *(a)* The corner of the small flap, ie, the intersection of the crestal incision line and the releasing incision(s), is secured first. *(b)* Because this is a large flap, the first suture is placed in the middle of the crestal incision.

Fig 3-5 Continuous locking suture.

Table 3-1	Healing by primary intention*	
Phase	**Duration**	**Characteristics**
Inflammation	3 to 7 days	Increased blood vessel permeability; presence of leukocytes
Proliferative	3 to 12 days	Contraction of wound area; neodeposition of fibrinogen
Remodeling	12 days to months	Reorganization of new tissue

*Reprinted from Siervo[18] with permission.

Table 3-2	Healing by secondary intention*	
Phase	**Duration**	**Characteristics**
Hemorrhagic	Up to 15 days	Presence of polymorpho-nucleate cells and macrophages; migration of epithelial cells
Proliferative	Up to 20 days	Formation of granulation tissue
Remodeling	Months	Scarring

*Reprinted from Siervo[18] with permission.

Table 3-3	Common suturing techniques in oral surgery*
Suture technique	**General indications**
Interrupted	Interproximal suturing where the flap is not under tension
Figure eight	Restricted areas (ie, lingual to mandibular molars)
Vertical mattress	Resistant to muscle movement; close adaptation of flaps to bone, teeth, or implants
Horizontal mattress	Resistant to muscle movement; adaptation of flaps to teeth or implants
Continuous unlocking	Long edentulous areas, tuberosities, or retromolar areas
Continuous locking	Long edentulous areas, tuberosities, or retromolar areas (see Fig 3-5)

*Data from Silverstein.[19]

Materials

The ideal suture material should possess all of the following features[20]:

- *Easy to handle.* The suture material should have virtually no elastic memory. Nylon has a high level of elastic memory; the memory of silk filaments is low, and that of polytetrafluoroethylene (PTFE) (eg, Gore-Tex, W. L. Gore) is minimal.
- *Easy to glide.* Materials that easily absorb biologic fluids do not glide freely through tissue. Silk, a braided natural material, is absorbent and does not glide as well as any of the monofilament materials.
- *No cavities in the three-dimensional structure.* A filament with many surface irregularities will increase traction and consequently increase friction and the production of heat. Silk sutures are highly cavitated.
- *Knot securely.* Sutures that glide easily through tissue tend to form knots that accidentally loosen. This drawback may be resolved by increasing the number of clockwise and counterclockwise half-knots to ensure that the knot is properly secure.
- *Resistant to traction.* The *tensile strength* of a filament is the force required to bring it to its breaking point. This property is directly proportional to the diameter of the filament and becomes weaker as the diameter decreases. The tensile strength of the tissue determines the size and tensile strength of the suture material.

- *Atraumatic.* The traumatic effect of a suture material is a function of its three-dimensional structure and the speed at which it moves through the tissue. Certain structure types cause more friction in the tissue as they glide through it. Slow movement of the suture through tissue prevents microburns along the line of the suture. The microburns may leave small defects in the tissue and facilitate bacterial colonization of both superficial and deep tissue planes.
- *No bacterial wicking or colonization.* Monofilaments have a lower incidence of bacterial colonization than other materials.
- *Small diameter.* The smaller the suture is in cross-section, the less damage it produces in the tissues and the less foreign body material it disperses within the tissues; however, the tensile strength of the suture may be compromised.

Suture tension

Burkhardt et al[21] evaluated various suture and needle characteristics in relation to the tearing characteristics of mucosal tissue. The authors of the study concluded that tissue trauma can be reduced by choosing finer-diameter sutures such as sizes 6-0 and 7-0 because they lead to filament breakage rather than tissue breakage under tension.

The author recommends PTFE (eg, Gore-Tex) suture material for all applications in implant surgery. Moreover, the smallest-diameter suture that will adequately hold the healing tissues should be selected.

Nontension flap closure

Nontension flap closure is of particular importance when flaps are sutured over an augmented alveolar ridge after bone grafting procedures such as guided bone regeneration (GBR), veneer block grafting, or the split-ridge technique. The original volume of soft tissue will not be sufficient to cover the newly augmented alveolar ridge, and nontension flap closure will require a flap-releasing technique.

Flap-releasing technique

The flap can be released to allow nontension closure by scoring the periosteal layer of the flap with a sharp blade (Figs 3-6a and 3-6b). One, two, or even three incisions can be made in the periosteal layer. If this is insufficient to produce a tension-free suture line, a muscle-layer release can be performed by inserting closed blunt-tip scissors such as Metzenbaum scissors into the score lines, opening the scissors within the muscle layer, and closing the scissors before removing them to be inserted in a different location for further release (Figs 3-6c and 3-6d). Figure 3-7 demonstrates the proper performance of this technique in a case of alveolar ridge expansion.

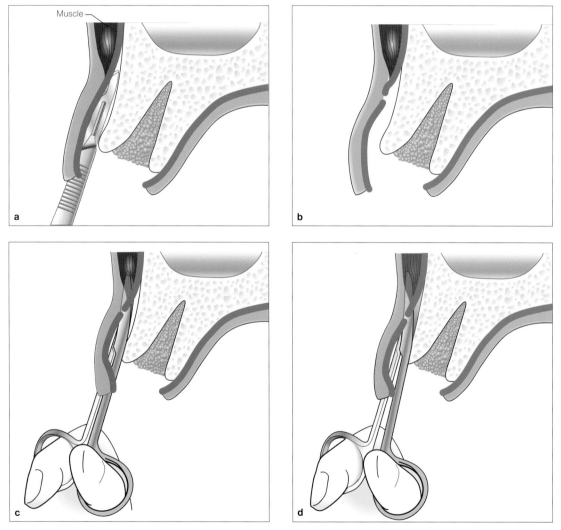

Fig 3-6 *(a and b)* The periosteum layer of the flap is scored for tension-free closure. *(c and d)* Muscle-layer release is performed after scoring of the periosteum for additional tension release in an extensive augmentation procedure.

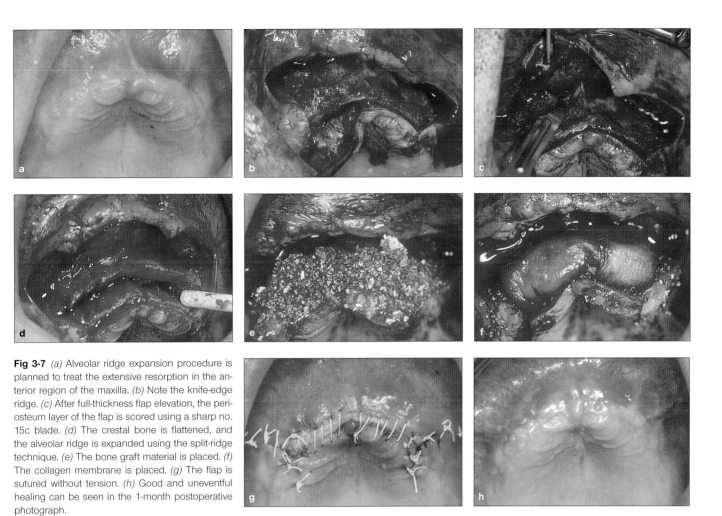

Fig 3-7 *(a)* Alveolar ridge expansion procedure is planned to treat the extensive resorption in the anterior region of the maxilla. *(b)* Note the knife-edge ridge. *(c)* After full-thickness flap elevation, the periosteum layer of the flap is scored using a sharp no. 15c blade. *(d)* The crestal bone is flattened, and the alveolar ridge is expanded using the split-ridge technique. *(e)* The bone graft material is placed. *(f)* The collagen membrane is placed. *(g)* The flap is sutured without tension. *(h)* Good and uneventful healing can be seen in the 1-month postoperative photograph.

Prosthesis use

Removable partial or full dentures should not be worn for 14 days following implant surgery. A provisional fixed prosthesis can be inserted if it does not compromise access for hygiene or place pressure on the surgical area.

Postoperative medications and home care instructions

Certain medications and postoperative home care instructions help to minimize swelling and consequently reduce the incidence of postoperative incision line reopening, some of which follow.

Selected home care instructions that minimize postoperative swelling
- Do not raise the lip to inspect the sutures.
- Use an ice pack for up to 12 hours after surgery.
- Eat a soft diet.

Selected medications that minimize postoperative swelling
- Ibuprofen, 600 mg
- Dexamethasone, 1.5 mg

Treatment of a reopened incision line

- Determine the cause. For example, if an interim removable prosthesis is the cause of incision reopening, the area over the implant should be relieved.
- If the incision reopening is minor, no attempt should be made to close the tissue. The incision line will heal by secondary intention (Fig 3-8). If the formation of granulation tissue continues for more than 2 weeks, trimming the epithelial margins of the wound with coarse diamond burs will encourage the granulation process.

- Incision line reopening increases the risk of infection; thus, maintaining good oral hygiene is very important. The patient should keep the area clean and use a 0.12% chlorhexidine oral rinse (eg, Peridex, Zila) at least twice a day.
- Sloughing of the mucosal flap is common when incisions reopen (Fig 3-9) and not problematic because granulation tissue will eventually cover the defect.

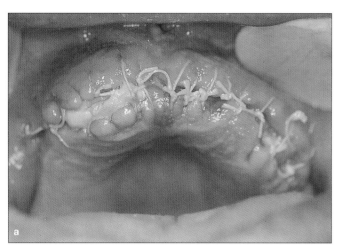 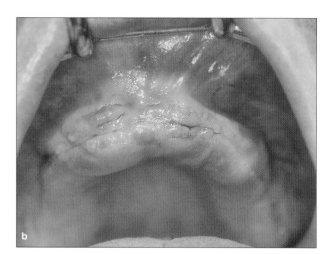

Fig 3-8 Minor incision line reopening *(a)* and its healing by secondary intention *(b)*.

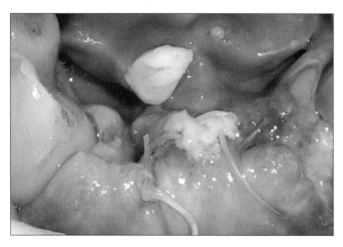

Fig 3-9 Sloughing of the mucosal flap due to improper suturing technique.

Cover Screw Exposure During the Healing Period

When the cover screw is exposed to the oral cavity (Fig 3-10), the implant is at a higher risk of infection and premature loading. When this happens, proper monitoring during the healing period and proper home care can minimize the risk of infection.

The cover screw can become exposed for several reasons:

- Pressure from the interim prosthesis
- Thin mucosa
- Shallow implant placement
- Immediate implant placement in an extraction site

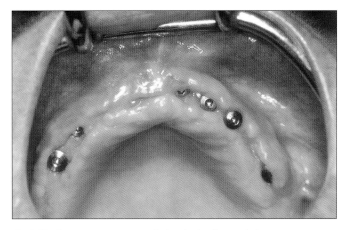

Fig 3-10 Cover screw exposure during the healing period.

Management

When a cover screw is partially or completely exposed, recovering of the screw is not necessary, but contributing factors should be identified. If impinging on the exposed screw, the interim prosthesis must be relieved to ensure no occlusal forces are applied onto the implant. The prosthesis can also be relined to prevent any further damage to the mucosa.

When a cover screw is exposed, the following steps should be taken:

- More frequent follow-up appointments should be scheduled during the healing period to allow close monitoring for potential infection in the exposed cover screw area. When there is no cover screw exposure, the patient is not seen again until 4 months after suture removal in the mandible or 6 months after suture removal in the maxilla. When a cover screw has been exposed, the patient should have at least one additional follow-up appointment between suture removal and placement of the healing abutment.
- At the follow-up appointment, the screw should be checked for looseness (Fig 3-11a) and the area rinsed with Peridex (Fig 3-11b).
- Hygiene compliance should be confirmed. A schedule of rinsing with Peridex and gentle brushing of the cover screw at least once a day should be maintained.
- If heavy plaque and/or calculus covers the screw (Fig 3-12), an ultrasonic scaler should not be used; instead, the screw should simply be replaced with a new one.
- The patient should be advised to eat soft foods in the area of the exposed cover screw to prevent any premature loading of the implant.

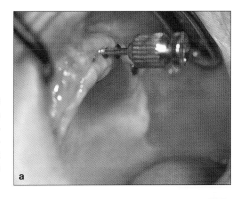
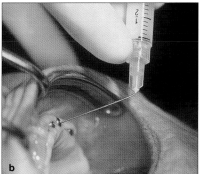

Fig 3-11 (a) When the cover screws are exposed, they need to be checked frequently to make sure that they are not loose because plaque and bacteria can develop between the cover screw and the implant platform and trigger infection. (b) Rinsing the areas between the gingiva and the cover screws should be done to keep it clean of food and plaque that might accumulate in this area.

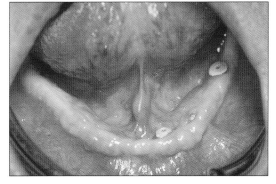

Fig 3-12 Heavy plaque and calculus completely cover the surface of the cover screws.

Bone Growth over the Cover Screw

During *stage-two surgery,* ie, the uncovering of the implant for cover screw removal and placement of the healing abutment, bony overgrowth may be observed on top of the cover screw (Fig 3-13). This can happen when the implant is placed slightly below the level of the crestal bone and is allowed an extended healing period of 8 months or longer. The bony overgrowth must be removed to allow for removal of the cover screw and proper seating of the healing abutment. Care should be taken to avoid damage to the implant platform during this procedure.

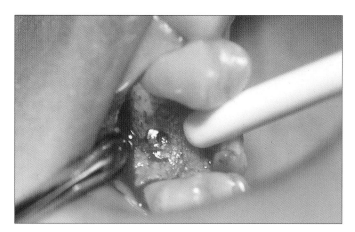

Fig 3-13 Bony overgrowth is noted on top of the cover screw during stage-two surgery.

Management

A bone mill (Fig 3-14) can be used if one is available for the implant system in use; otherwise, small hand chisels can be used to remove the bone.

After placement of the healing abutment, a periapical or bitewing radiograph should always be taken to ensure that no gap exists between the healing abutment and the implant platform. If the healing abutment is not seated properly, the impression coping and the definitive prosthetic abutment will not be seated properly either.

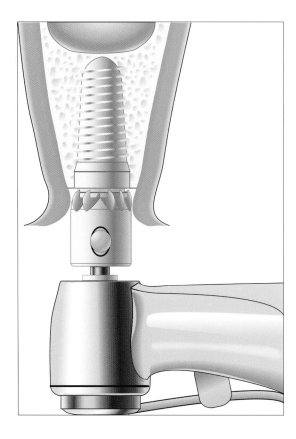

Fig 3-14 A specially designed bone mill is available for certain implant brands to remove bone overgrowth from the top of the implant without causing damage to the implant platform.

<table>
<tr><td>COMPLICATION 35</td><td></td></tr>
</table>

Soft Tissue Growth Between Implant Platform and Cover Screw

If the cover screw becomes loose during the healing period, soft tissue can grow to occupy the space between the cover screw and the implant platform. This tissue will prevent proper seating of the healing abutment, impression coping, and definitive prosthesis if not detected and removed during stage-two surgery.

Detection of the soft tissue overgrowth can be made visually or on the radiograph taken to confirm seating of the healing abutment or the impression coping. If the radiograph shows a gap between the prosthetic component and the implant platform (Fig 3-15a), soft tissue overgrowth should be assumed. A second radiograph should be taken after removal of the tissue to confirm proper seating of the prosthetic component (Fig 3-15b).

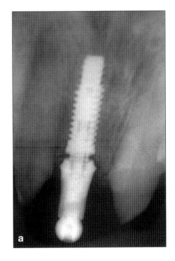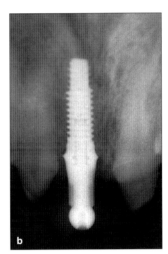

Fig 3-15 *(a)* Radiograph showing a gap between the implant platform and the impression coping due to soft tissue overgrowth. *(b)* Radiograph taken after removal of the soft tissue verifies the complete seating of the impression coping.

Management

The soft tissue overgrowth can be excised with a disposable tissue punch of an appropriate diameter (Fig 3-16) or with a hand instrument such as a small, spoon-shaped excavator (Fig 3-17). Care should be taken to avoid damage to the implant platform during removal of the soft tissue overgrowth.

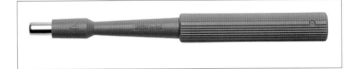

Fig 3-16 Disposable tissue punch.

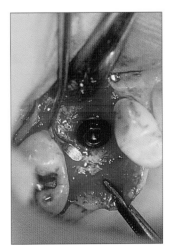

Fig 3-17 A spoon-shaped excavator can be used to remove soft tissue overgrowth from the top of and around the implant head.

Bone Loss or Thread Exposure During the Healing Period

Excessive bone loss during the healing period prior to stage-two surgery can occur for a variety of reasons. Infection and premature loading by an interim prosthesis are two primary causes of bone loss prior to placement of the definitive restoration. Recognition of the exact etiologic factor in the early bone loss or thread exposure is not always possible and, moreover, in many cases there is more than one etiologic factor involved.

Factors causing bone loss

The purpose of this section is to analyze possible factors responsible for bone loss that occurs between the insertion of the implant and the restorative phase. Prosthetic-related complications that arise after the delivery of the implant restorations are not within the scope of this text. Some of the factors below cause limited bone loss; others, such as infection, can cause major bone loss in a short period of time and lead to implant failure.

Microgap

When an abutment is connected to an implant, a microgap forms at the interface. As discussed in complication 22, part 2, the implant platform should never be placed below the crestal bone level; instead, it should be placed at least 0.25 mm higher than the alveolar crest, depending on the thickness of the soft tissue, so that the microgap will be supracrestal.[22] Another viable option is to move the microgap away from the bone and toward the center of the implant using the platform-switching concept.

In the past, implants were submerged to prevent micromovement during the healing period[23] and to enhance the emergence profile of the implant restoration. This practice was done at the expense of the crestal bone. The existence of microbial contamination at the implant-abutment microgap and at the inner threads of submerged implants is well documented in the literature.[24,25] The leakage of this microbial contamination is related to the development of peri-implantitis.

During the healing period, there is generally no bone loss around the collar of the implant in either a submerged or a nonsubmerged position. After connection of the abutment and loading of the prosthesis, up to 2 mm of bone loss apical to the microgap is observed around submerged implants as the tissues establish the peri-implant biologic width. If the microgap is moved coronally, away from the alveolar crest, less bone is resorbed; if the microgap is moved apically, toward the alveolar crest, a greater amount of bone resorption will occur. The amount of bone loss, therefore, depends on the location of the microgap. Moreover, this remodeling is not dependent on early or immediate loading of the implants or on immediate postextraction implant placement.[26]

Infection and peri-implantitis

Peri-implantitis is an infective process that leads to bone loss and implant failure if not addressed.

- *Periodontopathic bacteria.* The relation between plaque accumulation and peri-implantitis is well documented in the literature. One cause of peri-implantitis is the transmission of periodontopathic bacteria from natural teeth to the implants. Aoki et al[27] have identified *Actinobacillus actinomycetemcomitans*, *Prevotella intermedia*, *Porphyromonas gingivalis*, *Treponema denticola*, and *Fusobacterium nucleatum* in the gingival crevice of adjacent teeth as the source of peri-implant colonization. To reduce the risk of peri-implantitis, these pathogens should be eliminated from the oral cavity by preventive periodontal treatment before implant placement.[28]
- *Oral hygiene.* Poor oral hygiene has a negative impact on the prognosis of an implant. Plaque-induced periodontitis that exists during the healing period can infect the implant. Early detection and prompt management of infected implants can stop the process of bone resorption and prevent the possible consequence of implant loss.
- *Contamination of the implant body prior to placement.* This might lead to peri-implantitis and should be avoided to minimize this risk.
- *Existing bacteria prior to the insertion of the implant.* Infection can arise even with good oral hygiene because of preexisting bacteria at the time of surgery (retrograde peri-implantitis).

Surgical trauma

- *Generation of heat.* Overheating of the bone at the time of surgery will result in bone cell death and resorption. The temperature threshold for bone cell death is 1 minute at 47°C or 7 minutes at 40°C.[29] Bone resorption because of overheating can be localized, limited to the platform or apex of the implant, or more extensive. Techniques to minimize heat production during implant placement are described in detail in complication 16, part 2.

- *Compression necrosis.* Overtightening the implants during insertion can cause bone compression and subsequent bone necrosis and resorption. See complication 28, part 2, for prevention and management of this cause of early implant failure.

Histologic examination of implants removed for failure due to surgical trauma showed the presence of a fibrous connective tissue interposed between the implant and the bone. This tissue contained epithelial cells, even in the most apical part of the implant.[30]

Wide implants placed in narrow alveolar ridges

Placement of implants that are excessively wide relative to the width of the alveolar ridge can lead to gross bone resorption over a short period of time. If the implants are too wide for the available bone, the bone will resorb, accompanied by gingival recession.

A minimum of 1 mm of bone should be maintained to the buccal and lingual of the implant (Fig 3-18) to ensure sufficient bone thickness and blood supply for predictable implant survival. If necessary, a wider ridge can be created by alveoloplasty, a split-ridge technique, GBR, or veneer block grafting. Bone grafting can be done simultaneously with implant placement or as the first procedure in a staged approach that ensures adequate bone volume before implant placement.

The survival rate of implants falls significantly if buccal bone thickness is less than 1 mm. In narrow ridges for which bone grafting is not possible or desirable, narrow-diameter implants with an adequate implant-bone surface area are preferable to implants that are too wide for the available alveolar bone.

Fig 3-18 A minimum of 1 mm should exist on each side of the implant for successful long-term osseointegration.

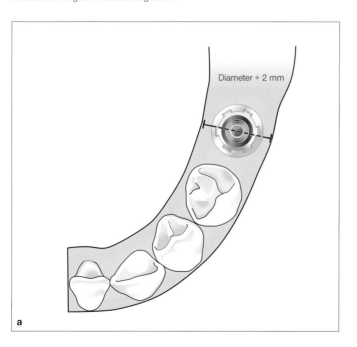

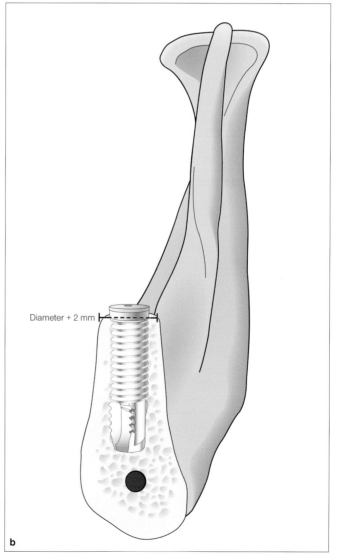

Pressure during the healing period

- *Pressure from interim dentures.* Use of an ill-fitting interim denture during the healing phase can put undesirable pressure or trauma on the implants and surrounding tissues and can induce bone loss. The clinician must ensure that removable dentures worn during the healing phase do not act as an irritant that becomes destructive to tissue and bone surrounding the implants.
- *Pressure from hard food.* Eating hard foods during the early healing period puts an excessive occlusal load on the implants.
- *Inadequate placement of implants into the bone itself.* The full length of the implant must be secured in bone unless a simultaneous GBR procedure is to be performed. For this purpose, implants come in various widths and lengths to accommodate the amount of bone available for placement. An exception to this rule occurs when there is thick soft tissue present at the implant site. In this case, the implant can be placed 1 to 2 mm coronal to the alveolar crest (as long as sufficient length of the implant is within bone for adequate stability), given that it is well submerged in the soft tissue and not exposed to the oral cavity.

Systemic disease

Certain systemic diseases, including uncontrolled diabetes and osteoporosis, can affect the osseointegration of implants and lead to bone loss during the healing phase.

Patient factors

Patient failure to follow postoperative instructions, take recommended medications, notify the clinician immediately upon noticing a problem, and keep postoperative appointments deny the doctor the opportunity to intervene in a timely manner and change the fate of a failing implant or bone graft.

Other causes

Other reasons for early bone resorption during the healing period include inadequate interimplant distance and use of implants with a smooth *crest module* (ie, smooth neck design). Bone loss in these situations is not significant but should be avoided.

Management

The course of action in early bone resorption depends on its cause and degree. The author has developed a classification system for bone loss patterns around dental implants that occur during the healing period. The five classes (Fig 3-19) are explained below and followed by a recommended course of treatment for each class.

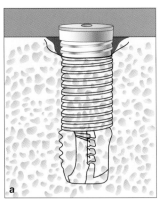 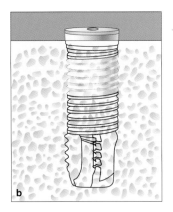 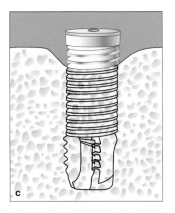

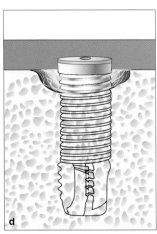 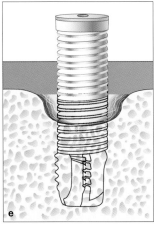

Fig 3-19 Al-Faraje classification of bone loss during the healing period. *(a)* Class I: Minimal bone loss with a self-containing configuration at the buccocoronal aspect of the implant with no infection and no exposure of the implant into the oral cavity (ie, the implant is well covered by soft tissue). *(b)* Class II: Minimal bone loss at the midbuccal surface of the implant with no infection and no exposure of the implant into the oral cavity. *(c)* Class III: Circumferential bone loss around the coronal aspect of the implant with implant stability, no infection, and no exposure of the implant into the oral cavity. *(d)* Class IV: Minimal bone loss accompanied by infection with no exposure of the implant into the oral cavity. *(e)* Class V: Gross bone and soft tissue loss accompanied by infection. Part of the implant is exposed to the oral cavity.

Al-Faraje classification of bone loss during the healing period

Class I

Minimal bone loss with a self-containing configuration at the buccocoronal aspect of the implant with no infection and no exposure of the implant into the oral cavity (ie, the implant is well covered by soft tissue). The cause of this pattern of bone loss is surgical trauma that led to minimal bone loss. It is usually discovered during second-stage surgery.

Management

Debridement of any possible granulation tissue in the defect, perforation of the cortical layer of the bone around the defect to create bleeding points, and placement of bone graft material and a membrane is recommended (Fig 3-20).

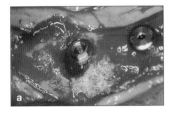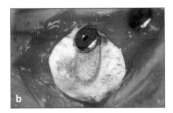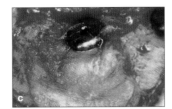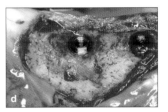

Fig 3-20 *(a)* Minimal bone loss at the buccocoronal aspect of the implant with no infection and no exposure of the implant into the oral cavity (Class I), discovered during stage-two surgery. *(b)* Placement of a membrane after debridement and creation of bleeding points. *(c and d)* Newly regenerated bone can be seen 4 months postoperatively.

Class II

Minimal bone loss at the midbuccal surface of the implant with no infection and no exposure of the implant into the oral cavity (ie, the implant is well covered by soft tissue). The cause of this pattern of bone loss is the placement of implants in a narrow ridge with less than 1 mm of bone on the buccal side of the implant preoperatively. This type of bone loss might not jeopardize the osseointegration or longevity of the implant; however, if the gingival tissue is thin, the esthetic appearance of the soft tissue in this area will be compromised.

Management

If the bone loss is minimal and few implant threads are visible through the buccal plate, conservative intervention will consist of elevation of a partial- or full-thickness flap for soft tissue augmentation with a connective tissue graft or an acellular dermal matrix allograft (eg, Alloderm, LifeCell) (Figs 3-21 and 3-22). The clinician may also elect to perform GBR (creating bleeding points and adding bone graft material before membrane placement).

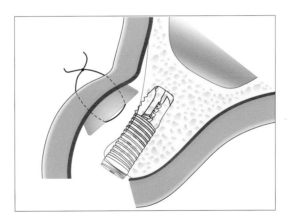

Fig 3-21 Placement of a connective tissue graft against the inner surface of the buccal flap to improve the esthetic outcome of an implant displaying Class II bone loss.

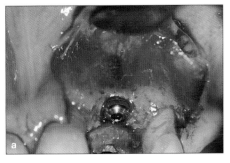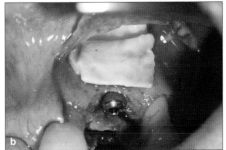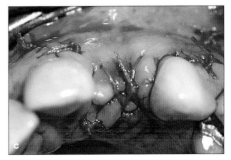

Fig 3-22 *(a)* Minimal bone loss at the midbuccal surface of the implant with no infection and no exposure of the implant into the oral cavity (Class II). *(b)* Placement of an acellular dermal matrix allograft. *(c)* Primary closure.

Class III

Circumferential bone loss around the coronal aspect of the implant with implant stability, no infection, and no exposure of the implant into the oral cavity (ie, the implant is well covered by soft tissue). The cause of this pattern of bone loss is either the placement of implants in a narrow ridge with less than 1 mm of bone on the buccal and lingual surfaces of the implant during placement or pressure from the interim prosthesis during the healing period.

Management

A full-thickness flap should be reflected and GBR performed. Figure 3-23 shows a case of Class III bone loss and the GBR procedure used to manage it.

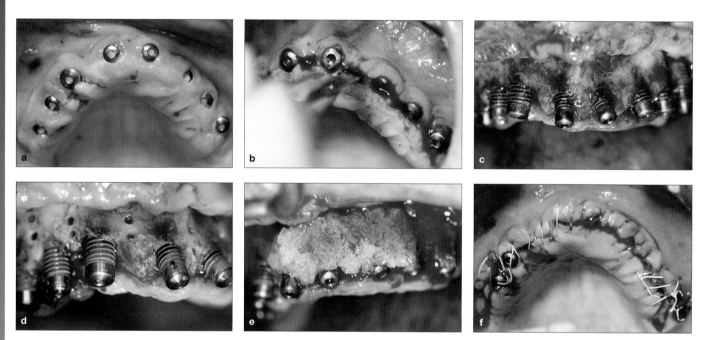

Fig 3-23 *(a)* Clinical view of implants found radiographically to display Class III bone loss. *(b and c)* Surgical intervention starts with full-thickness mucoperiosteal flap elevation to access the implants and bone. *(d)* The surface of the implants is cleaned, and bleeding points are created between the implants. *(e)* Placement of bone graft and a resorbable membrane. *(f)* Primary closure is obtained.

Class IV

Minimal bone loss accompanied by infection with no exposure of the implant into the oral cavity. The cause of this pattern of bone loss is infection. The degree of the infection will dictate the course of treatment.

Management

The implant should be removed or, if removal of all infected tissues is possible, GBR can be performed after antibiotic treatment of the implant's surface (Figs 3-24 and 3-25).

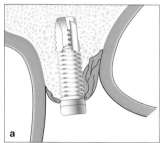 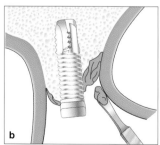 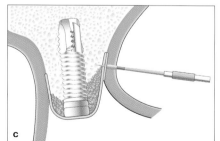 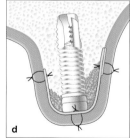

Fig 3-24 Minimal bone loss accompanied by infection with no exposure of the implant into the oral cavity (Class IV). *(a)* Treatment starts by elevating a full-thickness mucoperiosteal flap. *(b)* The infected tissues should be completely removed. *(c)* The implant surface is cleaned, bleeding points are created, and then bone graft material and a membrane are placed. *(d)* The flap is reapproximated and released for closure without tension for a healing period of 6 to 9 months.

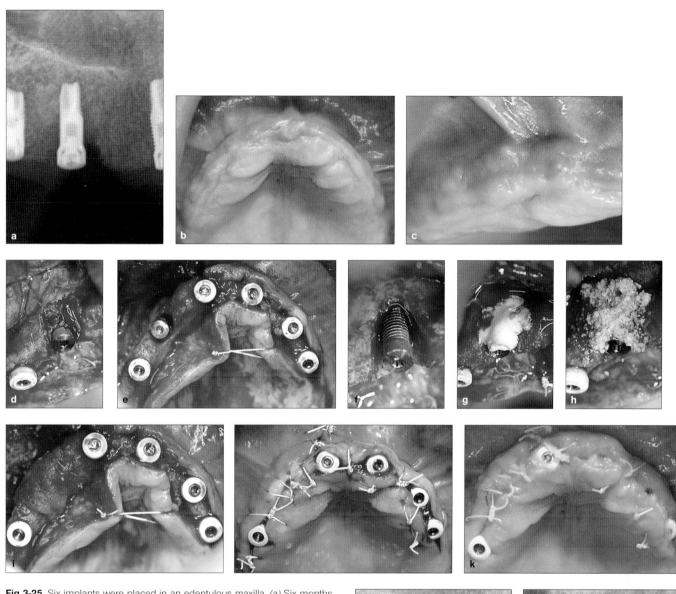

Fig 3-25 Six implants were placed in an edentulous maxilla. *(a)* Six months postoperatively (upon stage-two surgery), an infection was noted around one of the implants (Class IV). *(b and c)* There were no clinical symptoms except a small darkened area of the gingiva. *(d)* A full-thickness flap was reflected. All other implants received healing abutments, and a decision was made to save the infected implant. *(e and f)* The infected tissues were removed from around the implant. *(g)* Tetracycline paste (made from mixing 250 mg tetracycline in 5 mL of sterile saline or water) was placed for 1 minute on the surface of the implant, which was then thoroughly flushed with sterile saline. This procedure can be repeated twice. *(h)* After creating bleeding points, Bio-Oss (Geistlich) was placed. *(i)* The bone graft material was covered by two layers of Bio-Gide (Geistlich) membrane. *(j)* The flap was released and sutured without tension. *(k and l)* Two weeks after surgery. *(m)* Two-month postoperative radiograph shows no radiolucency around the treated implant (on the right).

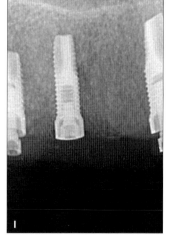

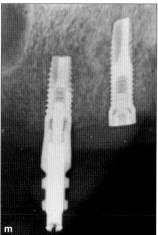

Class V

Gross bone and soft tissue loss accompanied by infection. Part of the implant is exposed to the oral cavity. The cause of this pattern of bone loss is prolonged history of infection.

Management

Complete elimination of infection is usually not possible. Therefore, removal of the implant is recommended even if the implant is not mobile, followed by delayed bone grafting (ie, after a healing period of 6 to 9 months, depending on the volume and type of bone graft material used), with or without simultaneous implant placement.

Implant Mobility During Stage-Two Surgery

Risk factors

Smoking habit

There is a conflict in the literature regarding the role of smoking in early implant failure and survival rates. While some studies, including Wallace,[31] Kumar et al,[32] and Sverzut et al,[33] have not found a statistically significant difference in early implant failure rates between smokers and nonsmokers, other studies, including De Bruyn and Collaert,[34] reported early implant failure prior to loading of 9% in smokers versus 1% in nonsmokers. Similarly, Gorman et al[35] reported a higher early implant failure rate of 6.5% for smokers versus 3.31% for nonsmokers. In a retrospective study by Alsaadi et al[36] of 6,946 implants placed in 2,004 patients, a significant difference in early implant failure between heavy smokers (more than 20 cigarettes per day) and nonsmokers was found.

On the other hand, a large prospective study by Lambert et al[37] did not support the influence of smoking on early implant failure but did find a greater number of failures in smokers during the interval between uncovering of the implant and insertion of the prosthesis.

Stability at the time of placement

Primary stability of implants at the time of placement is generally an important, but not an absolute, requirement for successful osseointegration. Many studies have shown superior survival rates for implants with high stability at the time of placement. However, other studies[38,39] have shown that implants that are mobile at the time of placement can osseointegrate and that hydroxyapatite (HA) coating significantly improves the survival rate of implants up to 3 years postsurgery, whether they are mobile or immobile at the time of placement.

Bone type

Good bone density is essential for predictable osseointegration and long-term survival of implants.[40] Type 1 and type 2 bone allow for a more homogenous distribution of stress along the entire bone, while type 3 and type 4 bone are weaker and less resistant to deformation because of their greater trabeculation.[41] Therefore, stress magnitudes are greater for types 3 and 4 bone. However, based on the author's considerable experience with implant placement in different bone density types, implants can have a similar rate of survival in all bone densities if the surgical technique and the healing period are modified accordingly.

Modifications of the surgical technique

For types 1 and 2 bone, microfracture or overheating of the bone during drilling or implant insertion can be avoided by a gradual increase in the diameter of the osteotomy and the use of sharp drills, copious irrigation, and tapping drills.

For types 3 and 4 bone, conservative drilling and/or the use of osteotomes is essential to increase the density of the bone during implant placement rather than remove bone.

Healing period

Early implant failure can be attributed to an insufficient healing period. Table 3-4 is a healing schedule for optimal osseointegration results. However, the level of primary stability of the implant also needs to be taken into consideration.

Table 3-4	Healing period for optimal osseointegration results according to bone type
Type of bone	**Minimum integration and healing time**
Type 1	5 months
Type 2	4 months
Type 3	6 months
Type 4	8 months
Bone-grafted site	9 months

Pressure from interim prosthesis

Pressure from the interim prosthesis may lead to bone loss in osseointegrated implants (see complication 36) or may prevent successful osseointegration.

Implant features

Some implant features such as thread design and surface texture enhance osseointegration. Numerous studies[42–45] have shown higher torque removal force for implants with certain surface texture characteristics, ie, a rough surface compared with a smooth machined surface. *Torque removal force* is the force required to remove an implant and is a measure of its stability or osseointegration. A higher torque removal force indicates a higher level of bony integration.

Systemic medical conditions

Certain systemic conditions such as diabetes and osteoporosis may negatively affect osseointegration.

Treatment of some systemic conditions

Certain treatments such as immunosuppressive therapies following transplantation, radiotherapy, or cancer treatment, and intravenous bisphosphonates for advanced osteoporosis can negatively influence the outcome of implant treatment.

Infection

Early infection may lead to unsuccessful osseointegration. A proper medication protocol should be followed to minimize the possibility of infection.

Conclusion

With the exception of infection, all of the above factors influencing the early survival of dental implants are considered to be risk factors. The presence of one risk factor is not necessarily a contraindication to implant treatment. However, the presence of several risk factors might represent a contraindication. The patient must be informed about the particular risk factors associated with his or her implant treatment and to what degree they may influence the surgical outcome and the implant survival rate.

COMPLICATION 38

Implant Periapical Lesion (IPL) and Retrograde Peri-implantitis

The term *retrograde peri-implantitis* refers to a rare lesion or radiolucency at the periapical aspect of an osseointegrated implant that usually develops within a few months after the surgical insertion of the implant.[46,47]

Predisposing conditions that might lead to retrograde peri-implantitis

Although the exact etiology and pathogenesis are not clear and are subject to speculation, many studies have suggested that retrograde peri-implantitis is provoked by bacteria from a previous infection that remain at the recipient site.

Proposed etiologic factors for retrograde peri-implantitis include:

- Infection from activation of residual bacteria in sites with a history of endodontic pathology in a previously extracted tooth
- Infection from scar tissue following removal of an impacted tooth
- Contamination from adjacent teeth with obvious endodontic pathology
- Infection from adjacent teeth with periodontal conditions[48]
- Infection at sites of previous tooth loss due to periodontitis, where bacteria may remain in the bone and initiate retrograde peri-implantitis despite thorough and vigorous debridement and irrigation of extraction sockets and a sufficient healing time[49]

- Apical entrapment of gingival epithelial cells during implant insertion[50]
- Necrosis from excessive heating of the bone during osteotomy drilling[51]

In a study by Quirynen et al,[52] the incidence of retrograde peri-implantitis was significantly higher for TiUnite (Nobel Biocare) implants (8 cases in 80 implants), which have a moderately rough surface, as compared with machined-surface implants (2 cases in 459 implants). The machined-surface implants, however, showed a higher failure rate (6.8%) than the TiUnite implants (2.5%).

It is important to note that there are two types of IPL: the infected type and the noninfected or inactive type. The noninfected, inactive lesion is usually created by the placement of implants that are shorter than the prepared osteotomy site. The treatment for this type of IPL consists of regular radiographic monitoring.

Prevention

Encapsulation is a bacterial survival mechanism. The bone at the implant site may contain residual encapsulated bacteria that can be activated by the implant osteotomy, reinstating the infection at the apex of the implant. Therefore, the use of bactericidal antibiotic at the time of extraction and implant placement may prevent retrograde peri-implantitis and should be considered as routine prophylaxis at implant surgery, especially after an endodontic failure.

Symptoms of infected IPL

Generally, clinical findings are pain, redness, tenderness upon touching the face over the apical area of the implant, swelling, periapical radiolucency at the apex of the implant, and possibly the presence of a fistulous tract.

Management of infected IPL

Any periapical implant radiolucency should be addressed as soon as possible to prevent acute exacerbation of the lesion and total loss of implant integration. Surgical exploration and debridement is the treatment of choice in retrograde peri-implantitis.

The following are steps in the surgical protocol for management of an infected IPL:

1. *Flap elevation.* A sulcular incision and two vertical releasing incisions are made buccal to the area of the affected implant and a full-thickness flap is elevated to expose the apex of the affected implant.
2. *Creation of a bony window.* Using a round bur on a high-speed surgical handpiece, the buccal cortical bone at the apex of the implant is removed to provide access to the apex of the implant.
3. *Debridement and curettage.* The granulation tissue and any purulent material are removed.
4. *Removal of the apical portion of the infected implant.* Depending on the length of the implant, the clinician may elect to resect the apex of the implant with a tapered fissure bur under copious irrigation. This is indicated primarily in cases where the implant extends into the maxillary sinus or nasal cavity, or in situations where retention of the apical part of the implant could obstruct complete mechanical debridement of the granulation tissue, resulting in failure to eliminate the infection and eventual loss of the implant.[53,54]
5. *Surface treatment.* The surface of the implant apex and the bony defect can be treated with a paste of 250 mg of tetracycline powder mixed with sterile water. The tetracycline paste should be applied for approximately 1 minute; the area is then rinsed and flushed. This procedure can be repeated twice. Several other chemical techniques for disinfecting implant surfaces have been proposed in the literature, including citric acid, chlorhexidine gel, and hydrogen peroxide.[55-57] In a case report with a successful outcome, a paste of calcium hydroxide and water (TempCanal, Pulpdent) was left in direct contact with the implant surface after debridement without surface detoxification.[58] Calcium hydroxide has been shown to inhibit the growth of bacterial species commonly involved in endodontic infections.[59]
6. *Grafting.* A membrane such as Bio-Gide is applied with or without bone grafting material such as Bio-Oss according to the principles of GBR.[60-62]
7. *Medication.* Systemic antibiotics such as penicillin G or amoxicillin (500 mg three times a day for 7 days) along with chlorhexidine 0.12% oral rinse for 3 weeks are recommended after the surgical intervention.

COMPLICATION 39	Cement Left in the Pocket

Although prosthetic complications are beyond the scope of this book, cement left in the pocket has been included because in the case of cement-retained prostheses on immediately loaded implants, its symptoms can arise very soon after surgery.

Cement-retained prostheses have become more popular than screw-retained prostheses because of the many advantages that they offer over the latter[63-68] (Box 3-1). However, one of their disadvantages is the possibility that excess cement may remain below the free gingival margin, which has been associated with peri-implant disease. Cement retained in the pocket can lead to serious consequences, including severe bone loss and implant failure.

A study by Wilson[69] explored the relationship between excess dental cement and peri-implantitis. A dental endoscope was used to evaluate 42 test implants with clinical signs of peri-implant disease and 12 control implants exhibiting no signs of inflammation. Excess cement was not found on any of the control implants but was present on 34 test implants. At 30 days after cement removal, 33 of the test implants were reevaluated. At this time, 25 implants no longer exhibited signs of inflammation. The results of the study—excess dental cement associated with clinical and endoscopic signs of peri-implantitis in 81% of the cases and removal of excess cement resulting in resolution of peri-implantitis in 74% of the cases—support the conclusion that excess dental cement contributes to peri-implantitis.

Box 3-1	A comparison of cement-retained and screw-retained prostheses*	
Type of prosthesis	**Advantages**	**Disadvantages**
Cement-retained	• More biomechanically sound in the anterior region of the mouth because the forces of occlusion are directed along the long axis of the implant • Superior esthetically because the abutment screw is concealed under the crown • Better hygiene without ridge lap pontics. • Less expensive to fabricate • Simpler to fabricate; technically more forgiving • Prosthesis screw loosening occurs less often • Easier to achieve passive fit • The porcelain in cement-retained crowns is more fracture-resistant without the screw access opening • Implant parallelism is not critical • Immediate chairside provisionalization is easier	• Potential for cement to be left in the pocket • Harder to retrieve • After cementation, signs of problems are difficult to identify • Cement failure on an abutment may not be detected and may lead to an unfavorable distribution of force • Recommended use is limited to areas where biomechanical risk factors are low
Screw-retained	• Provides better retention when excessively short (3- to 4-mm) abutments are needed, ie, for compromised vertical restorative space • Recommended in areas with a deep subgingival margin because they do not require cement • Easier to retrieve, if necessary	• Esthetically less acceptable • The prosthesis is bulky on the palatal surface when used in the anterior region • More expensive to fabricate • Biomechanically less sound in the anterior region because the forces of occlusion are not directed along the long axis of the implant • Higher risk of nonpassive fit of the framework, especially in multi-unit cases

*Data compiled from multiple sources.[63-68]

Anatomical considerations

Unlike natural teeth, implants do not develop perpendicular fiber attachments to alveolar bone. Histologic analysis[70–72] of healthy peri-implant mucosa and free marginal gingiva reveals that both tissues have a keratinized oral epithelium and a junctional epithelium. However, because the titanium implant lacks root cementum, collagen fiber bundles are generally oriented parallel to the implant surface and originate from the bone surface. This anatomical relationship may not provide enough protection against excess cement forced into the peri-implant sulcus.[73]

Note that peri-implantitis and severe bone loss can develop within a relatively short period of time, ie, 2 to 4 weeks. In part, this could be related to the impaired defense capacity of the peri-implant soft tissue against exogenous irritation, as suggested by Buser et al in 1992.[74] The gingiva adjacent to teeth is supplied with rich vascularization by supraperiosteal vessels lateral to the alveolar process and by vessels from the periodontal ligament; however, peri-implant mucosa is supplied only by the terminal branches of larger vessels originating from the periosteum of the bone at the implant site[75] (Fig 3-26).

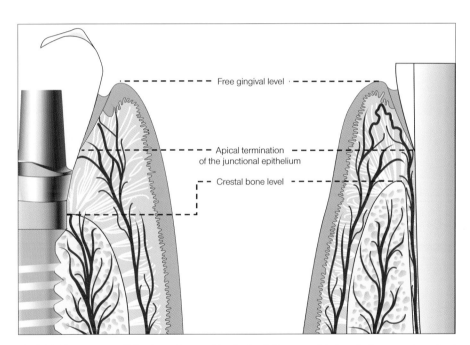

Fig 3-26 The sources of blood supply to peri-implant soft tissues and to the gingiva around a natural tooth. The blood supply to the peri-implant soft tissue is diminished because it lacks the periodontal source, which leads to an impaired defense capacity.

Case presentation 1

Figure 3-27 shows a case of excess residual cement in the pocket. The patient had one implant placed according to the two-stage surgery protocol with a healing period of 4 months (Figs 3-27a and 3-27b). At the delivery visit (Figs 3-27c and 3-27d), the prosthesis was cemented and the excess cement removed, but a radiograph was not taken to verify the complete removal of the excess cement. Two weeks after the cementation of the definitive prosthesis, the patient returned to the office complaining of soreness and swelling in the area (Fig 3-27e). The radiograph taken at this visit clearly showed excess cement left in the pocket and mild bone resorption (Fig 3-27f).

Management

In this case, because the problem was discovered early, implant failure was prevented by reflection of a full-thickness envelope flap, removal of the excess cement and infected tissues, and a GBR procedure (Figs 3-28g to 3-28j).

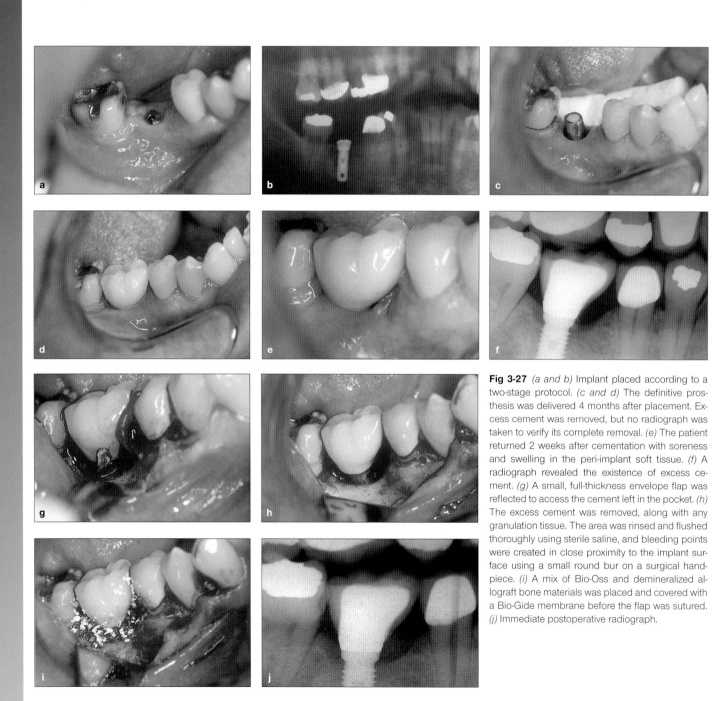

Fig 3-27 *(a and b)* Implant placed according to a two-stage protocol. *(c and d)* The definitive prosthesis was delivered 4 months after placement. Excess cement was removed, but no radiograph was taken to verify its complete removal. *(e)* The patient returned 2 weeks after cementation with soreness and swelling in the peri-implant soft tissue. *(f)* A radiograph revealed the existence of excess cement. *(g)* A small, full-thickness envelope flap was reflected to access the cement left in the pocket. *(h)* The excess cement was removed, along with any granulation tissue. The area was rinsed and flushed thoroughly using sterile saline, and bleeding points were created in close proximity to the implant surface using a small round bur on a surgical handpiece. *(i)* A mix of Bio-Oss and demineralized allograft bone materials was placed and covered with a Bio-Gide membrane before the flap was sutured. *(j)* Immediate postoperative radiograph.

Case presentation 2

Figure 3-28 shows a case in which the problem of excess cement was not dealt with in a timely manner, and thus bone loss was extensive. A radiograph at the surgical appointment revealed a radiopaque material that was found to be excess cement during surgery. A decision was made to remove the implants and perform a GBR procedure to prepare the bone for future replacement of the two failed implants.

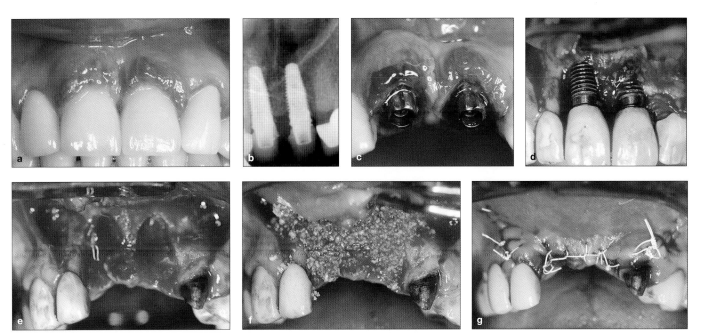

Fig 3-28 *(a)* Cement left in the pocket in a patient who did not bring the problem to the clinician's attention in a timely manner. *(b)* The radiograph displayed extensive bone loss and radiopaque material that was found to be cement upon removal. *(c)* The crowns were removed. *(d)* A full-thickness flap was reflected, and the excess cement was removed along with granulation tissue. It was determined that the implants would have to be removed. *(e)* The implants were removed. *(f and g)* A GBR procedure was performed.

Case presentation 3

In some cases, excess cement is not detected on radiographs but becomes a consideration if no other apparent etiology can account for the bone loss. Figure 3-29a shows a radiograph of peri-implantitis with no apparent cause. The patient had good oral hygiene, was a nonsmoker, had no occlusal trauma such as premature or heavy loading, and lacked any signs of peri-implant pathology prior to the insertion of the implant prosthesis. When a flap was reflected so that the area could be explored surgically, a piece of cement was discovered on the buccal side of the implant abutment. It was removed, and GBR was performed. Figure 3-29b shows the improvement of the peri-implant tissue health 4 months postsurgery.

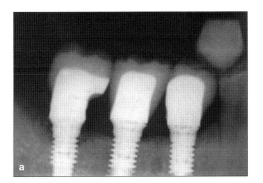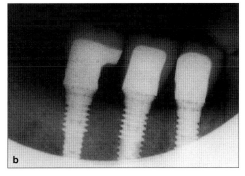

Fig 3-29 *(a)* Peri-implantitis with bone loss due to cement left in the pocket. *(b)* Four months after the excess cement was removed and a GBR procedure was performed, improvement of the peri-implant tissues can be observed.

Case presentation 4

In this case, the implant was placed too deep (Fig 3-30a). Figure 3-30b shows the top of the 4.5-mm-high healing abutment at the level of the highest free gingival margin of the adjacent natural crowns; removal of excess cement would be difficult because of the depth of the subgingival implant-abutment interface. A full-thickness flap was reflected at the prosthesis-delivery visit to verify the complete removal of the excess cement (Figs 3-30c to 3-30e).

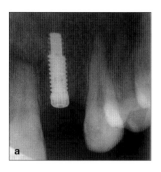
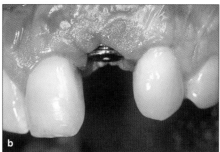
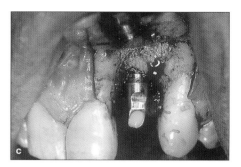

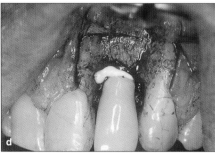
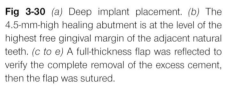
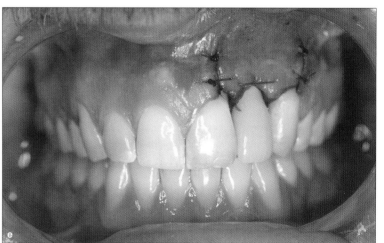

Fig 3-30 *(a)* Deep implant placement. *(b)* The 4.5-mm-high healing abutment is at the level of the highest free gingival margin of the adjacent natural teeth. *(c to e)* A full-thickness flap was reflected to verify the complete removal of the excess cement, then the flap was sutured.

Cement- vs screw-retained prostheses

Despite the problem of excess cement removal, overall, cement-retained prostheses have many advantages over screw-retained prostheses (see Box 3-1). Screw-retained prostheses are often subjected to off-axis loading that causes screw loosening.[76] A 2006 in vivo study by Assenza et al[77] demonstrated an increase in vascular endothelial growth and microvessel density, both signs of inflammation, around loosely screwed abutments as compared to tightly screwed and cement-retained restorations.

Moreover, Keller et al[78] found that microbial leakage into the gap between the restoration and the abutment contributes to bacterial colonization of the internal surface of screw-retained prostheses. This finding was supported by a 2001 study by Piattelli et al,[79] which found bacterial penetration at the implant-abutment interface of all screw-retained implant assemblies studied. No bacteria were detected in the internal cavity of implants with cement-retained abutments.

The author recommends screw-retained prostheses for situations with deep subgingival margins and in areas with limited or compromised interarch distance and recommends cement-retained prosthesis in all other clinical situations, with emphasis on the importance of complete excess cement removal during the delivery of the definitive prosthesis.

Radiotherapy, Osteoradionecrosis, and Dental Implants

The effect of the presence of dental implants in patients receiving radiotherapy in the head and neck region has been studied. The concern has centered around three possible consequences[80]:

1. Osteoradionecrosis of the bone surrounding the implant
2. Implant failure and loss of osseointegration
3. Reduced dose of irradiation to a tumor that is essentially blocked by the implant

Postoperative and definitive radiotherapy doses in the head and neck region are substantially higher (65 to 70 Gy) than those applied preoperatively (approximately 50 Gy); therefore, it is in cases of the former that there is the greatest risk of bone necrosis.[80] (Gy is an abbreviation for gray, which is a unit of absorbed radiation equal to the dose of one joule of energy absorbed per kilogram of matter, or 100 rad.)

Radiation causes *endarteritis*, inflammation of the tunica intima of an artery (Fig 3-31), leading to tissue hypoxia, hypocellularity, and hypovascularity, which may lead to chronic nonhealing wounds.[81] Irradiated bone may not be capable of proper remodeling because damage to osteoclasts occurs earlier than vascular alterations.[82] Moreover, there is an increased risk of osteoradionecrosis in irradiated bone.

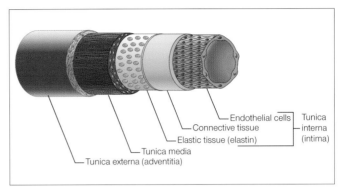

Fig 3-31 Anatomy of a human artery.

Osteoradionecrosis

It is believed that trauma related to dental, periodontal, or surgical procedures in irradiated tissue may be a factor in the development of osteoradionecrosis.[83] Osteoradionecrosis occurs secondary to radiation damage in the bone, which is affected by how much radiation is absorbed, how much tissue is irradiated, and how the radiation is administered over time (called the *fractionation pattern*). Factors that increase the risk of osteoradionecrosis include higher doses of radiation, a longer time period since radiotherapy (as a result of progressive endarteritis), and surgery performed 1 month or less prior to radiation treatment.[80,84] The mandible, which is highly compact, of low vascularity (which may be further reduced by previous head and neck surgery), and difficult to access for radiation treatment, appears to be especially susceptible to osteoradionecrosis.[80]

Ben Slama et al[85] reported a case of bilateral osteoradionecrosis in a patient who had dental implants inserted 10 years before cancer therapy. The first lesion appeared 3 months after the end of radiotherapy and was treated by mandibular resection. The second lesion appeared as a result of peri-implantitis on the opposite side of the mandible 40 months after radiotherapy and led to pathologic fracture.

Management of implants in the irradiation zone

Granström et al[80] do not advise removal of implants within 1 month before irradiation, suggesting that it might result in osteoradionecrosis. In addition, they point out that the removal of implants by a trephine drill can cause significant trauma to the bone. On the other hand, when abutments and titanium bars have been left in place during irradiation, some patients have shown soft tissue complications such as skin dehiscence as a consequence of the backscatter irradiation effects. Therefore, the authors of the study[80] recommend leaving implants in place during irradiation, as long as they are submerged in skin or mucosa, but removing all prostheses, frameworks, and abutments before initiating radiation treatment.

Osseointegration in irradiated bone

Several studies have associated implant insertion in irradiated bone with a higher failure rate. However, in a study by Jisander et al,[86] oral cancer patients were treated with external radiation in the region of planned implant sites. Between 18 and 228 months after radiation therapy, 103 implants were placed. The 1-year survival rate of the implants was 97% in the mandible and 92% in the maxilla. While the irradiation dose used did not affect implant survival, these results may have been influenced by the addition of hyperbaric oxygen treatment for patients receiving more than 50 Gy.

The conflicting results of various studies in the literature regarding the survival of dental implants in patients after radiation therapy can be attributed to several variables, including the timing of the radiation therapy, the dose levels, the anatomical location, adjunctive hyperbaric oxygen therapy, and the materials and size of the inserted implants.

Timing of radiation therapy

Titanium implants can be integrated in the facial bones even in highly irradiated tissues.[80] However, the failure rate of implants over time is higher in previously irradiated bone, generally within the first 3 years after implant surgery.

An atraumatic surgical technique when placing the implants, intensive cooling of the bone, and consequent preservation of the blood vessels in the implant area can minimize the possibility of osteoradionecrosis in irradiated bone. A higher rate of implant failure can be prevented by the adjunctive use of hyperbaric oxygen.[87,88]

Dose level of the radiation

Increasing the dose of radiation has been shown to increase its effect on osseointegration. In a study by Ohrnell et al,[89] animals receiving a 30- or 35-Gy dose of radiation had noticeably less bone formation around their implants than on their control side or in animals receiving 10- or 20-Gy doses.

A study by Visch et al[90] comparing implant survival rates at 10 years in patients receiving a radiation dose either greater or less than 50 Gy reported an association between improved implant survival in lower-dose patients as compared with higher-dose patients.

Anatomical location

Implants in some anatomical areas are at greater risk of failure because of radiation than others. In general, implants in narrow ridges have a tendency to fail at a higher rate.

Adjunctive hyperbaric oxygen therapy

Several studies have described the positive role of hyperbaric oxygen therapy in revitalizing the bone by stimulating angiogenesis, leading to an improved survival rate of dental implants in irradiated jawbone.

Hyperbaric oxygen treatment has been shown to increase the torque necessary to remove implants in both control and irradiated bone. The effects of hyperbaric oxygen on implant integration seem to be primarily the result of increased bone formation at the implant-bone interface.[91]

In a study[92] of the effects of hyperbaric oxygen treatment on the strength of the implant-bone interface with and without preceding irradiation, the results showed that the postradiation use of hyperbaric oxygen treatment for 21 days increased the biomechanical force necessary to remove the implants by 44% in irradiated bone and by 22% in nonirradiated bone.

Materials

Stainless steel and titanium are the metals most often used in maxillofacial reconstruction. Metal implants may modify radiation doses, causing an overdose because of the buildup of backscatter of primary and secondary irradiation, while the region behind the implant is underdosed.

Diagnostic radiation for immediate postsurgical assessment of dental implants

Because of the possible detrimental effects of ionizing radiation on the healing and remodeling of bone, immediate postsurgical diagnostic radiographs of dental implants have been discouraged. However, the results of an in vitro study[93] that investigated the effect of ionizing radiation on the growth and differentiation of osteoblasts indicated that a single 400-mGy dose of ionizing radiation does not induce significant changes in cell growth. Thus, diagnostic-level radiation doses should not have a significant effect on the proliferation and differentiation of osteoblasts.

| COMPLICATION 41 | # Shallow Vestibule Secondary to Ridge Augmentation |

As alveolar ridge resorption takes place, the attachment of mucosa and muscles near the denture-bearing area exerts a greater influence on the retention and stability of dentures, and the amount and quality of fixed tissue over the denture-bearing area may be decreased.

In *vestibuloplasty*, the soft tissue and mentalis muscle attachments are surgically detached and allowed to heal in a more apical position, exposing more of the basal bone. A greater surface area of basal bone will prevent dislodgment of the denture by the abnormal muscle insertions into the residual alveolar ridge. Vestibuloplasty may also be necessary after ridge augmentation procedures such as alveolar ridge expansion by the split-ridge technique, GBR, and veneer block grafting.

When treatment planning vestibuloplasty, three conditions must be present:

1. Inadequate labial vestibular depth from mucosal and muscular attachments in the anterior mandible
2. Presence of an adequate vestibular depth on the lingual aspect of the mandible
3. Adequate anterior mandibular height (at least 15 mm)[94]

Vestibuloplasty by secondary epithelialization (Kazanjian technique)

In vestibuloplasty by secondary epithelialization, also called the *Kazanjian technique*,[95] a mucosal flap pedicled from the alveolar ridge is elevated from the underlying tissue and sutured to the depth of the vestibule, and the inner portion of the lip is allowed to heal by secondary epithelialization.

Step-by-step protocol

1. A superficial incision is made in the labial mucosa anterior to the mental foramina (at about the vermilion border of the lip), and a thin mucosal flap is dissected from the underlying tissue. This dissection is done with a blade.
2. Supraperiosteal dissection is also performed on the anterior aspect of the mandible to release the mentalis muscle attachments from the labial aspect of the mandible. The muscular attachments are filleted from the periosteum. An attempt should be made to dissect as close to the periosteum as possible. Perforations in the periosteum will not cause significant problems but should be avoided.
3. The flap of labial mucosa is sutured to the greatest depth of the vestibular periosteum. Exposed labial tissue heals by secondary intention.

4. A surgical splint or modified relined denture may be used to maintain the depth of the newly formed vestibule during the healing phase.

Note: Extending the vestibuloplasty into the molar region is not recommended because of the risk of damage to the mental neurovascular bundle during supraperiosteal dissection.

The disadvantages of the Kazanjian operation include scarring in the depth of the vestibule, which can lead to a reduction in lower lip height, flattening of the labiomental fold, an unpredictable amount of vestibular depth relapse, and a drooping chin (referred to as a "witch's chin") because of the lower insertion of the mentalis muscle. The clinician should not be aggressive when releasing this muscle to lower its position; however, a chin reduction procedure can be performed later, if necessary.

Relapse rates are as high as 50% to 100% because of contraction of the granulation tissue during healing and reattachment of muscles released during the surgical procedure. Thus, a modification of this technique using a transpositional flap, called the *lip switch technique*, was introduced in 1978 and has since become popular.[96]

The lip switch technique

Step-by-step protocol

1. Anesthesia can be accomplished by bilateral inferior alveolar blocks and by local infiltration on the ridge and lower lip for hemostasis.
2. The desired depth is determined, and an incision is made on the lower lip at a distance from the attached mucosa that is 1½ times[97] the proposed vestibular depth (Fig 3-32a).

3. A flap is elevated until the alveolar crest is reached using a blade and blunt dissection with Metzenbaum scissors (Fig 3-32b).
4. A second incision is placed through the submucosa and periosteum below the pedicle near the crest, and a subperiosteal flap is elevated inferiorly to the desired vestibular

depth. This periosteal flap is scored with a blade at the intended vestibular depth to permit the placement of sutures (Fig 3-32c).

5. The superior portion of the periosteal flap is sutured to the incised lip margin with interrupted resorbable sutures, and the free mucosal flap is sutured inferiorly to the base of the dissection (Fig 3-32d).

6. Soft relining of the denture is necessary for a few weeks, after which a hard reline can be done.

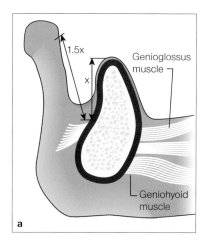
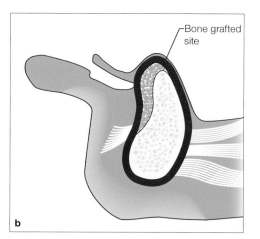
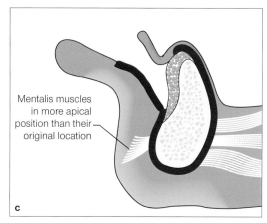
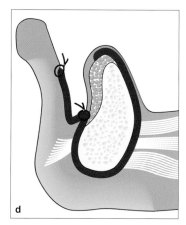

Fig 3-32 The lip switch technique. Ridge augmentation has led to a shallow vestibule. *(a)* The initial incision on the labial mucosa starts at a distance from the attached mucosa that is 1½ times the proposed vestibular depth. *(b)* A thin mucosal flap is dissected from the underlying tissue until it reaches the periosteum layer on the alveolar bone. *(c)* An incision is placed through the periosteum below the pedicle near the crest, and a subperiosteal flap is elevated inferiorly to the desired vestibular depth. The periosteum is scored at the intended vestibular depth to allow placement of sutures. *(d)* The superior margin of the periosteal flap is sutured to the incised lip margin, and the free mucosal flap is sutured to the base of the periosteum flap (at the scored depth).

Postoperative instructions

- A pressure dressing such as 0.5-inch surgical tape should be applied to the chin for 48 hours.
- The patient should not pull on the lip, which might cause opening of the incision line.
- The patient should be limited to a liquid diet for a minimum of 72 hours.
- Antibiotics and anti-inflammatory medications are recommended.
- The patient should rinse with a chlorhexidine oral rinse after each meal for 3 to 4 weeks.

COMPLICATION 42 | # Medicolegal Issues

The best way a dental practitioner can protect against the occurrence and success of malpractice lawsuits is by taking every measure to ensure that the treatment provided is appropriate to the patient's needs and carried out with the utmost care and precision.

Diagnosis

Good treatment begins with an accurate diagnosis. Therefore, the dental practitioner must use all diagnostic tools available to determine the best treatment approach and identify any potential risk factors (see appendix A).

Patient consultation and informed consent

Another important step is making time for a thorough patient consultation before treatment is begun. During this consultation, the patient should be given at least two different treatment options, with all possible risks and outcomes as well as cost for each option fully explained. Once a treatment approach has been chosen, the patient should be provided with informed consent forms that fully explain in writing the treatment and the expected outcome and associated risks. The patient should be allowed to take the forms home and given ample time to read them. A second consultation should be scheduled to allow the patient to ask questions before signing the forms. Fully informed patients better understand the risks and possibilities for untoward outcomes and therefore have more realistic expectations going into treatment. See appendix B for sample informed consent forms for various procedures related to implant dentistry.

Documentation

It is essential that the dental practitioner have thorough documentation of all aspects of diagnosis and treatment. The patient's complaint, diagnostic findings, the details of the procedures performed (eg, anesthesia, specifications of materials used, surgical techniques), the outcome, and follow-up should all be documented in detail, both in writing and through other records such as diagnostic casts, photographs, radiographs, and CT images.

Referral

The timely referral of patients to the emergency room or specialists when needed is absolutely essential. Dental practitioners should never try to manage a complication that is beyond their clinical abilities and experience.

Malpractice insurance

It is also very important to have a good malpractice (liability) insurance policy and an attorney who specializes in representing medical/dental practitioners. Any complications should be reported immediately to the malpractice insurance provider.

References

1. Hashem AA, Claffey NM, O'Connell B. Pain and anxiety following the placement of dental implants. Int J Oral Maxillofac Implants 2006;21:943–950.

2. Al-Khabbaz AK, Griffin TJ, Al-Shammri KF. Assessment of pain associated with the surgical placement of dental implants. J Periodontol 2007;78:239–246.

3. Gonzalez-Santana H, Penarrocha-Diago M, Guarinos-Carbo J, Balaguer-Martinez J. Pain and inflammation in 41 patients following the placement of 131 dental implants. Med Oral Patol Cir Bucal 2005;10:258–263.

4. Muller E, Ríos Calvo MP. Pain and dental implantology: Sensory quantification and affective aspects. Part I: At the private dental office. Implant Dent 2001;10:14–22.

5. Fortin T, Bosson JL, Isidori M, Blanchet E. Effect of flapless surgery on pain experienced in implant placement using an image-guided system. Int J Oral Maxillofac Implants 2006;21:298–304.

6. Leckel M, Kress B, Schmitter M. Neuropathic pain resulting from implant placement: Case report and diagnostic conclusions. J Oral Rehabil 2009;36:543–546.

7. Siervo S. Suturing Techniques in Oral Surgery. Chicago: Quintessence, 2008:212.

8. Monsour PA, Savage NW. Cervicofacial emphysema following dental procedures. Aust Dent J 1989;34:403–406.

9. McKenzie WS, Rosenberg M. Iatrogenic subcutaneous emphysema of dental and surgical origin: A literature review. J Oral Maxillofac Surg 2009;67:1265–1268.

10. Bergendal T, Forsgren L, Kvint S, Löwstedt E. The effect of an airbrasive instrument on soft and hard tissues around osseointegrated implants. A case report. Swed Dent J 1990;14:219–223.

11. Frühauf J, Weinke R, Pilger U, Kerl H, Müllegger RR. Soft tissue cervicofacial emphysema after dental treatment: Report of 2 cases with emphasis on the differential diagnosis of angioedema. Arch Dermatol 2005;141:1437–1440.

12. Karras SC, Sexton JJ. Cervicofacial and mediastinal emphysema as the result of a dental procedure. J Emerg Med 1996;14:9–13.

13. Rossiter JL, Hendrix RA. Iatrogenic subcutaneous cervicofacial and mediastinal emphysema. J Otolaryngol 1991;20:315–319.

14. Davies DE. Pneumomediastinum after dental surgery. Anaesth Intensive Care 2001;29:638–641.

15. Silverstein P. Smoking and wound healing. Am J Med 1992;93:22S–24S.

16. Baig MR, Rajan M. Effects of smoking on the outcome of implant treatment: A literature review. Indian J Dent Res 2007;18:190–195.

17. Heitz-Mafield LJ, Huynh-Ba G. History of treated periodontitis and smoking as risks for implant therapy. Int J Oral Maxillofac Implants 2009;24(suppl):39–68.

18. Siervo S. Suturing Techniques in Oral Surgery. Chicago: Quintessence, 2008:211.

19. Silverstein LH. Principles of Dental Suturing. Mahwah, NJ: Montage Media, 1999:10–11.

20. Siervo S. Suturing Techniques in Oral Surgery. Chicago: Quintessence, 2008:53–57.

21. Burkhardt R, Preiss A, Joss A, Lang NP. Influence of suture tension to the tearing characteristics of the soft tissues: An in vitro experiment. Clin Oral Implants Res 2008;19:314–319.

22. Adell R, Lekholm U, Brånemark P-I. Surgical procedures. In: Brånemark P-I, Zarb GA, Albrektsson T (eds). Tissue-Integrated Prostheses: Osseointegration in Clinical Dentistry. Chicago: Quintessence, 1985:211–240.

23. Oh TJ, Yoon J, Misch CE, Wang HL. The causes of early implant bone loss: Myth or science? J Periodontol 2002;73:322–333.

24. Quirynen M, van Steenberghe D. Bacterial colonization of the internal part of two-stage implants. An in vivo study. Clin Oral Implant Res 1993;4:158–161.

25. Persson LG, Lekholm U, Leonhardt A, Dahlen G. Lindhe J. Bacterial colonization on internal surfaces of Brånemark system implant components. Clin Oral Implant Res 1996;7:90–95.

26. Piattelli A, Vrespa G, Petrone G, Iezzi G, Annibali S, Scarano A. Role of the microgap between implant and abutment: A retrospective histologic evaluation in monkeys. J Periodontol 2003;74:346–352.

27. Aoki M, Takanashi K, Matsukubo T, et al. Transmission of periodontopathic bacteria from natural teeth to implants [epub ahead of print 11 Dec 2009]. Clin Implant Dent Relat Res.

28. Sumida S, Ishihara K, Kishi M, Okuda K. Transmission of periodontal disease-associated bacteria from teeth to osseointegrated implant regions. Int J Oral Maxillofac Implants 2002;17:696–702.

29. Eriksson AR, Albrektsson T. Temperature threshold levels for heat-induced bone tissue injury: A vital-microscopic study in the rabbit. J Prosthet Dent 1983;50:101–107.

30. Piattelli A, Scarano A, Piattelli M. Microscopical aspects of failure in osseointegrated dental implants: A report of five cases. Biomaterials 1996;17:1235–1241.

31. Wallace RH. The relationship between cigarette smoking and dental implant failure. Eur J Prosthodont Restor Dent 2000;8:103–106.

32. Kumar A, Jaffin RA, Berman C. The effect of smoking on achieving osseointegration of surface-modified implants: A clinical report. Int J Oral Maxillofac Implants 2002;17:816–819.

33. Sverzut AT, Stabile GA, de Moraes M, Mazzonetto R, Moreira RW. The influence of tobacco on early dental implant failure. J Oral Maxillofac Surg 2008;66:1004–1009.

34. De Bruyn H, Collaert B. The effect of smoking on early implant failure. Clin Oral Implants Res 1994;5:260–264.

35. Gorman LM, Lambert PM, Morris HF, Ochi S, Winkler S. The effect of smoking on implant survival at second-stage surgery: DICRG Interim Report No. 5. Dental Implant Clinical Research Group. Implant Dent 1994;3:165–168.

36. Alsaadi G, Quirynen M, Komarek A, van Steenberghe D. Impact of local and systemic factors on the incidence of oral implant failures, up to abutment connection. J Clin Periodontol 2007;34:610–617.

37. Lambert PM, Morris HF, Ochi S. The influence of smoking on 3-year clinical success of osseointegrated dental implants. Ann Periodontol 2000;5:79–89.

38. Orenstein IH, Tarnow DP, Morris HF, Ochi S. Three-year post-placement survival of implant mobile at placement. Ann Periodontol 2000;5:32–41.

39. Morris HF, Ochi S. Survival and stability (PTVs) of six implant designs from placement to 36 months. Ann Periodontol 2000;5:15–21.

40. Sevimay M, Turhan F, Kiliçarslan MA, Eskitascioglu G. Three-dimensional finite element analysis of the effect of different bone quality on stress distribution in an implant-supported crown. J Prosthet Dent 2005;93:227–234.

41. Lekholm U, Zarb GA. Patient selection and preparation. In: Brånemark P-I, Zarb GA, Albrektsson T (eds). Tissue-Integrated Prostheses: Osseointegration in Clinical Dentistry. Chicago: Quintessence, 1985:199–210.

42. Gotfredsen K, Nimb L, Hjörting-Hansen E, Jensen JS, Holmén A. Histomorphometric and removal torque analysis for TiO2-blasted titanium implants. An experimental study on dogs. Clin Oral Implants Res 1992;3:77–84.

43. Klokkevold PR, Johnson P, Dadgostari S, Caputo A, Davies JE, Nishimura RD. Early endosseous integration enhanced by dual acid etching of titanium: A torque removal study in the rabbit. Clin Oral Implants Res 2001;12:350–357.

44. Gotfredsen K, Berglundh T, Lindhe J. Anchorage of titanium implants with different surface characteristics: An experimental study in rabbits. Clin Implant Dent Relat Res 2000;2:120–128.

45. Le Guéhennec L, Soueidan A, Layrolle P, Amouriq Y. Surface treatments of titanium dental implants for rapid osseointegration. Dent Mater 2007;23:844–854.

46. Meffert RM. Periodontitis and peri-implantitis: One and the same? Pract Periodontics Aesthet Dent 1993;5:79–80.

47. Ayangco L, Sheridan PJ. Development and treatment of retrograde peri-implantitis involving a site with a history of failed endodontic and apico-ectomy procedures: A series of reports. Int J Oral Maxillofac Implants 2001;16:412–417.

48. Tözüm TF, Sençimen M, Ortakoğlu K, Ozdemir A, Aydin OC, Keleş M. Diagnosis and treatment of a large periapical implant lesion associated with adjacent natural tooth: A case report. Oral Surg Oral Med Oral Pathol Oral Radiol Endod 2006;101:e132–e138.

49. Schou S, Holmstrup P, Worthington HV, Esposito M. Outcome of implant therapy in patients with previous tooth loss due to periodontitis. Clin Oral Implants Res 2006;17(suppl 2):104–123.

50. Scarano A, Di Domizio P, Petrone G, Iezzi G, Piatelli A. Implant periapical lesion: A clinical and histologic case report. J Oral Implant 2000;26:109–113.

51. Eriksson AR, Adell R. Temperatures during drilling for the placement of implants using the osseointegration technique. J Oral Maxillofac Surg 1986;44:4–7.

52. Quirynen M, Vogels R, Alsaadi G, Naert I, Jacobs R, van Steenberghe D. Predisposing conditions for retrograde peri-implantitis, and treatment suggestions. Clin Oral Implants Res 2005;16:599–608.

53. Dahlin C, Nikfarid H, Alsén B, Kashani H. Apical peri-implantitis: Possible predisposing factors, case reports, and surgical treatment suggestions. Clin Implant Dent Relat Res 2009;11:222–227.

54. Bousdras V, Aghabeigi B, Hopper C, Sindet-Pedersen S. Management of apical bone loss around a mandibular implant: A case report. Int J Oral Maxillofac Implants 2006;21:439–444.

55. Meffert RM. How to treat ailing and failing implants. Implant Dent 1992;1:25–33.

56. Artzi Z, Tal H, Chweidan H. Bone regeneration for reintegration in peri-implant destruction. Compend Contin Educ Dent 1998;19:17–30.

57. Mellonig JT, Griffiths G, Mathys E, Spitznagel J Jr. Treatment of the failing implant: Case reports. Int J Periodontics Restorative Dent 1995;15:385–395.

58. Flanagan D. Apical (retrograde) peri-implantitis: A case report of an active lesion. J Oral Implantol 2002;28:92–96.

59. Podbielski A, Boeckh C, Haller B. Growth inhibitory activity of gutta percha points containing root canal medications on common endodontic bacterial pathogens determined by an optimized quantitative in vitro assay. J Endodontol 2000;26:398–403.

60. Ataullah K, Chee LF, Peng LL, Lung HH. Management of retrograde peri-implantitis: A clinical case report. J Oral Implantol 2006;32:308–312.

61. Bretz WA, Matuck AN, de Oliveira G, Moretti AJ, Bretz WA. Treatment of retrograde peri-implantitis: Clinical report. Implant Dent 1997;6:287–290.

62. Tseng CC, Chen YH, Pang IC, Weber HP. Peri-implant pathology caused by periapical lesion of an adjacent natural tooth: A case report. Int J Oral Maxillofac Implants 2005;20:632–635.

63. Taylor T. Prosthodontic problems and limitations associated with osseointegration. J Prosthet Dent 1998;79:74–78.

64. Hebel K, Gajjar R. Cement-retained vs screw-retained implant restoration: Achieving optimal occlusion and esthetics in implant dentistry. J Prosthet Dent 1997;77:28–35.

65. Cicciu M, Beretta M, Risitano G, Maiorana C. Cemented-retained vs screw-retained implant restorations: An investigation on 1939 dental implants. Minerva Stomatol 2008;57:167–179.

66. Vigolo P, Givani A, Majzoub Z, Cordili G. Cemented versus screw-retained implant-supported single-tooth crowns: A 4-year prospective clinical study. Int J Oral Maxillofac Implants 2004;19:260–265.

67. Zarone F, Sorrentino R, Traini T, Di Iorio D, Caputi S. Fracture resistance of implant-supported screw- versus cement-retained porcelain fused to metal single crowns: SEM fractographic analysis. Dent Mater 2007;23:296–301.

68. Rosen H, Gornitsky M. Cementable implant-supported prosthesis, serial extraction, and serial implant installation: Case report. Implant Dent 2004;13:322–327.

69. Wilson TG. The positive relationship between excess cement and peri-implant disease: A prospective clinical endoscopic study. J Periodontol 2009;80:1388–1392.

70. Palacci P. Esthetic Implant Dentistry. Soft and Hard Tissue Management. Chicago: Quintessence, 2001:34–35.

71. Berglundh T, Lindhe J. Dimension of the peri-implant mucosa: Biological width revisited. J Clin Periodontol 1996;23:971–973.

72. Cochran DL, Hermann JS, Schenk RK, Higginbottom FL, Buser D. Biologic width around dental implants. A histometric analysis of the implanto-gingival junction around unloaded and loaded non-submerged implants in the canine mandible. J Periodontol 1997;68:186–198.

73. Gapski R, Neugeboren N, Pomeranz A, Reissner M. Endosseous implant failure influenced by crown cementation: A clinical case report. J Oral Maxillofac Implants 2008;23:943–946.

74. Buser D, Weber HP, Donath K, Fiorellini J, Paquette DW, Williams R. Soft tissue reactions to nonsubmerged unloaded titanium implants in beagle dogs. J Periodontol 1992;63:226–236.

75. Berglundh T, Lindhe J, Jonsson K, Ericsson I. The topography of the vascular systems in the periodontal and peri-implant tissues in the dog. J Clin Periodontol 1994;21:189–193.

76. Assenza B, Scarano A, Leghissa G, et al. Screw- vs cement-implant-retained restorations: An experimental study in the beagle. Part 1. Screw and abutment loosening. J Oral Implantol 2005;31:242–246.

77. Assenza B, Artese L, Scarano A, et al. Screw- vs cement-implant-retained restorations: An experimental study in the beagle. Part 2. Immunohistochemical evaluation of the peri-implant tissue. J Oral Implantol 2006;32:1–7.

78. Keller W, Bragger U, Mombelli A. Peri-implant microflora of implants with cemented and screw retained suprastructures. Clin Oral Implants Res 1998;9:209–217.

79. Piattelli A, Scarano A, Paolantonio M, et al. Fluids and microbial penetration in the internal part of cement-retained versus screw-retained implant-abutment connections. J Periodontol 2001;72:1146–1150.

80. Granström G, Tjellström A, Albrektsson T. Postimplantation irradiation for head and neck cancer treatment. Int J Oral Maxillofac Implants 1993;8:495–501.

81. Ihde S, Kopp S, Gundlach K, Konstantinović VS. Effects of radiation therapy on craniofacial and dental implants: A review of the literature. Oral Surg Oral Med Oral Pathol Oral Radiol Endod 2009;107:56–65.

82. Teng MS, Futran ND. Osteoradionecrosis of the mandible. Curr Opin Otolaryngol Head Neck Surg 2005;13:217–221.

83. Marx RE. Osteoradionecrosis of the jaws. Review and update. HBO Rev 1984;5:78–126.

84. Marx RE, Johnson RP. Studies in the radiobiology of osteoradionecrosis and their clinical significance. Oral Surg Oral Med Oral Pathol 1987;64:379–390.

85. Ben Slama L, Hasni W, De Labrouhe C, Bado F, Bertrand JC. Osteoradionecrosis and dental implants. Rev Stomatol Chir Maxillofac 2008;109:387–391.

86. Jisander S, Grenthe B, Alberius P. Dental implant survival in the irradiated jaw: A preliminary report. Int J Oral Maxillofac Implants 1997;12:643–648.

87. Granström G, Tjellström A, Brånemark P-I, Fornander J. Bone-anchored reconstruction of the irradiated head and neck cancer patient. Otolaryngol Head Neck Surg 1993;108:334–343.

88. Granström G, Jacobsson M, Tjellström A. Titanium implants in irradiated tissue: Benefits from hyperbaric oxygen. Int J Oral Maxillofac Implants 1992;7:15–25.

89. Ohrnell LO, Brånemark R, Nyman J, Nilsson P, Thomson P. Effects of irradiation on the biomechanics of osseointegration. An experimental in vivo study in rats. Scand J Plast Reconstr Surg Hand Surg 1997;31:281–293.

90. Visch LL, van Waas MA, Schmitz PI, Levendag PC. A clinical evaluation of implants in irradiated oral cancer patients. J Dent Res 2002;81:856–859.

91. Nilsson P, Albrektsson T, Granström G, Röckert HO. The effect of hyperbaric oxygen treatment on bone regeneration. An experimental study using the bone harvest chamber in the rabbit. Int J Oral Maxillofac Implants 1988;3:43–48.

92. Johnsson K, Hansson A, Granström G, Jacobsson M, Turesson I. The effects of hyperbaric oxygenation on bone-titanium implant interface strength with and without preceding irradiation. Int J Oral Maxillofac Implants 1993;8:415–419.

93. Dare A, Hachisu R, Yamaguchi A, Yokose S, Yoshiki S, Okano T. Effects of ionizing radiation on proliferation and differentiation of osteoblast-like cells. J Dent Res 1997;76:658–664.

94. Peterson LJ, Ellis E, Hupp JR, Tucker MR. Contemporary Oral and Maxillofacial Surgery. St Louis: Mosby, 1998:340–342.

95. Kazanjian VH. Surgical operations as related to satisfactory dentures. Dent Cosmos 1924;66:387.

96. Kethley JL Jr, Gamble JW. The lipswitch: A modification of Kazanjian's labial vestibuloplasty. J Oral Surg 1978;36:701–705.

97. Dym H, Ogle OE. Atlas of Minor Oral Surgery. Philadelphia: Saunders, 2001:202–204.

Anatomical Considerations of the Maxillary Sinus

To avoid complications associated with lateral window sinus elevation, it is crucial that the implant dentist have a clear understanding of the anatomy of the sinuses. There are four pairs of paranasal sinuses: frontal, ethmoid, sphenoid, and maxillary (Figs 4-1 and 4-2). Of these, only the maxillary sinuses are of significant interest to the implant surgeon.

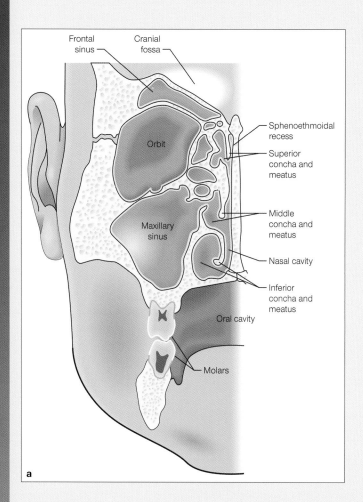

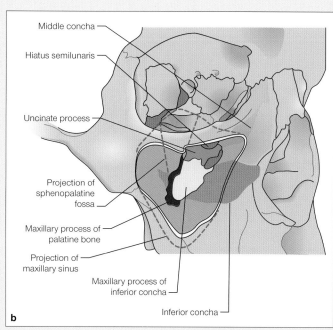

Fig 4-1 Anatomy of the paranasal sinuses. (a) Coronal view. (b) Lateral view.

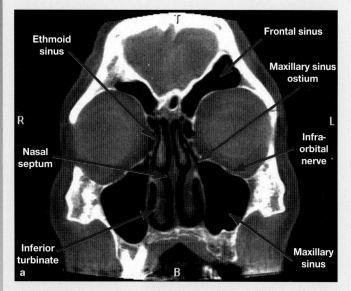

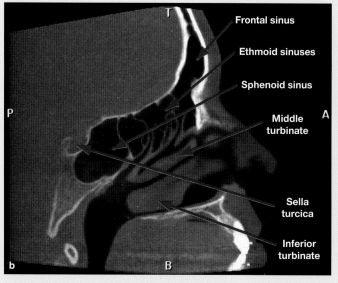

Fig 4-2 Computed tomography (CT) scans of the paranasal sinuses. (a) Coronal view. (b) Sagittal view.

The maxillary sinus reaches adult size by approximately 12 to 14 years of age.[1] Periods of more rapid expansion correspond to eruption of the primary and permanent teeth and the corresponding growth of the alveolar process.[2] In children, there is considerable space between the floor of the sinus and the apices of the maxillary teeth. By 12 years of age, the floor of the sinus is usually approximately level with the floor of the nasal cavity; however, there is often continued inferior expansion of the sinus.[3] This is frequently associated with other dental events, such as eruption of the third molars and extraction or loss of the maxillary molars (Fig 4-3). Continued inferior pneumatization of the sinus can eventually result in extreme resorption of the alveolar bone, leaving inadequate support for dental implants[1] (Fig 4-4).

The roots of the maxillary incisors and canines are not typically in close proximity to the sinus. The roots of the maxillary premolars and molars, however, are consistently just inferior to the maxillary sinus floor, with the roots of the second molar nearest the sinus cavity, followed by those of the first and third molars.[4]

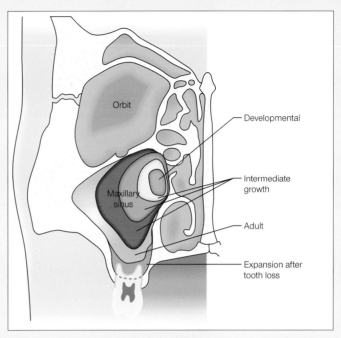

Fig 4-3 Development of the maxillary sinus.

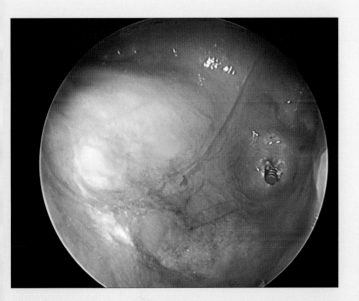

Fig 4-4 Endoscopic photograph of a dental implant penetrating into the maxillary sinus.

The adult maxillary sinus is roughly a laterally directed pyramid, averaging 37.5 × 25 × 30 mm.[5] The average volume is approximately 15 to 20 mL.[6] The sinus usually has a single communication to the nasal cavity, found in the medial wall of the sinus, which is also the lateral wall of the nasal cavity. This wall often contains several areas of incomplete bone formation, which may lead to the formation of additional nasal cavity–sinus communications called *accessory ostia,* which are of questionable physiologic significance. The natural ostium of the maxillary sinus averages 2.4 mm in diameter but can range from 1 to 17 mm.[5] Considered from an intranasal perspective, this opening is found in the *middle meatus,* the space above the inferior turbinate (concha) and the middle turbinate; from within the sinus, the opening is high on the medial wall. The posterior wall separates the sinus from the structures of the infratemporal and pterygomaxillary fossae. The lateral wall is formed by the zygoma. The anterior wall includes the canine fossa and the infraorbital foramen (through which the infraorbital nerve, a branch of the maxillary nerve, exits into the soft tissues of the face).

Bony septa rising from the floor of the sinus and extending in a mediolateral orientation are frequently encountered and can become a significant cause of membrane perforation during flap elevation if not recognized (Fig 4-5). These septa, first described by Underwood[7] in 1910, have been reported in the literature to have an incidence of 16% to 58%. In an analysis of 312 sinuses in 156 patients, Velasquez-Plata et al[8] noted an incidence of bony septa in 24% of sinuses and in 33% of patients. Kim et al[9] reported on 200 sinuses in 100 patients and found 53 sinuses (26.5%) to contain one or more septa. Ulm et al[10] noted that in an edentulous population, the incidence of septa may be as high as 32%. Maxillary septa may arise from the anterior, middle, or posterior portions of the sinus floor but most commonly are found in the middle third.[8,9] Maxillary sinus septa are discussed further in complication 53.

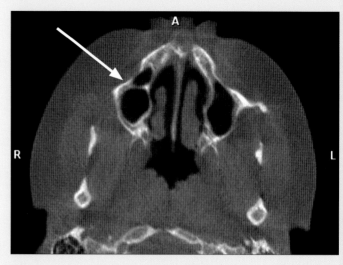

Fig 4-5 Axial CT demonstrating a right maxillary sinus septum *(arrow)*.

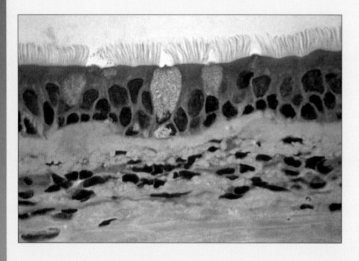

Fig 4-6 Histologic view of the sinus membrane.

The roof of the sinus is also the floor of the orbit and contains the infraorbital canal, through which the infraorbital nerve runs in a posteroanterior direction before exiting through the infraorbital foramen. In up to 14% of sinuses, the nerve may be located on a bony mesentery or may even be dehiscent.[11] Because of its superior location, this rarely presents a concern for the implant surgeon. The floor of the maxillary sinus comprises the hard palate, alveolus, and dental portion of the maxilla and may be 1 to 10 mm below the level of the floor of the nasal cavity.

The maxillary sinus derives its blood supply predominantly from the external carotid circulation via branches of the internal maxillary artery. Sensory innervation is via branches of the maxillary nerve, while autonomic innervation is via branches of the sphenopalatine nerve.

A rare but significant anatomical variation is maxillary sinus hypoplasia. The hypoplastic sinus cavity is much smaller than normal and often features considerable bony thickening of the inferior and lateral walls. The etiology of a hypoplastic sinus is uncertain but is theorized to be related to deficient bone absorption or an inability to adequately aerate the sinus cavity.[12] A history of childhood facial trauma is not uncommon for patients with maxillary sinus hypoplasia.

The physiology of the maxillary sinus is closely related to its microanatomy. The mucosal lining of the maxillary sinus, the sinus membrane, is respiratory mucosa: pseudostratified, ciliated, columnar epithelieum (Fig 4-6). Healthy sinus lining is 0.2 to 0.8 mm thick, with a relatively thin basement membrane. Coating the sinus lining is a bilayered secretory blanket. The inner layer, called the *sol*, is thin, serous, and rich in proteins, immunoglobulin, and complement. The surface layer, called the *gel*, is a viscous mucus that floats on the thinner sol layer. The cilia of the cells lining the sinus reach up through the sol layer and sweep the gel layer along, so that any surface materials are swept toward the sinus ostium at a rate of 3 to 25 mm per minute.[13] The mucus flows in a predictable, stellate pattern beginning at the inferior and lateral portion of the sinus and ending at the superior and medial sinus opening. Because of this system of mucus flow, the normally functioning sinus is nearly sterile.

| # Preoperative Acute Sinusitis

Differential diagnosis

While viral illnesses such as the common cold can cause some sinus inflammation, true sinus infections are generally bacterial in origin. Because of the small size of the natural ostium of the maxillary sinus, swelling of the nasal lining due to a viral illness can easily compromise its drainage. This leads to a breakdown of the ciliary transport within the sinus and allows bacteria present in the nasal cavity to invade and infect the sinus. The bacteria most commonly responsible include *Haemophilus influenzae, Moraxella catarrhalis,* and *Streptococcus pneumoniae.*[14]

The symptoms of acute sinusitis include fever, foul rhinorrhea or postnasal drainage, and facial pain/swelling. Because of the proximity of the roots of the molars to the sinus cavity, dental pain is common and often leads patients to see their dentist before their physician. Untreated, the symptoms may last more than 3 weeks. The diagnosis of acute sinusitis is made clinically, and while laboratory tests (such as a white blood cell count) or imaging (showing an "air-fluid level" from pus in the sinus) may be helpful, they are not generally required (Fig 4-7).

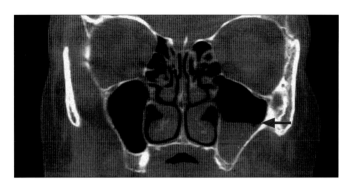

Fig 4-7 Coronal CT scan demonstrating an air-fluid level (*arrow*) in the left maxillary sinus.

Acute sinusitis that is a direct result of dental disease, called *odontogenic sinusitis,* is thought to account for up to 10% of sinus infections. It is different from standard acute sinusitis in that these infections are typically polymicrobial, with a predominance of anaerobes.

Medical management

Sinus surgery in the presence of active sinusitis is strongly contraindicated. If purulence is encountered intraoperatively, prudence would dictate aborting the procedure until after resolution of the infection.

Standard medical treatment for acute sinusitis is 14 to 21 days of oral antibiotics to cover the most common offending bacteria supplemented with oral decongestants and other symptomatic care such as antipyretics and analgesics (Table 4-1). First-line antibiotics include amoxicillin or trimethoprim-sulfamethoxazole. Patients likely to have resistance to these medications or those for whom treatment with first-line drugs has failed can be treated with amoxicillin + clavulanic acid or a fluoroquinolone (eg, ciprofloxacin, levofloxacin, or moxiflox-

acin). Rarely, a short course of oral steroids such as a methyl-prednisolone pack may be used to reduce swelling.

Resolution of an odontogenic sinusitis infection requires treatment of both the sinus infection and the dental source and thus represents an opportunity for coordination of care between the dental professional and the patient's physician.[1,4,6] Because of the frequent presence of anaerobic bacteria, odontogenic sinusitis may respond well to antibiotics such as clindamycin or metronidazole.

The surgeon should delay sinus grafting until there has been complete resolution of the infection and the inflammatory changes associated with it. Six weeks from initiation of therapy should be adequate.

Table 4-1 Recommended treatment for acute bacterial sinusitis in adults

Indication	Drug	Dose/length of therapy
Acute bacterial sinusitis	Amoxicillin	500 mg orally three times daily for 10 to 14 days
Acute bacterial sinusitis with allergy to penicillin	Trimethoprim-sulfamethoxazole OR	1 double-strength tablet (160/800 mg) twice daily for 10 to 14 days
	Macrolide: Azithromycin Clarithromycin	500 mg orally once daily for 7 to 10 days 500 mg orally twice daily for 10 to 14 days
Acute bacterial sinusitis with antibiotic use in the past 4 to 6 weeks (or failure of above-listed medications)	Amoxicillin-clavulanate OR	875 mg orally twice daily for 14 to 21 days
	Fluoroquinolone: Ciprofloxacin Levofloxacin Moxifloxacin	750 mg orally twice daily for 10 to 14 days 500 mg orally once daily for 10 to 14 days 400 mg orally once daily for 10 to 14 days
Acute bacterial sinusitis with suspected odontogenic origin	Clindamycin OR	300 mg orally four times daily for 14 to 21 days
	Metronidazole (+ a penicillin/macrolide)	500 mg orally twice daily for 14 to 21 days

Preoperative Chronic Sinusitis

Differential diagnosis

In contrast to acute sinusitis, chronic sinusitis is primarily a disease of inflammation, not infection. While the cause of the disorder is unknown, many of the chemical mediators are similar to those found in certain forms of asthma and allergic disorders. Studies have shown, however, that the incidence of allergy and asthma in patients with chronic sinusitis is about 50% and 60%, respectively, suggesting that the underlying diseases are not identical.[15] Chronic sinusitis is diagnosed by history, examination, and imaging. For the diagnosis to be made, a patient must have had symptoms for at least 12 weeks. The most common symptoms of chronic sinusitis include congestion, nasal obstruction, sinus pressure, postnasal drainage, fatigue, and decreased sense of smell. Dental pain, fever, and severe headache are relatively uncommon. Examination through anterior rhinoscopy (direct visualization through the nostrils) or fiberoptic endoscopy (Fig 4-8) demonstrates evidence of mucosal inflammation: swelling, thick drainage, or polyps.

Nasal polyps, unlike polyps elsewhere in the body, are not neoplastic. Instead, they represent severe, persistent mucosal inflammation. When the nasal or sinus lining is severely inflamed, mucosal tears or cracks occur, which are then covered with granulation tissue and remucosalized. Repetition of this process eventually leads to the well-defined soft tissue structures recognized as polyps. On examination, nasal polyps are pale, soft, and insensate (Fig 4-9). While nasal polyps are not invasive, years of pressure from extensive polyp disease can lead to bone thinning or displacement.

The imaging study of choice for diagnosis of chronic sinusitis is a CT scan (Fig 4-10). Conventional radiographs are inadequate to demonstrate appropriate detail, and magnetic resonance imaging (MRI), while highly effective for evaluating soft tissue, tends to overemphasize mucosal inflammatory changes. Dental imaging, such as panoramic radiographs, may demonstrate partial or complete maxillary sinus opacification and may be suggestive of a problem but does not show enough of the sinuses or have the detail necessary to make the diagnosis of chronic sinusitis. The standard for diagnosis has been a helical CT scan, but cone beam CT scanners are now approaching the same level of detail and are an excellent choice for imaging of chronic sinusitis because of their much lower radiation levels compared with helical CT scans.

While sinus augmentation will not initiate chronic sinusitis, it may exacerbate the condition. It has been suggested that patients with chronic sinusitis have a higher incidence of postoperative acute sinus infection associated with sinus augmentation.[16,17] Unrecognized sinus inflammatory disease may also be a cause of graft or implant failure. Galli et al[18] reported 14 cases of sinus disease presenting 4 to 24 months after sinus grafting, all of which required endoscopic sinus surgery (ESS; described in the next section) to resolve. Six of the sinuses

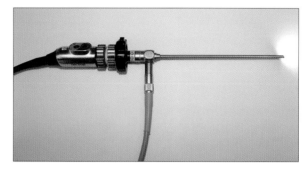

Fig 4-8 Rigid nasal endoscope and camera.

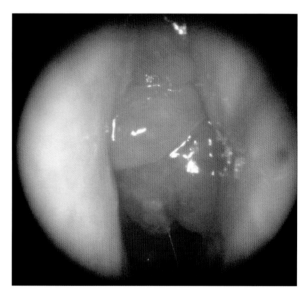

Fig 4-9 Endoscopic photograph of nasal polyps.

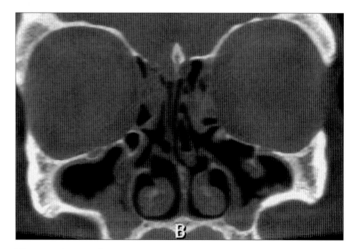

Fig 4-10 Coronal CT scan demonstrating chronic inflammatory changes of the maxillary and ethmoid sinuses. Note the absence of air-fluid levels.

demonstrated extrusion of graft material into the sinus cavity. Despite aggressive medical and surgical therapy, six patients required removal of some or all of the implants.

Medical management

While chronic sinusitis cannot be eliminated before surgery, optimizing control of the disease prior to grafting procedures will help ensure success. The treatment of chronic sinusitis is aimed at controlling inflammation. Corticosteroids such as prednisone are probably the most effective medical treatment available. Unfortunately, they carry significant potential for adverse effects, in both the short term (eg, mood changes, indigestion, insomnia, weight gain, hyperglycemia) and the long term (eg, hypothalamus-pituitary-adrenal axis suppression, osteoporosis, cataracts). Consequently, corticosteroids are usually given sparingly and in short bursts that are rapidly tapered. For example, a typical course of prednisone might start at 40 mg daily for 3 days, followed by 30 mg daily for 3 days, 20 mg daily for 3 days, 10 mg daily for 3 days, and finally 5 mg daily for 3 days. Contraindications to oral steroid use may include diabetes, peptic ulcer disease, osteoporosis, or psychiatric disorders. While steroids may slow wound healing, the benefit of suppression of inflammation in the chronic sinusitis patient probably outweighs this risk. Intramuscular or injected intranasal steroids such as triamcinolone carry many of the same risks as oral steroids; therefore, the only long-term steroid therapy generally used is steroid nasal sprays. While the sprays are thought to have very low absorption (and thus a low risk of side effects), they are also modest in their effects. Nasal steroid sprays will rarely make any significant impact on nasal polyps. Other medical therapies used include antihistamines, decongestants, leukotriene blockers, and antibiotics (when bacterial infection occurs). Buffered saline rinses of the nasal cavity with a syringe or Neti pot are often helpful in controlling symptoms as well.

If attempts at medical therapy fail to control sinus complaints, the patient may be a candidate for ESS. Performed through the nostrils in a surgical setting, the goal of ESS is to remove irreversibly inflamed tissue (polyps) and expand the natural opening of the sinus to allow better aeration and mucus flow. In the past, the swollen lining of the maxillary sinus might have been stripped off and allowed to remucosalize, but studies have found that the regenerated epithelium lacks the same quantity of healthy cilia. Consequently, in an effort to restore the normal mucus flow, current medical practice is to preserve the inflamed lining in hopes that it will heal on its own. This is why this type of surgery is sometimes referred to as *functional endoscopic sinus surgery* (FESS), reflecting a desire for the sinus to retain normal function postoperatively. Although individual healing times vary, augmentation often can be performed 6 to 8 weeks after an ESS procedure. Patients reporting a history of chronic sinusitis or ESS with signs of inflammation on preoperative imaging should be considered for referral to an otolaryngologist.

Neither medical therapy nor ESS can cure chronic sinusitis. Consequently, all therapy is aimed at symptom control, which is significant considering that chronic sinusitis sufferers may have a lower quality of life than patients with chronic back pain, emphysema, or even congestive heart failure.[19]

COMPLICATION 45 # Preoperative Fungal Sinusitis

Differential diagnosis

There are three main forms of fungal sinus disease that may appear on diagnostic imaging. The first form is known as a *fungal ball*. Fungal balls may occur in any of the sinuses and are not uncommon in the maxillary sinus. These represent simple collections of fungal hyphae and mucous concretions within the lumen of the sinus without mucosal invasion (Fig 4-11). They occur for unknown reasons in otherwise healthy, immunocompetent individuals. Generally asymptomatic until they become sizable enough to begin a slow expansion of the sinus, they occasionally serve as a nidus of inflammation, leading to chronic sinus drainage and recurrent bacterial sinusitis. Radiographically, they appear as an opacity filling all or part of the sinus with mixed densities. The speckles of high density within the fungal collection are thought to be caused by heavy metals such as manganese and iron.[20]

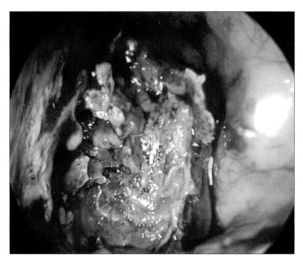

Fig 4-11 Endoscopic photograph of a fungal ball of the right maxillary sinus.

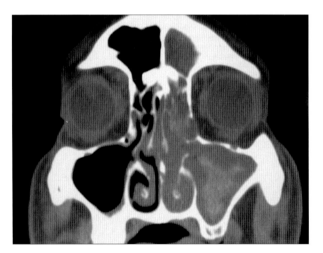

Fig 4-12 Coronal CT scan demonstrating changes consistent with AFRS of the left sinuses.

The second form of fungal sinusitis is known as *allergic fungal rhinosinusitis* (AFRS). Generally considered a form of chronic sinusitis, AFRS is thought to be a severe inflammatory reaction to inhaled fungal elements. Extensive polyps are common, with thick mucus containing fungal elements, eosinophils, and their breakdown products trapped between the polyps. This disease can demonstrate extensive bony remodeling on CT scans, with the same mixed densities found in fungal balls noted (Fig 4-12). Although there has been some debate regarding diagnostic criteria, most experts agree that there must be nasal polyps, typical CT findings, allergy to fungus, eosinophilic mucin, and fungus demonstrated by culture or pathology.[21]

The third and most severe form of fungal sinusitis is *invasive fungal sinusitis*, often referred to as *rhinocerebral mucormycosis* because many of the invasive organisms belong to the order *Mucorales*. Invasive fungal disease occurs nearly exclusively in the immunocompromised patient, most commonly presenting in patients with diabetic ketoacidosis. Any immunocompromised patient with facial pain, fever, and evidence of a cranial neuropathy (such as loss of sensation in the face, lips, or palate) should be considered to have invasive fungal sinusitis until proven otherwise and sent directly to the emergency room. Other findings include pallor or necrosis of the palate and/or gingiva (Fig 4-13) and mobile teeth.

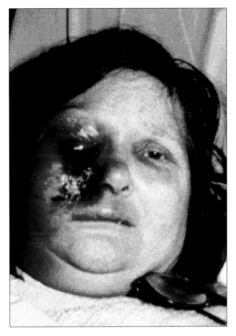

Fig 4-13 Photograph of a woman with extensive right facial necrosis due to invasive fungal sinusitis. (Reprinted from Rupp[22] with permission.)

Medical management

Signs of fungal sinusitis on preoperative imaging are an indication for referral to an otolaryngologist for evaluation. Medical therapy is often inadequate to prepare the sinus for grafting in these patients.

Treatment of a fungal ball is through ESS. The natural sinus opening is widely expanded, and all fungal elements and concretions are flushed out or removed from the sinus. Leaving residual portions of the fungal ball may result in recurrence.

The treatment of AFRS is usually surgical: ESS techniques are used to remove all polyps and mucin. Recurrence is common and has led to attempts at therapy with oral or intranasal antifungals, with limited success. As a result, many patients with AFRS require repeated surgical procedures. With invasive fungal sinusitis, survival is predicated on prompt initiation of treatment, which generally includes aggressive extirpative surgery and systemic antifungals.

| COMPLICATION 46 | Preoperative Cystic Structures and Mucoceles |

Differential diagnosis

In radiologic evaluation of dental disease or in preparation for sinus augmentation, patients are often found to have areas of soft tissue opacification within the maxillary sinuses. As opposed to the opacities seen with acute sinusitis or mucus stasis, which have a perfectly flat superior border demonstrating an air-fluid level (see Fig 4-7), these opacities usually are small and dome-shaped in appearance (Fig 4-14). Although a radiologist may refer to these as *polyps*, they are not a sign of inflammation. Rather, these are thought to represent cystic structures within or beneath the sinus membrane. Up to 20%

of adults have asymptomatic dome-shaped opacities, often found on the floor of the maxillary sinus.[23] The more common variety are *pseudocysts*, which are subperiosteal accumulations sometimes referred to as *nonsecreting cysts*. The less common *retention cysts* are true epithelium-lined cysts within the membrane (sometimes called *secreting cysts*).[16] Rarely will either of these structures change significantly; in fact, it is not uncommon to see these opacities unchanged on images spanning several years.

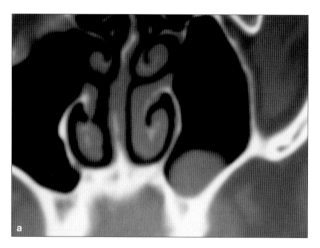

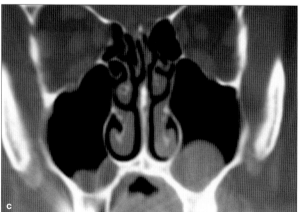

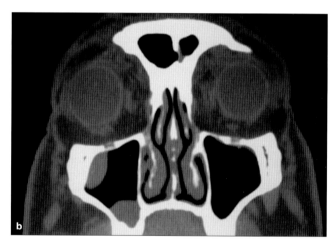

Fig 4-14 *(a)* Coronal CT scan demonstrating a small dome-shaped opacity of the floor of the left maxillary sinus. *(b)* Coronal CT scan demonstrating two dome-shaped opacities of the right maxillary sinus. *(c)* Coronal CT scan demonstrating dome-shaped opacities of the floor of both maxillary sinuses. Note the bilobed nature of the opacity on the right.

Much of the confusion regarding preoperative management of noninflammatory maxillary lesions concerns the inappropriate use of the term *mucocele*. A true obstructive mucocele of the maxillary sinus (sometimes referred to as an *antral mucocele* or a *postoperative maxillary cyst*) is usually related to prior surgical trauma such as a Caldwell-Luc procedure, inferior antrostomy (in which an opening is created intranasally beneath the inferior turbinate), or orthognathic surgery.[24] Radiographically, these lesions demonstrate either complete opacification of the sinus or bony septations preventing drainage of a portion of the sinus (Fig 4-15).

When evaluating maxillary sinus opacities on dental or panoramic radiographs or CT scans, the key is to first identify whether the lesion is of inflammatory origin. Inflammatory changes within the maxillary sinus are diffuse and often associated with similar changes in the other paranasal sinuses. A sinus with 2 to 3 mm of mucosal thickening is at risk of postoperative exacerbation of inflammatory disease and possible infection; a sinus with a single 1-cm dome-shaped opacity and no other visible mucosal thickening is not.

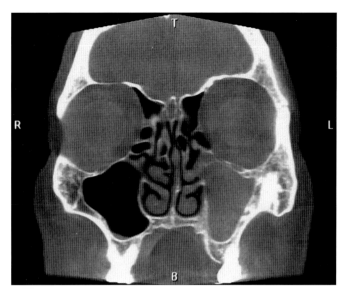

Fig 4-15 Coronal CT scan demonstrating complete opacification of the left maxillary sinus and bony changes consistent with an obstructive mucocele.

Medical management

The concern for the surgeon considering lateral window sinus elevation is whether cystic structures must be dealt with preoperatively to prevent intraoperative or postoperative complications. While some have suggested that these lesions should be removed or aspirated prior to mucosal elevation and grafting, most surgeons have found that these lesions can be easily elevated with the rest of the sinus membrane without adverse consequences.[25] Potential exceptions include cysts that are located at or very near the natural opening of the sinus and very large cysts (Fig 4-16). While some have suggested that a cyst occupying more than 50% of the sinus should be addressed preoperatively, a more practical measure is to estimate whether the graft material will lift the cyst enough to compromise drainage of the sinus.

Medical treatment is rarely helpful in mucocele management, and preoperative referral to an otolaryngologist is prudent.

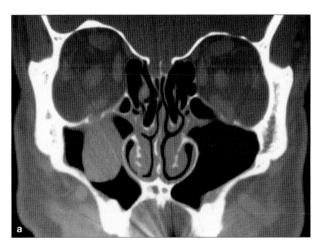 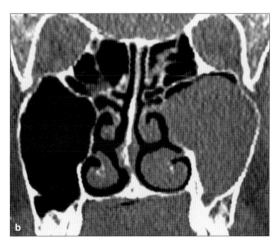

Fig 4-16 *(a)* Coronal CT scan demonstrating a large dome-shaped opacity of the right maxillary sinus originating from the roof of the sinus. Note the slight mucosal thickening throughout the sinus, possibly related to the lesion's proximity to the natural ostium. *(b)* Coronal CT scan demonstrating a very large dome-shaped opacity that nearly fills the left maxillary sinus.

Other Preoperative Sinus Lesions

Differential diagnosis

Neoplasms of the maxillary sinuses occur but are uncommon. One of the most frequently encountered tumors is the *inverted papilloma*, a benign growth associated with human papillomavirus (HPV) infection. While not malignant, an inverted papilloma can be locally expansile and has a high rate of recurrence if not completely excised. A small percentage (about 10%) may eventually degenerate into carcinoma.[26]

Squamous cell carcinoma is the most common malignant tumor of the maxillary sinus, although a variety of other cancers (including lymphoma, plasmacytoma, adenocarcinoma, and sarcoma) are rarely found. Malignant tumors of the maxillary sinus are suggested by imaging that reveals bony destruction rather than expansion, maxillary nerve numbness, or mobile teeth (Fig 4-17).

Diseases of abnormal bone metabolism can occur in the maxillary sinus. Fibrous dysplasia, Paget disease of bone, and similar disorders are occasionally encountered and are easily detected using sinus imaging (Fig 4-18).

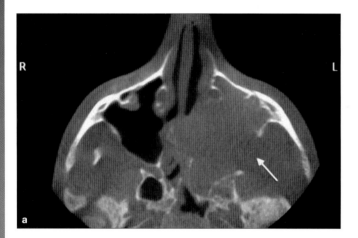
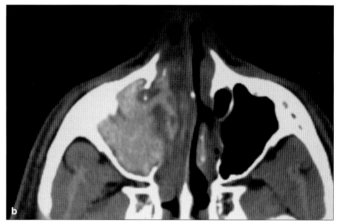

Fig 4-17 *(a)* Axial CT scan demonstrating a neoplasm of the left maxillary sinus. Note the bony erosion of the posterior and medial *(arrow)* bony walls. *(b)* Axial CT scan demonstrating a neoplasm of the right maxillary sinus.

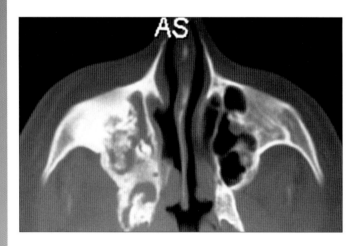

Fig 4-18 Axial CT scan demonstrating bony disease of both maxillary sinuses.

Medical management

Signs, symptoms, or imaging suggestive of a sinus neoplasm require prompt referral as well as communication with the patient's primary care physician to ensure timely work-up and treatment.

Summary of Preoperative Sinus Complications

Table 4-2 provides a summary of the parameters for differential diagnosis of preoperative sinus complications. Guidelines for presurgical referral of patients with specific sinus conditions are provided in Table 4-3.

Table 4-2 Differential diagnosis of maxillary sinus disease

Diagnosis	Symptoms	Physical findings	CT findings
Acute sinusitis	Fever, pain, swelling, purulent drainage	Tenderness over sinus, purulent drainage	Air-fluid levels (although CT is not usually required)
Chronic sinusitis	Congestion, nasal obstruction, anosmia, postnasal drainage	Nasal inflammation, polyps, no tenderness/swelling	Mucosal thickening or sinus opacification without air-fluid levels
Pseudocyst/retention cyst	None	No abnormal findings	Dome-shaped opacity without associated mucosal thickening
Mucocele	Occasional facial pain or pressure	Occasional sinus drainage prior to trauma/surgery	Total opacification, bony thickening
Fungal ball	Often none Chronic drainage	Occasional sinus drainage	Mixed densities, expansion of sinus
Allergic fungal sinusitis	Congestion, nasal obstruction, anosmia, postnasal drainage	Severe inflammation, polyps, thick mucous secretions	Extensive opacification (often unilateral) and expansion of the sinus
Invasive fungal sinusitis	Facial pain, fever, loss of sensation	Facial, intranasal, palate numbness; pallor; mobile teeth	Varies from minimal mucosal thickening to extensive destruction
Sinus tumors	Nasal obstruction, pain, bleeding, facial numbness	Intranasal mass, expansion of maxilla, mobile teeth	Sinus opacification with bony erosion rather than expansion
Bony diseases	Pain, recurrent infections	Bony expansion, sinus drainage	Thickened, abnormal bony changes

Table 4-3 Referral guidelines for sinus conditions

Diagnosis	When to refer
Acute sinusitis	Failure of antibiotic therapy or complications
Chronic sinusitis	Preoperatively for control of inflammatory disease
Pseudocyst/retention cyst	Only if large enough to become obstructive
Mucocele	Preoperatively for ESS
Fungal ball	Preoperatively for ESS
Allergic fungal sinusitis	Preoperatively for ESS
Invasive fungal sinusitis	Emergency referral to nearest tertiary-level medical facility
Sinus tumors	As soon as diagnosis suspected
Bony diseases	Preoperatively

Lateral Window Sinus Elevation Surgical Protocol

Before discussing the complications that may occur during the lateral window sinus elevation, it is important to present the surgical protocol that should be followed to minimize the risk of complications.

The lateral window sinus elevation surgical protocol consists of the following eight steps (Fig 4-19):

1. Anesthesia
2. Incision and full-thickness flap reflection
3. Osteotomy and window infracture or removal
4. Sinus membrane elevation

5. Bone graft placement
6. Incision closure
7. Postoperative provisionalization
8. Postoperative instructions and care

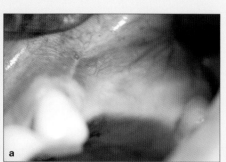
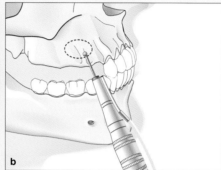

Fig 4-19 Lateral window sinus elevation surgical protocol. *(a)* Preoperative view of surgical site. *(b)* Anesthesia delivery. *(c and d)* Adequate flap size is important for surgical access. The flap is reflected at least 10 mm beyond the corners of the window.

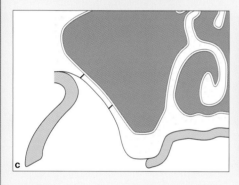
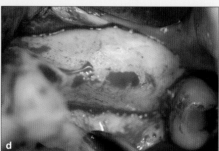

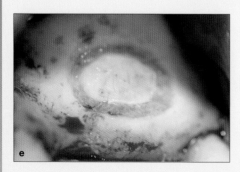
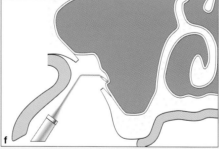
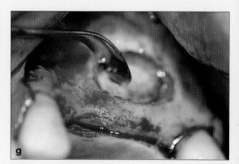

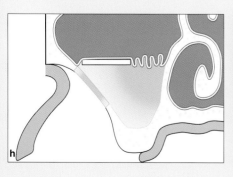
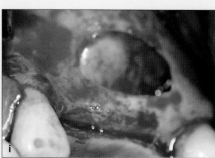

The window is outlined *(e)* and then pushed inward after being completely separated from the surrounding bone *(f to i)*.

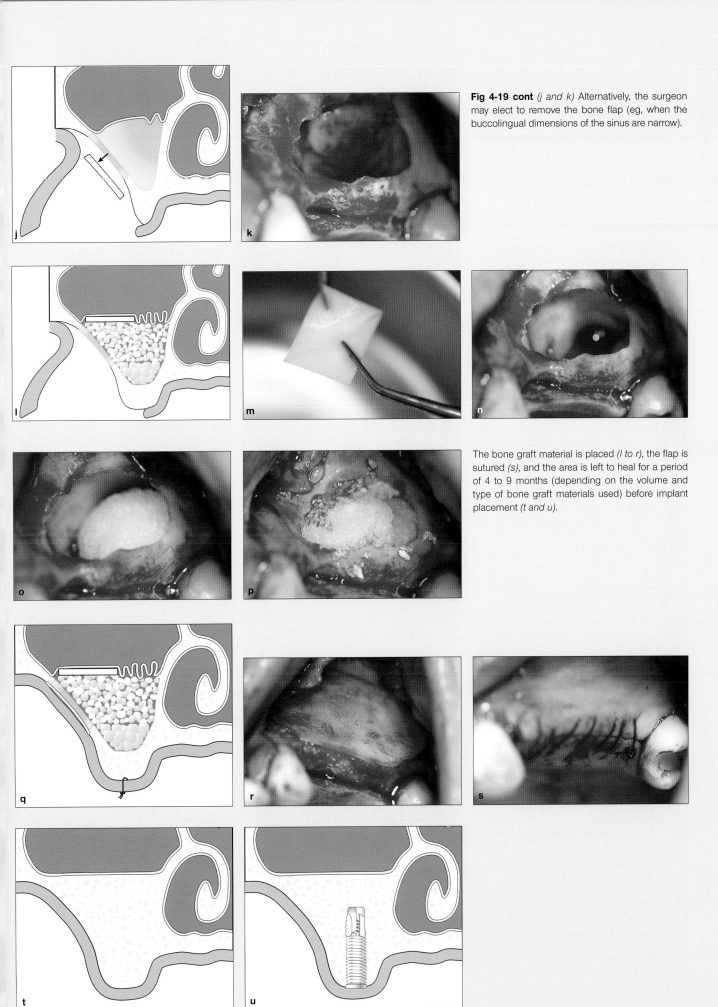

Fig 4-19 cont *(j and k)* Alternatively, the surgeon may elect to remove the bone flap (eg, when the buccolingual dimensions of the sinus are narrow).

The bone graft material is placed *(l to r)*, the flap is sutured *(s)*, and the area is left to heal for a period of 4 to 9 months (depending on the volume and type of bone graft materials used) before implant placement *(t and u).*

Anesthesia

Maxillary, infraorbital, and greater palatine nerve blocks are recommended. For this purpose, long-acting anesthetics such as bupivacaine hydrochloride with 1:200,000 epinephrine should be used. Infiltration anesthesia in the labial mucosa, buccal mucosa, and palatal region is also recommended and can be accomplished by administering lidocaine hydrochloride with 1:100,000 epinephrine. Oral triazolam and/or other oral sedative medications are optional but highly recommended to guarantee optimal patient comfort during surgery.

Incision and flap reflection

Using a no. 15 or 15C blade, a midcrestal incision is made from the maxillary tuberosity forward to the canine area, where an anterior vertical oblique releasing incision is made. The flap should have a broad base to ensure proper blood supply, and the anterior vertical incision should be at least 10 to 15 mm anterior to the wall of the sinus to ensure soft tissue closure over the bone (Fig 4-20a).

Full-thickness reflection is achieved using a periosteal elevator to allow access to the canine fossa just below the infraorbital foramen, the buttress of the zygomatic arch, and the posterolateral maxillary wall. The periosteal elevator should adhere to the bone surface at all times during flap elevation to avoid damaging the periosteum. If the tuberosity is not to be included in the flap, then a second distal beveled releasing incision should be made.

To enhance visibility, silk suture can be used to tie the flap back to the cheek in two or three places, but care should be taken not to damage the parotid duct. When performing two sinus lifts at the same time, the palatal flaps of both sides can be connected with a couple of sutures to keep them out of the way (Fig 4-20b).

When retracting the facial flap for the sinus graft, care should be taken not to apply pressure on the infraorbital bundle with the retractor.

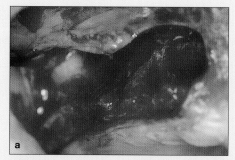

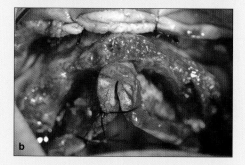

Fig 4-20 (a) Midcrestal and releasing incisions are made for accessing the right maxillary sinus in the edentulous patient. (b) Sutures are used to tie back the palatal and the buccal flaps for improved surgical access.

Osteotomy and window infracture or removal

The lateral window's location and size are outlined on the lateral wall of the maxillary bone based on measurements made from the CT scan.

Osteotomy technique

The osteotomy is initiated using a no. 6 or 8 diamond round bur on a surgical straight handpiece (Fig 4-21a) to outline the window until a bluish hue is visible (Fig 4-21b) or hemorrhage occurs. (Note that a carbide bur will more readily tear the sinus membrane when it comes in contact with it.) The osteotomy should be performed under copious irrigation with cooled sterile saline to avoid overheating the bone, using a paintbrush stroke to score the bone.

The window is made of inferior, superior, and two (anterior and posterior) vertical walls.

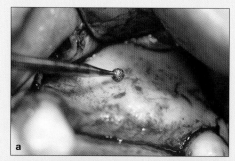

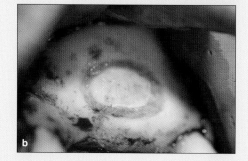

Fig 4-21 (a) A diamond bur is used to outline the window until the bluish hue of the maxillary sinus membrane becomes visible (b). Note the rounded corners of the window.

Inferior border

The inferior osteotomy should be created approximately 2 to 3 mm superior to and parallel with the floor of the sinus (not the crest of the ridge). The total length of the inferior osteotomy is approximately 20 mm.

Anterior border

The anterior vertical line is scored 5 mm distal to the anterior vertical wall of the antrum. Note that by placing the anterior border of the window close to the anterior wall of the sinus, the clinician can better free the membrane from the anterior wall. The height of the vertical anterior osteotomy should be approximately 15 mm.

Posterior border

The posterior vertical line should be made 15 to 20 mm distal to the anterior one. The height of the vertical posterior osteotomy should be approximately 15 mm.

Superior border

The superior osteotomy connects the two vertical osteotomies, completing the window.

Window corners

The corners of the access window should be rounded to facilitate the introduction of the surgical curette into the corners without risk of tearing the membrane. The window can be square or rectangular with rounded corners, oval, or round.

Window infracture or removal

Once the bone scoring is complete, the bony window is either gently infractured, ie, lifted into the sinus and used as the future sinus floor, using bone tampers and a mallet (Fig 4-22), or completely removed. Criteria for both methods are described in Box 4-1.

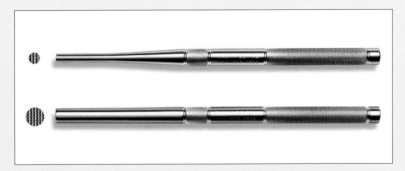

Fig 4-22 Bone tampers are used to infracture the sinus bony access window.

Box 4-1	Indications for infracture versus removal of the bony window	
Infractured bony window (lifting it inside as the future sinus floor)		**Complete removal of the bony window**
• Good surgical access		• Difficult surgical access
• No septa		• Presence of septa
• Wide sinus*		• Narrow sinus*

*Based on the distance from the lateral wall to the medial wall of the sinus.

Sinus membrane elevation

A sinus elevation curette of appropriate offset angle is slid along the bone 360 degrees around the margin of the access window, and then the sinus membrane is carefully separated from the anterior and medial walls of the sinus to a height at least 15 mm from the crest of the ridge (not from the sinus floor). Distally, the elevation is limited to the extent needed to place the planned number of implants. When pushing the sinus membrane superiorly with the sinus freer and other sinus membrane instruments, it is important that the sharp edges of these instruments remain on the bone and that the curved portion of these instruments is placed against the window. The surgeon should confirm visually and tactilely that the sinus instruments are held against the antral floor or walls at all times. At this point, the bony window can be lifted inside the sinus to act as the new floor of the sinus or it can be completely removed (see Box 4-1). If needed, a Kerrison rongeur can be used to enlarge the access window.

Bone graft placement

Technique

Grafting the sinus cavity consists of the following steps:

1. Placement of a resorbable collagen membrane on the new ceiling of the sinus cavity (on the sinus membrane)
2. Placement of the bone graft materials
3. Placement of the second resorbable collagen membrane to cover the bony window

1. Placement of the resorbable membrane

The corners of the collagen membrane are cut and rounded, and 1-cm releasing cuts are made to ease the manipulation of the membrane. The collagen membrane can be moistened with blood or sterile saline with antibiotics such as tetracycline prior to placement. Moisture will also ease the manipulation of the material and improve adherence to the surface of the tissue. The collagen membrane is then placed on the medial and superior walls of the sinus. The placement of this membrane will also repair any perforation that might occur during the membrane's elevation. The author recommends the OraMem membrane (Salvin) because it is long lasting and has the ideal level of memory for easy handling inside the sinus cavity.

2. Placement of the bone graft materials

A variety of bone graft materials and combinations can be used, such as:

- 100% autogenous bone
- 50% demineralized freeze-dried bone allograft (DFDBA) + 50% xenograft (eg, Bio-Oss, Geistlich)
- DFDBA-xenograft mix with autogenous bone layer at the bottom half or one-third
- Platelet-rich plasma (PRP) alone or as an addition to bone grafting materials
- Recombinant human bone morphogenetic protein 2/acellular collagen sponge (rhBMP-2/ACS; eg, Infuse, Medtronic) alone or with xenograft material

All the materials and combinations listed above are reported in the literature to have a high degree of success.

Guidelines for proper bone graft placement include:

- Packing should be accomplished using only a small amount of the graft material at a time and in an inferior and anterior (not superior) direction.
- The graft material should be placed in the least accessible areas first.
- The sinus should be packed until the graft material reaches the bone flap superiorly and reconstitutes the maxillary wall contour laterally.
- Packing should be firm but not excessive because perforation of the medial wall is possible and because blood vessels must be able to grow into the graft to form new bone. Tight packing restricts the supply of blood, oxygen, and other osteogenic components to the graft site, compromising the graft's opportunity to integrate.
- Overfilling may increase the amount of time required for the graft to mature.
- Placement of an autogenous bone layer at the bottom one-third of the elevated sinus cavity is highly recommended. Most investigators agree that a greater amount of bone is found close to the intact sinus floor and less as the distance from the sinus floor increases.
- Autogenous bone remains the best grafting material because of its highly osteogenic, osteoinductive, and osteoconductive properties. This allows bone to form more rapidly and in conditions where significant bone augmentation or repair is required. However, it is important to add xenograft to the autogenous bone, especially if it is cancellous bone, because the osteoconductive material increases bone density and helps to maintain the volume of the graft during the faster remodeling and resorption processes of the cancellous bone.

3. Placement of the second resorbable membrane

In the final step, a second membrane is placed over the window. If the membrane is nonresorbable (such as expanded polytetrafluoroethylene [e-PTFE]), it should be secured with two titanium tacks or screws. However, the author recommends the Bio-Gide membrane (Geistlich) for its pliability, ease of handling, and adherence capacity that allows it to be placed without fixation screws. Placement of this membrane is important because it delays the invasion of fibrous tissue into the graft and permits the lateral bony wall to be restored. Studies by Tawil and Mawla[27] in 2001 and by Wallace et al[28] in 2005 showed higher percentages of vital bone and greater implant survival rates when this second membrane was placed.

Simultaneous implant placement

Implants can be placed simultaneously with the bone graft if the alveolar bony ridge will allow the placement of stable implants. Usually 5 mm or more of alveolar height is required for simultaneous implant placement.

During this procedure, it is important to protect the sinus membrane by placing a collagen membrane on it (Fig 4-23a). After the implant sites are prepared, the bone graft is placed in the sinus and packed against the intact medial and anterior walls (Figs 4-23b and 4-23c). The implants then are placed (Fig 4-23d), and the bone is packed against the posterior maxillary wall and in between the implants, leaving no voids (Fig 4-23e). During this part of the procedure it is important to maintain the implant in the proper position so that subsequent prosthetic restoration is not compromised. Next, the lateral portion of the surgical site should be firmly packed with the bone graft material, and finally a resorbable membrane is placed to cover the window (Fig 4-23f).

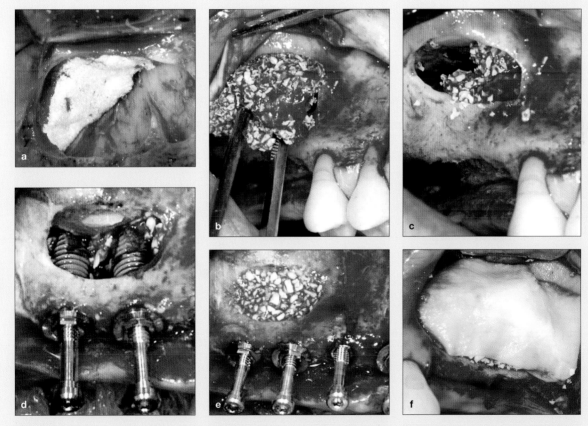

Fig 4-23 Simultaneous implant placement procedure. *(a)* After complete elevation of the maxillary sinus membrane for its protection from laceration during graft placement, a collagen membrane is placed over it. *(b and c)* The implant osteotomies are then completed, and the bone graft material is placed against the medial and anterior walls of the sinus. The implants are placed *(d)*, and the graft material is packed *(e)*. *(f)* Finally, the second resorbable collagen membrane is placed, and the flap is laid down and sutured. (Reprinted from Testori and Wallace[29] with permission.)

Incision closure

Good surgical technique dictates wound closure over intact bone without tension. Releasing the periosteum for passive closure is necessary only if a ridge augmentation procedure is performed simultaneously with the sinus graft surgery. However, in the maxilla, the crestal incision should always be made a little more toward the palatal side (to lengthen the buccal flap as much as possible) because the palatal flap cannot be released and pulled. The first suture should be placed at the corner between the crestal incision and the oblique releasing incision, then the operator can proceed to close the crestal and the releasing incisions. PTFE (eg, Gore-Tex, W. L. Gore) is the author's preferred suture material because, among other features, it has minimal elastic memory, making it easy to handle.

Postoperative provisionalization

It is highly recommended to delay placement of a provisional prosthesis for 2 weeks or longer if possible; however, if a removable denture must be worn during the healing period, the buccal flanges need to be adjusted by shortening them significantly.

Postoperative instructions and care

The following guidelines should be observed during the postoperative period:

- Medications (eg, antibiotics, analgesics, anti-inflammatory medications, chlorhexidine rinse, oxymetazoline nasal spray, and pseudoephedrine) should be taken as directed.
- Smoking should be avoided.
- For 2 weeks, the patient should avoid nose blowing, which could create positive pressure in the sinus.
- Sucking liquid through a straw, which creates negative intrasinus pressure, should be avoided.
- Sneezing or coughing should be avoided if possible; otherwise, it must be done with the mouth open to decrease internal antral pressure.
- Some nasal bleeding (oozing of blood through the nose) is normal during the first day.
- Swelling, pain, and ecchymosis are to be expected.
- Rest is recommended for 3 to 7 days.
- For 24 hours after surgery, light pressure and ice should be placed on the surgical site.
- On the first night after surgery, the head should be elevated on two or more pillows. This will prevent airway obstruction and aspiration of blood and heavy saliva and will diminish edema.
- Liquid diet (systemic enteral nutrition formulas) is recommended for 2 days, then soft foods (the consistency of mashed potatoes or scrambled eggs) should be consumed for at least 2 weeks (until the mucosal incision has closed completely).
- A provisional prosthesis should not be worn for 2 weeks.
- The patient should not lift or pull on the lip to look at the sutures.
- The patient should be seen for a postoperative checkup in 1 week.
- The office should be notified if the patient feels granules in the nose, still has discomfort after taking prescribed medications, or has any questions.

A clinical case showing each step in this procedure is presented in Fig 4-24.

Fig 4-24 *(opposite page)* Simultaneous lateral window sinus floor elevation and alveolar ridge expansion by split cortical technique. *(a to c)* The patient is fully edentulous with thin alveolar ridges. *(d)* A full-thickness flap is elevated. *(e and f)* The alveolar ridge is expanded and the implants are placed. *(g to p)* Bilateral sinus floor elevation is then performed according to the steps described in the text. *(q)* Postoperative panoramic radiograph shows the height of the graft in both sinuses.

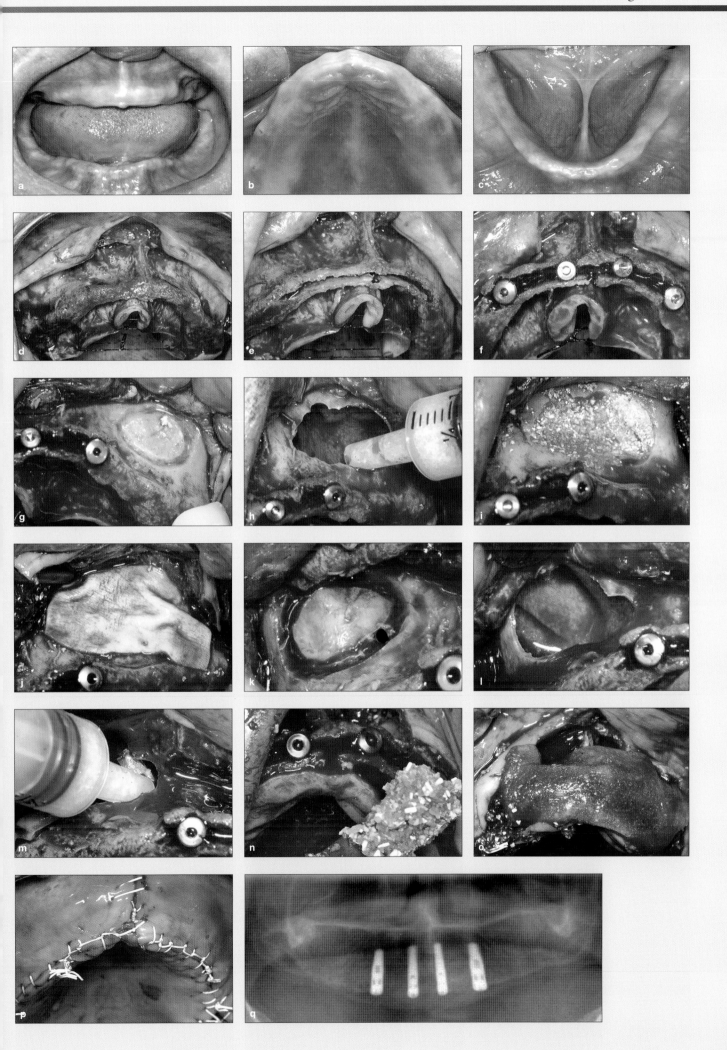

COMPLICATION 48 | Hematoma During Anesthesia

If the needle is overinserted during posterior superior alveolar nerve block, it may penetrate the pterygoid plexus of the vein and the maxillary artery in the infratemporal fossa (Fig 4-25) and thus cause hematoma.[30] This results in extraoral swelling a few minutes after the injection. The hematoma will cause tissue tenderness and discoloration that will last until the blood is broken down by the body. There is also a possibility of infection spreading to the cavernous venous sinus if the needle is contaminated. A hematoma can also develop during other blocks, such as the infraorbital and inferior alveolar nerve blocks. To avoid injection into blood vessels, aspiration should be attempted in all injections.

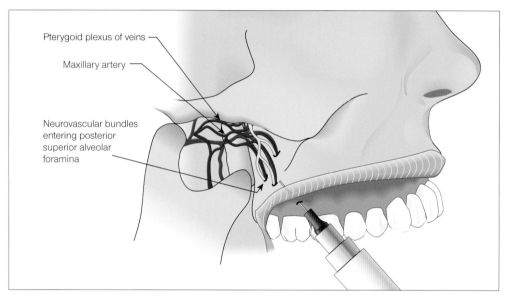

Fig 4-25 Note the proximity of the neurovascular bundle in the posterior area of the maxilla to the needle during anesthesia of the posterior maxilla.

COMPLICATION 49 | Bleeding During Incision and Flap Reflection

Because the incisions should be made midcrestal or on the attached gingiva where the blood vessels are very small, bleeding is normally minimal; however, if there is more bleeding than usual, management consists of:

• Biting pressure using 2 × 2 gauze for a few minutes
• Electrocautery
• Hemostatic liquids

Observing the following surgical guidelines will minimize soft tissue bleeding:

• Ensure that the flap size is sufficient for the procedure intended.
• Make a clean incision.
• Do not crush or tear the soft tissue.
• Smooth any sharp bony areas.
• Identify and manage small bleeding soft tissue arteries.

| COMPLICATION 50 | Bleeding During Osteotomy |

Hemorrhage during bony window osteotomy usually arises from damage to the intraosseous anastomosis between the posterior superior alveolar artery and the infraorbital artery,[31] both of which are branches of the maxillary artery (Fig 4-26). The bony vessels that cause bleeding are small in size, and hemostasis should be allowed to occur naturally, perhaps facilitated by the application of either light pressure with gauze or bone wax. An electrocoagulator is not recommended because it may cause membrane necrosis.[29]

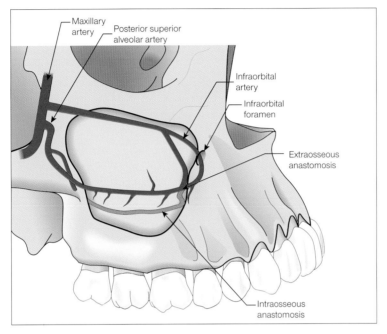

Fig 4-26 The infraorbital artery and the posterior superior alveolar artery often form an extraosseous anastomosis and almost always form an intraosseous anastomosis in an area located an average of 19 mm from the alveolar margin.

| COMPLICATION 51 | Damage to Adjacent Dentition |

Care must be taken when working in proximity to the natural dentition. An excessively large antral opening can devitalize adjacent teeth or reduce the bony support of the adjacent natural dentition, which may lead to dental loss or the need for endodontic therapy.

| COMPLICATION 52 | Perforation of the Sinus Membrane During Osteotomy |

Perforation of the sinus membrane is the most frequent intraoperative complication during sinus surgery. Factors that affect sinus membrane perforation during osteotomy include instrumentation and the thickness of the sinus membrane. Perforation can occur in up to 56% of cases in which rotary instruments are used and in as few as 3.8% in which piezoelectric instruments are used.[32,33] Thin membranes are more prone to tearing during elevation. A study by Cho et al[34] found that the rate of perforation of thin (< 1.5 mm) membranes is 31%, compared to 16.6% for thicker membranes. Choosing a diamond bur instead of a carbide bur when using rotary instruments, using a brush-stroke technique when working with the handpiece (so as not to apply excessive pressure on the window), and having good access to the surgical field (adequate flap reflection and lighting) can help significantly in reducing the incidence of membrane perforation during window osteotomy.

COMPLICATION 53	Perforation of the Sinus Membrane During Elevation

Factors that affect sinus membrane perforation during membrane elevation include the size of the access window, the width of the sinus, and the presence of maxillary sinus septa.

Size of the access window

A small access window can increase the probability of membrane perforation. To solve this problem, the bony window can be enlarged using a Kerrison rongeur (Fig 4-27) after separation of the sinus membrane around the margin of the complete access window.

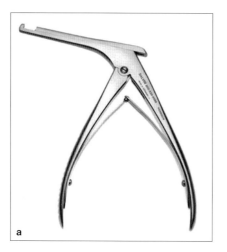
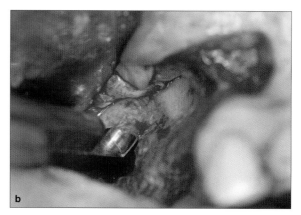

Fig 4-27 *(a)* Kerrison rongeur. *(b)* Enlargement of the access window by extending its anterior wall using a Kerrison rongeur. Because extension using rotary instrumentation might cause a large perforation from the air and irrigation that are generated, it is not recommended.

Width of the sinus

The distance between the lateral and medial walls of the sinus influences the incidence of perforations: The rate is higher in narrow sinuses than in wider ones.[35] Using cross-sectional CT scans, the implant dentist can evaluate presurgically the width of the sinus in the area of the entry window (ie, the bony oste- otomy). If the sinus is narrow (Fig 4-28a), removal of the bony window before membrane elevation is recommended. In the case of wide sinuses, the window can be pushed inward (Fig 4-28b).

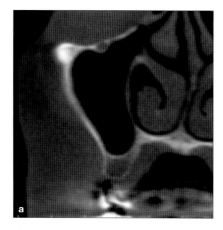
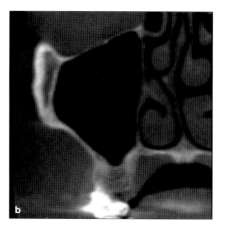

Fig 4-28 *(a)* Cross-sectional CT image demonstrating a narrow buccolingual dimension of the maxillary sinus. *(b)* Cross-sectional CT image demonstrating a wide buccolingual dimension of the maxillary sinus.

Maxillary sinus septa

The presence of septa can complicate the creation of the bony window in the lateral wall and increase the risk of tearing the sinus membrane during its elevation; therefore, it is important to analyze these septa with CT scans prior to surgery (Fig 4-29). Radiographs (panoramic or Waters projection) might not show septa, or they might falsely suggest that these formations are a pathologic condition.

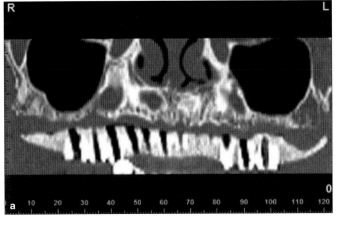

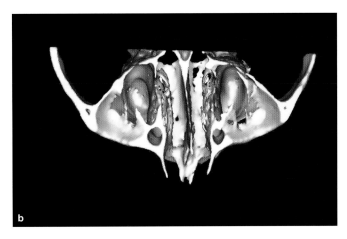

Fig 4-29 A panoramic CT image *(a)* and a 3D-generated image *(b)* showing no septa in the maxillary sinus.

Underwood (basal perpendicular) septa

Septa were first described by anatomist Underwood in 1910.[7] *Underwood septa*, as these maxillary sinus septa are often called, are osseous ridges delimiting the root compartments of the premolars and molars (Fig 4-30). The shape of septa has been described as resembling an inverted gothic arch arising from the inferior and lateral walls of the sinus and coming to a sharp edge along its most apical border.[36] They are encountered in 31% to 48% of cases[8–10] and appear to develop in one of two ways: primary (arising from the development of the maxilla) or secondary (as a result of tooth loss and remnant interseptal bone).[37] Tooth loss and pneumatization adjacent to either a primary or secondary septum may exaggerate the height or size of a septum. Depending on their type, size, and location, septa should be removed during a sinus grafting procedure because they can impede the view of the sinus floor and may limit placement of autogenous bone grafts or bone substitutes, thus preventing adequate filling of the sinus floor. In a study by Ulm et al,[10] no correlation was found between the six residual ridge classes described by Cawood and Howell[38] and the incidence of Underwood septa.

The scientific literature describes additional variations of the maxillary sinus septa, including partial perpendicular and horizontal[39] septa and complete septation of the maxillary sinus by a vertical septum.[40,41]

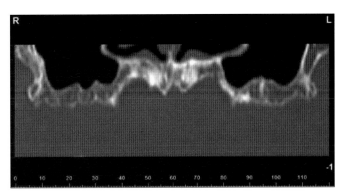

Fig 4-30 A panoramic CT image showing basal perpendicular (Underwood) septa in the maxillary right sinus.

Partial perpendicular septa

The upper margin of the maxillary hiatus is in contact anteriorly with the lacrimal bone and posteriorly with the ethmoid bone. The punctum convergii is located at the latter part of the convergence of these two parts of the margin. From this punctum, a partial perpendicular septum can develop into the maxillary sinus, dividing it into two incomplete compartments.

Partial horizontal septa

This type of septum is a horizontally located maxillary process from the palatine bone and the inferior concha. Neither process will follow the normal development of the sinus in the inferior-medial direction. Instead, they will maintain their primary horizontal positions while the level of the floor of the sinus becomes gradually lower during their development.

These septa can be disregarded if positioned higher than the area to be grafted. Otherwise, such horizontal septa will be an impediment to sinus drainage and will eventually lead to sinus graft failure (Figs 4-31a to 4-31c).

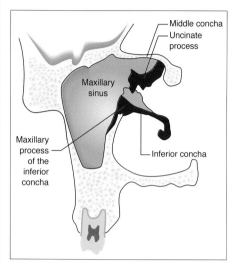

Fig 4-31a Typical infromedial position of the maxillary process of the inferior concha.

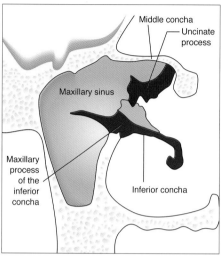

Fig 4-31b Atypical development of the maxillary process of the inferior concha, leading to the formation of partial horizontal septa. Depending on its height from the sinus floor, this type of septum can cause difficulties during lateral window sinus elevation and impede sinus drainage during planned antral punctures.

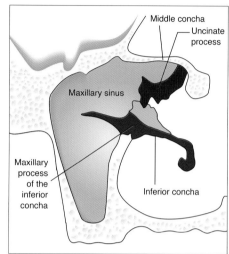

Fig 4-31c When the horizontal septum is positioned high in relation to the floor of the sinus, limited sinus elevation can be achieved, but when it is positioned low, the elevation should be avoided altogether.

Complete septa

A complete vertical septum (Fig 4-32) usually divides the sinus into a large anterior and smaller (accessory) posterior sinus. The anterior sinus drains into the middle meatus, while the posterior sinus opens into the superior or nasal meatus through a bony hiatus, which is delimited by structures similar to those of the normal semilunar hiatus (ie, the maxillary process of the middle concha and the posterior maxillary process of the palatine bone). Each of these sinuses can show isolated signs of pathology and thus must be treated separately. The accessory sinus either develops in the cartilaginous nasal capsule at the same time as the normal sinus or results from excessive pneumatization of the posterior part of the maxilla by a large ethmoid air cell. Note that in the latter case, a pathology involving the ethmoid bone will also involve the accessory sinus.

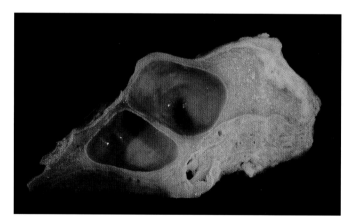

Fig 4-32 Cadaveric specimen in which a septum subdivides the maxillary sinus into two separate compartments. (Reprinted from Watzek et al[30] with permission.)

Al-Faraje classification of septa of the maxillary sinus

The author has developed a classification of possible variations of the septa of the maxillary sinus (Table 4-4):

Class I: Single basal perpendicular septa
Class II: Multiple basal perpendicular septa
Class III: Single partial perpendicular septa

Class IV: Multiple partial perpendicular septa
Class V: Partial horizontal septa
Class VI: Complete perpendicular septum

Table 4-4	Al-Faraje classification of maxillary sinus septa for assessment prior to sinus bone graft surgery		
Class	**Description**	**Form**	**Considerations**
I	Single basal perpendicular septum		Care should be taken when reflecting the maxillary sinus membrane off the floor of the sinus.
II	Multiple (two or more) basal perpendicular septa		Care should be taken when reflecting the maxillary sinus membrane off the floor of the sinus.
III	Single partial perpendicular septum		Making two separate windows is strongly recommended.
IV	Multiple (two or more) partial perpendicular septa		Presents a strong risk of membrane perforation and thus may be a contra-indication for sinus bone graft surgery.
V	Partial horizontal septum		Risk depends on location. When located superiorly, sinus bone graft surgery can usually proceed. When located inferiorly, sinus bone graft surgery is contraindicated.
VI	Complete perpendicular septum		Usually does not interfere with sinus bone graft surgery.

Management of maxillary septa

Following are basic principles for the management of maxillary septa during sinus elevation:

- Complete removal of the bony window, rather than pushing it inside the sinus cavity, is recommended in most scenarios.
- Identifying the exact location, extent, and size of the septa before sinus graft surgery is critically important.
- Class I or Class II septa do not complicate the sinus lift procedure; the surgeon should simply take the septa into consideration during reflection of the membrane off the floor of the sinus.
- In Class III septa, the surgeon can make two windows separated by the septum, and then, after the elevation of the sinus membrane off the septum, a Kerrison forceps or he-

mostat can be used to remove the septum (Fig 4-33). The exact location and size of the septum should be identified on CT scan images before surgery.
- Class IV septa significantly increase the risk of membrane perforation and may contraindicate surgery.
- In the case of Class V septa, the height of the septum dictates the course of action. If the horizontal septum is located significantly superior to the floor of the sinus, then the procedure can be performed. Otherwise, the close proximity of the horizontal septum to the floor of the sinus might be a contraindication for the sinus graft surgery.
- Class VI septa usually do not interfere with sinus graft surgery, which can still be performed in the anterior compartment for future implant placement.

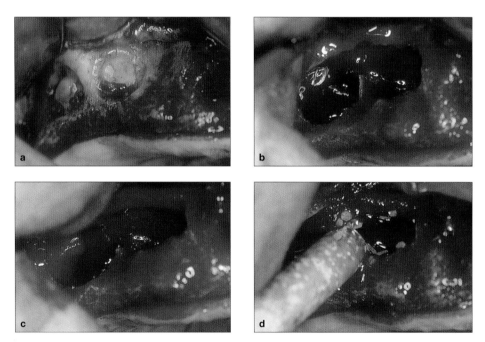

Fig 4-33 A case of a single partial perpendicular septum (Al-Faraje Class I). The recommended management is the creation of 2 separate windows *(a)* followed by the elevation of the maxillary sinus membrane off each side of the septum *(b)* and then the removal of the septum using a Kerrison rongeur *(c)* before the introduction of the bone graft material into the sinus cavity *(d)*.

Management of perforations during sinus membrane elevation

Perforation of the sinus membrane during elevation is the most frequent intraoperative complication that occurs during sinus graft surgery. In the event of a perforation (Fig 4-34), the surgeon should continue the elevation but at a distance from the perforation to release the tension along the perforation. Working near the perforation will usually cause its size to increase. In the case of one or more small perforations (less than 5 or 6 mm in diameter), the surgeon can place an absorbable collagen membrane to repair the perforation(s) and prevent the bone graft materials from invading the sinus cavity after the completed elevation (see Fig 4-34f). However, in the case of large perforations (10 mm or more in diameter), the operator can abort the procedure or use the Loma Linda pouch technique[42] (Fig 4-35).

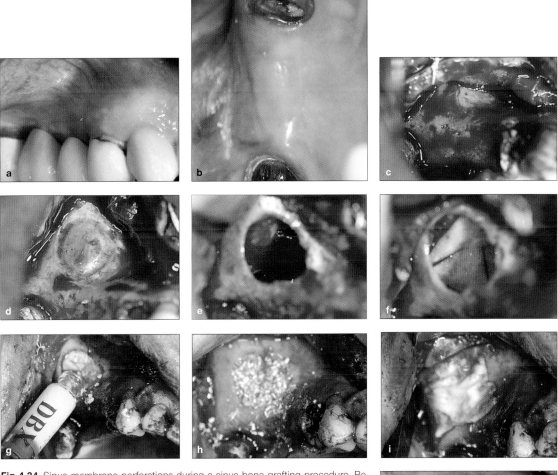

Fig 4-34 Sinus membrane perforations during a sinus bone grafting procedure. Removal of the existing fixed partial denture *(a and b)* and reflection of a full-thickness flap *(c)*. *(d)* Creation of an access bony window. *(e)* Two small perforations (< 5 mm each) are made. The perforations are managed by the placement of an absorbable collagen membrane *(f)* followed by the the bone grafting material *(g and h)* and finally a second outer collagen membrane *(i)*. *(j)* The procedure is completed by suturing the full-thickness flap back into place.

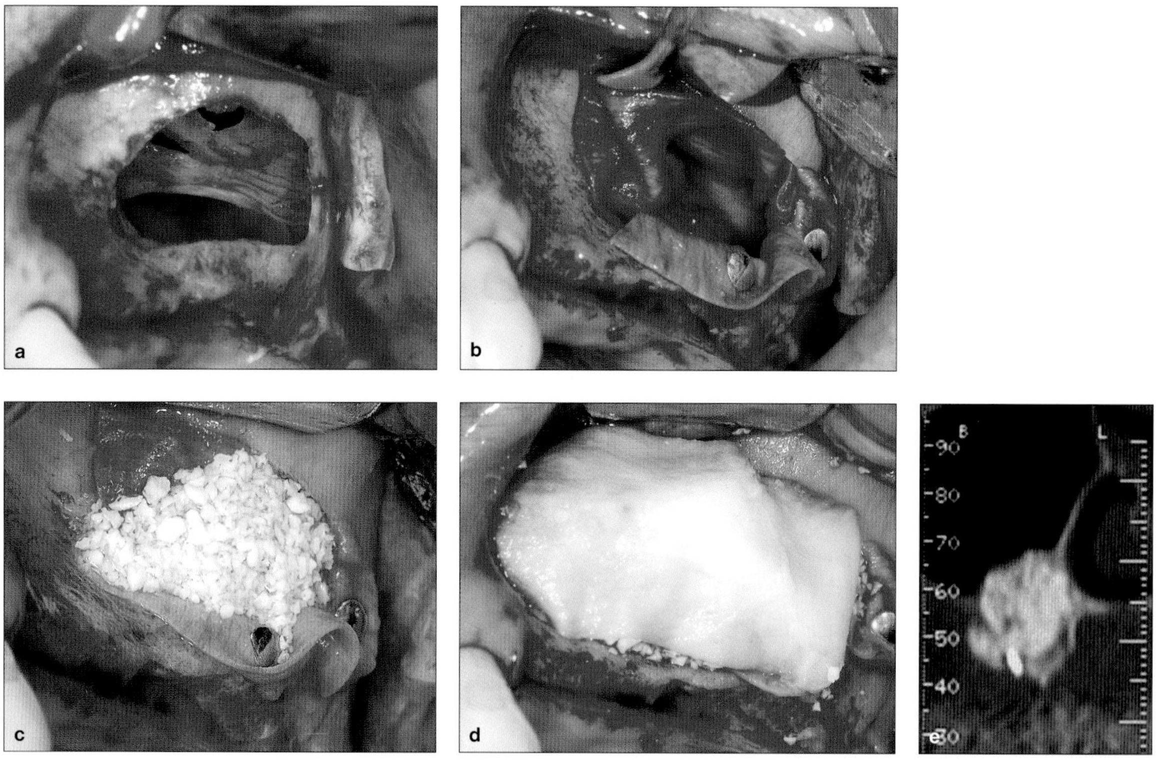

Fig 4-35 *(a)* A large membrane perforation is managed by the placement of an absorbable collagen membrane inside the sinus, which is *(b)* affixed with titanium pins on the outer surface. The bone graft material is then placed inside the formed pouch *(c)* before a second membrane is placed *(d)*. *(e)* The 6-month postoperative 3D image shows the level of bone graft fill. (Reprinted from Testori and Wallace[29] with permission.)

Incomplete Elevation

Complete elevation of the sinus membrane off the anterior and medial walls of the sinus to the desired height is important to prevent re-pneumatization of the sinus, to promote proper drainage, and to expose the graft material to greater bone surface area. Incomplete elevation will lead to partial augmentation with subsequent bone graft volume loss and possible complications with implant placement (Fig 4-36).

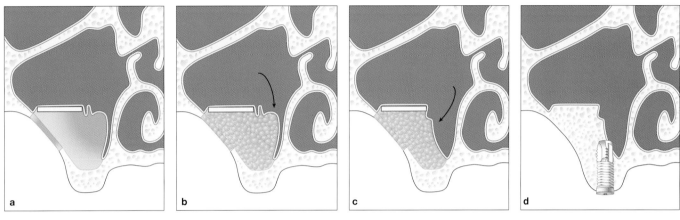

Fig 4-36 Partial sinus membrane elevation *(a)* can lead to an incomplete graft placement *(b)*, which can cause re-pneumatization and volume loss of the graft *(c)* and imperfect implant positioning in the grafted sinus *(d)*.

COMPLICATION 55 | Bleeding During Membrane Elevation

Suction cannot be used during elevation of the sinus membrane because it will cause a large perforation of the membrane. Therefore, the best way to remove blood from inside the sinus during the procedure is by temporarily packing the area with gauze saturated with anesthetic and epinephrine (1:100,000 or 1:50,000) for 1 to 2 minutes to facilitate hemostasis. This can be done a few times during the elevation procedure.

COMPLICATION 56 | Fracture of the Residual Alveolar Ridge

If fracture of the residual alveolar ridge occurs, implant placement must be aborted if it was planned to be performed simultaneously with the sinus elevation procedure.

COMPLICATION 57 | Excessive Elevation of the Membrane

Excessive elevation of the membrane, which can lead to excessive filling of the sinus, can be prevented with gentle elevation and meticulous manipulation of the sinus membrane and by taking measurements with a periodontal probe or ruler to avoid overfilling of the sinus cavity. The best way to handle this complication is to abort the procedure rather than overfilling the sinus. The membrane will gradually relapse toward the floor of the sinus over a period of several weeks, and then another attempt can be made. Overfilling can lead to membrane tear and improper sinus drainage with subsequent graft material loss. If this occurs, removal of all the graft material is indicated.

Presence of a Mucus Retention Cyst

Pathologies such as mucus retention cysts can be easily detected on CT scan images; therefore, it is important to evaluate the sinus membrane on the patient's CT scan before surgery (Fig 4-37). Mucus retention cysts are not a contraindication for the sinus augmentation procedure, but they need to be treated because, as a result of their weight, they might lead to membrane tear once elevated. They can be treated during sinus surgery (during or before elevation) by aspirating the serum content of the cyst using a 22-gauge needle to collapse the cyst walls.

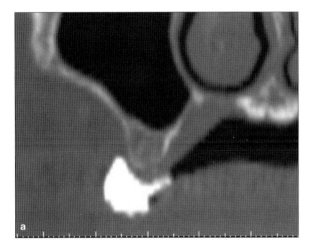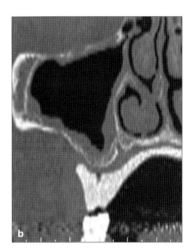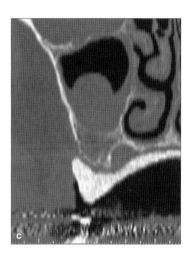

Fig 4-37 Cross-sectional CT images of the maxillary sinus showing that *(a)* no maxillary sinus membrane can be detected under healthy conditions because it is less than 1 mm thick. *(b)* Irregular sinus membrane thickening (indicating chronic sinusitis). *(c)* A mucus retention cyst on the floor of the sinus.

COMPLICATION 59   Blockage of the Maxillary Ostium

Any blockage of the ostium or disturbance of mucociliary action can lead to failure to clear secretions and bacteria from the sinus, resulting in infection. To prevent the occurrence of this complication, the surgeon should keep the augmentation below the level of the ostium. As a rule of thumb, the surgeon should limit augmentation to less than 2.5 cm above the floor of the antrum.

COMPLICATION 60   Unstable Implants

If implants placed simultaneously with the bone graft become unstable, they must be removed. The implants can be replaced after a 6- to 9-month healing period.

COMPLICATION 61   Wound Dehiscence

Etiology

Etiology of wound dehiscence may include poor flap design, inadequate suturing technique, mechanical overload from the removable prosthesis, and smoking.

Prevention and management

Flap design

The ideal flap is large enough with mesial and/or distal incisions, full thickness to preserve the periosteum, and trapezoidal in shape. These criteria are required for proper vascular supply to the flap. When the sinus graft procedure is performed by itself, obtaining tension-free primary closure is usually not difficult; however, when a ridge augmentation procedure is performed simultaneously, the flap's periosteum layer should be released before incision line closure.

Suturing technique

Increased suture tension should be avoided because it may cause a tourniquet effect and delay healing. In some instances, overtightened sutures may actually tear through the mucoperiosteal flap, exposing the underlying bone and graft.

Provisionalization

Removable prostheses should not be worn for 2 weeks. For the rest of the healing period, they can be worn, but only after the adjustment of the buccal flanges.

Smoking

Smokers should abstain from smoking 10 days prior to surgery and 2 weeks afterward because smoking increases the incidence of postoperative complications.[43]

| # Acute Graft Infection/Sinusitis

Acute sinusitis can occur as a complication of sinus augmentation procedures. Bhattacharyya[16] reported an incidence as high as 20% in 1998, while Barone et al[17] placed this figure at 5% in 2006. Others have reported an incidence less than 2%.[44] Whether this represents a trend of fewer postoperative infections or whether the discrepancy is reflective of differences between the dental and medical literature, it is now clear that acute sinusitis after sinus augmentation is not a frequent occurrence.

Etiology

Etiology of acute graft infection and sinusitis includes preexisting sinus disease, contamination intrasurgically from a bacteria present in the sinus or the oral cavity, infection from the extracted teeth that penetrate the sinus floor, perforation of the sinus membrane postoperatively, significant loss of graft material into the sinus during surgery, ostium obstruction due to overpacked graft material or postoperative edema, and poor aseptic conditions. It may also occur secondary to delayed healing as a result of incision line opening.

Symptoms

Symptoms include pain, swelling, suppuration, and flap dehiscence.

Prevention

The following measures can be taken to help prevent acute sinusitis and infection of the graft:

- Preexisting sinus disease should be diagnosed and treated before surgery. Patients presenting with preoperative sinusitis and sinuses with thick mucosa need to be informed of their increased risk.
- Preexisting periapical pathologies should be diagnosed and treated and hopeless teeth extracted prior to the sinus graft procedure. Extraction of teeth—even if they are not infected—simultaneously with sinus graft surgery presents a higher risk because of the difficulty in obtaining primary closure.
- The flap should be designed so that the incision lines (crestal and releasing) are placed directly over a barrier membrane.
- Prescribing the medications preoperatively can help prevent acute postoperative sinus infection.

- The sinus membrane should be elevated properly to avoid postoperative accumulation of antral secretions, which might cause sufficient pressure to perforate the sinus membrane and contaminate the graft.
- A staged surgical approach (ie, placing the implants after the healing period of the graft material) can be used to avoid the increased risk of infection that is associated with simultaneous sinus augmentation and implant placement because of the higher chances of bone graft contamination during preparation of the implant osteotomies.
- The risk of ostium obstruction can be reduced by taking care not to overpack the graft material.
- The patient should be strongly advised against smoking, and the use of an onlay bone graft in conjunction with sinus augmentation should be avoided, because both of these factors appear to significantly increase the rate of infective complications.[17]

Treatment

Postoperative sinusitis should be taken seriously because it may lead to graft or implant loss.[45] Moreover, acute sinusitis should be treated aggressively to prevent the spread of infection to the brain and the orbital regions. Broad-spectrum high-dose systemic antibiotics (eg, 375 mg of amoxicillin + clavulanic acid) should be administered, and surgical drainage of the infection should be performed, along with partial or complete removal of the infected graft material.[46–49] Thorough saline irrigation of the surgical site should follow. Once the infection is resolved and the radiographs show the sinus to be clear (usually 4 to 6 months later), the region can be regrafted.

When sinus graft infection occurs in the presence of implants, removal of the implants to ease the removal of the infected graft material is generally required. If the implants are not removed, the surface of the implants exposed to the infected region should be treated with antibiotic solutions or pastes (eg, tetracycline).

COMPLICATION 63

Exposure of the Bone Graft and/or Barrier Membrane

Etiology

Etiology of early bone graft and/or barrier membrane exposure includes insufficient soft tissue closure, flap necrosis, excessive postoperative swelling, and soft tissue dehiscence, largely due to smoking and overload from the removable prosthesis.

Treatment

The treatment of early exposure of the bone graft and/or membrane is difficult and has a poor prognosis. However, if there is no accompanying infection, the area should be cleaned with chlorhexidine rinse or gel three to four times per day and should be observed for closure by secondary intention. Resuturing is usually not recommended because it may lead to even greater exposure due to subsequent flap necrosis. Exposure of a membrane in the presence of infection necessitates removal of the membrane because it may act as a conduit for bacterial contamination, resulting in subsequent loss of the graft and/or implants.

COMPLICATION 64

Sinus Congestion

If sinus congestion occurs, it can be treated with decongestants and analgesics.

COMPLICATION 65

Early Implant Migration into the Sinus Cavity

Implants might become displaced into the sinus cavity in the early postoperative period if they were inserted simultaneously with the sinus augmentation procedure in low-density alveolar bone less than 5 mm in height. Prevention and management are covered in detail in complication 20, part 2.

COMPLICATION 66 | Insufficient Quality and/or Quantity of Healed Graft

Etiology

Etiology of insufficient quality and/or quantity of healed graft includes the use of insufficient bone graft material, improper sinus membrane elevation, and bone graft loss into the sinus cavity during or after surgery.

Prevention

Potential causes of insufficient quality and/or quantity of healed graft can be avoided by using a sufficient quantity of bone graft during surgery and by using proper sinus membrane elevation techniques. The sinus membrane should be elevated off the medial and anterior walls to the most superior position achieved on the lateral wall, and the graft material must have close contact with all bony walls of the elevated areas without any voids.

COMPLICATION 67 | Implant Failure in the Augmented Sinus

Progressive implant loading, which gradually converts less mineralized bone into bone more capable of bearing masticatory forces, has been suggested as a means to prevent implant failure.[50]

COMPLICATION 68 | Chronic Infection/Sinusitis

The etiology of chronic infection/sinusitis includes improperly treated acute infection (eg, treatment by antibiotics only without surgical intervention, treatment by nonspecific antibiotic therapy), significant loss of graft material into the sinus during surgery, and/or displacement of an implant into the sinus.

Chronic sinusitis is a cause for major concern and should be met with prompt management through administration of specific antibiotics based on the microbial culture, monitoring, and referral to an otolaryngologist when necessary to avoid potential life-threatening consequences, as described in complication 69.

Oroantral fistulas can present in chronic infection and may be treatable with antibiotics and irrigation with chlorhexidine rinse to encourage healing by secondary intention. In some cases, however, surgical reentry may be required to remove the infected part of the graft or the entire graft (Figs 4-38 and 4-39).

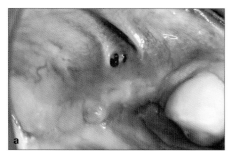 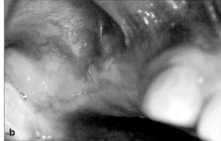

Fig 4-38 *(a)* Oroantral fistula at 2 months postoperative, treated with antibiotics and chlorhexidine oral rinse. *(b)* The infection was resolved 1 month later.

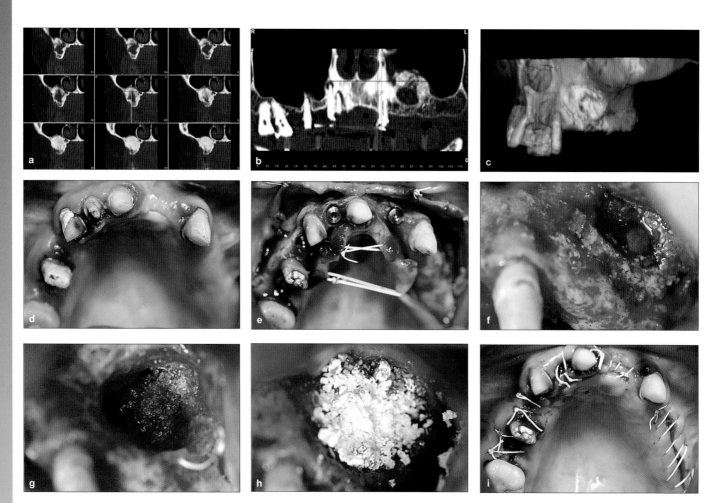

Fig 4-39 *(a to c)* Six-month postoperative CT scans of the right sinus showing a radiolucent area in the previously grafted left sinus. *(d to i)* The area is explored surgically for the complete removal of all infected tissue (around 30% of the graft) and regrafting.

| COMPLICATION 69 | Infection of All Paranasal Sinuses/ Intracranial Cavity |

Infection of all paranasal sinuses may develop as a result of untreated chronic sinusitis because of the proximity of these sinuses to the bone-augmented maxillary sinus. In addition, there is the possibility of the infection spreading into the intracranial space with a brain abscess as a potential result. The resulting infection might lead to orbital complications,[51] loss of vision,[52] and a severe neurologic deficiency or death.[53] The incidence of intracranial infection is extremely low and can be avoided by proper postoperative patient monitoring, appropriate medications, and prompt management and/or referral upon infection development.

| COMPLICATION 70 | Delayed Implant Migration into the Sinus Cavity |

Implants might be displaced into the sinus cavity late postoperatively for a variety of reasons, including loss of primary stability due to excessive compression from the removable prosthesis. Prevention and management are covered in complication 20, part 2.

| COMPLICATION 71 | Sinus Aspergillosis |

Aspergillosis is a fungal infection, usually of the lungs, caused by the fungus *Aspergillus*. A ball of fungal fibers, blood clots, and white blood cells may form in the lungs or sinuses.[54] Symptoms are similar to those of chronic sinusitis but difficult to resolve and can become invasive, resembling malignancy. Development of aspergillosis is most often related to endodontic filling material[55] but has also been observed following sinus grafting. Treatment consists of antifungal therapy and surgery by an otolaryngologist.

Implant Survival Rate in the Grafted Maxillary Sinus

Based on a systematic review of the literature from 1986 to 2002, Del Fabbro et al[56] sought to determine the survival rate of root-form dental implants placed in the grafted maxillary sinus and the effects of graft material, implant surface characteristics, and simultaneous versus delayed placement on survival rate. The reported overall implant survival rate was 91.49%. The database included 6,913 implants placed in 2,046 subjects with loaded follow-up times ranging from 12 to 75 months. Implant survival was 87.70% with grafts of 100% autogenous bone, 94.88% when autogenous bone was combined with various bone substitutes, and 95.98% with grafts consisting of bone substitutes alone. The survival rate for implants having smooth and rough surfaces was 85.64% and 95.98%, respectively. Simultaneous and delayed procedures displayed similar survival rates of 92.17% and 92.93%, respectively. When implants are placed in grafted maxillary sinuses, the performance of rough implants is superior to that of smooth implants. Bone substitute materials are as effective as autogenous bone when used alone or in combination with autogenous bone.

Summary of Postoperative Complications

Prevention is the best approach to managing postoperative complications associated with the lateral window technique. Although the complication rate following sinus bone graft surgery is low, it is important to take all possible precautions before, during, and after surgery to prevent complications. The following measures can help to reduce the incidence of postoperative infections and/or complications:

- Appropriate patient selection. Patients with sinus disease and smokers have a higher incidence of postoperative complications. If nasal or sinus disease is suspected, the patient should be referred to an otolaryngologist for clinical assessment, which should include nasal endoscopy and, if necessary, a CT scan of the maxillofacial area, particularly the ostiomeatal complex.[57]
- Appropriate treatment planning. Proper evaluation of the vertical restorative space during treatment planning can prevent insufficient or excessive restoration height, thus allowing for the proper crown-root ratio in the definitive prosthesis. The vertical restorative space will influence the type of the prosthesis and the need for bone grafting (eg, onlay bone grafting) in addition to, or in place of, a sinus graft procedure for proper restoration.
- Proper selection and use of the prophylactic and therapeutic antibiotics, antibacterial rinses, and anti-inflammatory medications to minimize postoperative infection (see part 5).
- Proper patient preparation for surgery (eg, sterile draping and chlorhexidine and/or betadine preparation of the mouth and face).
- Proper surgical protocol (eg, adequate extension of the incisions, passive wound closure, avoiding intraoperative surgical site contamination from the saliva or adjacent pathology, proper suturing technique; see appendix A).
- Taking extra care when combining sinus elevation with lateral augmentation for the treatment of the extremely atrophied maxilla. This approach has been shown to be a safe method that produces good and reliable clinical results[58]; however, it presents higher risk for wound dehiscence/incision line opening.
- Adequate postoperative instructions (eg, not to wear a prosthesis over the site until the mucosal incision heals, to eat a soft diet; see appendix C).
- Proper follow-up protocol to help detect complications early.
- Prescribing specific postoperative medications when complications arise to control infections as early as possible (see part 5).
- Adequate healing period of 6 months or more[59] (autogenous bone graft is ready for implant placement in 4 to 6 months; mixture of xenograft and autograft materials or rhBMP-2/ACS with xenograft are ready for implant placement in 8 to 12 months; and alloplastic materials alone require up to 18 months for complete consolidation).
- Referral to otolaryngologist in a timely manner when indicated.

References

1. Mehra P, Murad H. Maxillary sinus disease of odontogenic origin. Otolaryngol Clin North Am 2004;37:347–364.

2. Abubaker A. Applied anatomy of the maxillary sinus. Oral Maxillofac Clin North Am 1999;11:1–14.

3. Sicher H. The viscera of head and neck. In: Oral Anatomy. St Louis: Mosby, 1975:418–424.

4. Maloney PL, Doku HC. Maxillary sinusitis of odontogenic origin. J Can Dent Assoc 1968;34:591–603.

5. Schaeffer JP. The sinus maxillaris and its relations in the embryo, child, and adult man. Am J Anat 1910;10:313–367.

6. Brook I. Sinusitis of odontogenic origin. Otolaryngol Head Neck Surg 2006;135:349–355.

7. Underwood AS. An inquiry into the anatomy and pathology of the maxillary sinus. J Anat Physiol 1910;44:354–369.

8. Velasquez-Plata D, Hovey LR, Peach CC, Alder ME. Maxillary sinus septa: A 3-dimensional computerized tomographic scan analysis. Int J Oral Maxillofac Implants 2002;17:854–860.

9. Kim MJ, Jung UW, Kim CS, et al. Maxillary sinus septa: Prevalence, height, location, and morphology. A reformatted computed tomography scan analysis. J Periodontol 2006;77:903–908.

10. Ulm CW, Solar P, Krennmair G, Matejka M, Watzek G. Incidence and suggested surgical managment of septa in sinus-lift procedures. Int J Oral Maxillofac Implants 1995;10:462–465.

11. Donald PJ, Gluckman JL, Rice DH. The Sinuses. New York: Raven, 1995.

12. Bolger WE, Woodruff WW, Morehead J, Parsons DS. Maxillary sinus hypoplasia: Classification and description of associated uncinate hypoplasia. Otolaryngol Head Neck Surg 1990;103:759–765.

13. Amedee RG, Miller AJ. Sinus anatomy and function. In: Bailey BJ (ed). Otolaryngology Head & Neck Surgery, ed 4. Philadelphia: Lippincott, Williams & Wilkins, 2006:321–328.

14. Jousimes-Somer HR, Savolainen S, Ylikoski JS. Comparison of the nasal bacterial floras in two groups of healthy subjects and in patients with acute maxillary sinusitis. J Clin Microbiol 1989;27:2736–2743.

15. Pearlman AN, Chandra RK, Chang D, et al. Relationships between severity of chronic sinusitis and nasal polyposis, asthma, and atopy. Am J Rhinol Allergy 2009;23:145–148.

16. Bhattacharyya N. Bilateral chronic maxillary sinusitis after the sinus lift procedure. Am J Otolaryngol 1999;20:133–135.

17. Barone A, Santini S, Sbordone L, Crespi R, Covani U. A clinical study of the outcomes and complications associated with maxillary sinus augmentation. Int J Oral Maxillofac Implants 2006;21:81–85.

18. Doud Galli SK, Lebowitz RA, Giacchi RJ, Glickman R, Jacobs JB. Chronic sinusitis complicating sinus lift surgery. Am J Rhinol 2001;15:181–186.

19. Gliklich RE, Metson R. The health impact of chronic sinusitis in patients seeking otolaryngologic care. Otolaryngol Head Neck Surg 1995;113:104–109.

20. Mukherjig SK, Figueroa R, Ginsberg LE, et al. Allergic fungal sinusitis: CT findings. Radiology 1998;207:417–422.

21. Bent JP III, Kuhn FA. Diagnosis of allergic fungal sinusitis. Otolaryngol Head Neck Surg 1994;111:580–588.

22. Rupp ME. Images in clinical medicine. Rhinocerebral mucormycosis. N Engl J Med 1995;333:564.

23. Gordts F, Clement PA, Buisseret T. Prevalence of paranasal sinus abnormalities on MRI in a non-ENT population. Acta Otorhinolaryngol Belg 1996;50:167–170.

24. Gardner DG, Gullane PJ. Mucoceles of the maxillary sinus. Oral Surg Oral Med Oral Pathol 1986;62:538–543.

25. Mardinger O, Manor I, Mijiritsky E, Hirshberg A. Maxillary sinus augmentation in the presence of antral pseudocyst: A clinical approach. Oral Surg Oral Med Oral Pathol Oral Radiol Endod 2007;103:180–184.

26. Lawson W, Ho BT, Sharri CM, Biller HF. Inverted papilloma: A report of 112 cases. Laryngoscope 1995;105:282–288.

27. Tawil G, Mawla M. Sinus floor elevation using a bovine bone mineral (Bio-Oss) with or without the concomitant use of a bilayered collagen barrier (Bio-Gide): A clinical report of immediate and delayed implant placement. Int J Oral Maxillofac Implants 2001;16:713–721.

28. Wallace SS, Froum SJ, Cho SC, et al. Sinus augmentation utilizing anorganic bovine bone (Bio-Oss) with absorbable and nonabsorbable membranes placed over the lateral window: Histomorphometric and clinical analyses. Int J Periodontics Restorative Dent 2005;25:551–559.

29. Testori T, Wallace SS. Surgical procedures: Lateral window approach. In: Testori T, Del Fabbro M, Weinstein R, Wallace S (eds). Maxillary Sinus Surgery and Alternatives in Treatment. London: Quintessence, 2009:190–215.

30. Fehrenbach MJ, Herring SW. Illustrated Anatomy of the Head and Neck. Philadelphia: Saunders, 1996:222–223.

31. Watzek G, Ulm CW, Haas R. Anatomic and physiologic fundamentals of sinus floor augmentation. In: Jensen OT (ed). The Sinus Bone Graft. Chicago: Quintessence, 1999:31–47.

32. Jensen OT, Shulman LB, Block MS, Iacono VJ. Report of the sinus consensus conference of 1996. Int J Oral Maxillofac Implants 1998;13(suppl):11–45.

33. Wallace SS, Mazor Z, Froum SJ, Cho SC, Tarnow DP. Schneiderian membrane perforation rate during sinus elevation using piezosurgery: Clinical results of 100 consecutive cases. Int J Periodontics Restorative Dent 2007;27:413–419.

34. Cho SC, Yoo SK, Wallace SS, Froum SJ, Tarnow DP. Correlation between membrane thickness and perforation rates in sinus augmentation surgery. Presented at the Academy of Osseointegration Annual Meeting, Dallas, 14–16 March 2002.

35. Cho SC, Wallace SS, Froum SJ, Tarnow DP. Influence of anatomy on Schneiderian membrane perforations during sinus elevation surgery: Three-dimentional analysis. Pract Proced Aesthet Dent 2001;13:160–163.

36. McGowan DA, Baxter PW, James J. The Maxillary Sinus and Its Dental Implications. Oxford: Wright, 1993:1–25.

37. Krennmair G, Ulm GW, Lugmayr H, Solar P. The incidence, location, and height of maxillary sinus septa in the edentulous and dentate maxilla. J Oral Maxillofac Surg 1999;57:667–671.

38. Cawood JI, Howell RA. A classification of the edentulous jaws. J Oral Maxillofac Surg 1988;17:232–236.

39. Nemanic G. The reflection of some anatomical structures of the maxillary sinus on the clinical and x-ray diagnostic. Kongres UAJ Novi Sad 1968.

40. Schlungbaum G. Über die Bildung mehrerer Nebenräume der Nasenhohle im Oberkiefer und ihre Deutung, mit Berücksichtigung der Beziehungen der Zähne zu ihnen. Vierteljahrhundertsschrift für Zahnheilkunde 1921;43.

41. Perovic D. Beiträge zur Kenntnis der Engwicklung und des Baues des menschlichen Oberkiefers sowie des Sinus maxillaris. Bull Sci Cons Acad RPF (Yougosla) 1954;11:5.

42. Proussaefs P, Lozada J. The "Loma Linda pouch": A technique for repairing the perforated sinus membrane. Int J Periodontics Restorative Dent 2003;23:593–597.

43. Beaumont C, Zafiropoulos GG, Rohmann K, Tatakis DN. Prevalence of maxillary sinus disease and abnormalities in patients scheduled for sinus lift procedures. J Periodontol 2005;76:461–467.

44. Schwartz-Arad D, Herzberg R, Dolev E. The prevalence of surgical complications of the sinus graft procedure and their impact on implant survival. J Periodontol 2004;75:511–516.

45. Ziccardi VB, Betts NJ. Complications of maxillary sinus augmentation. In: Jensen OT (ed). The Sinus Bone Graft. Chicago: Quintessence, 1999:201–208.

46. Hong SB, Kim JS, Shin SI, Han JY, Herr Y, Chung JH. Clinical treatment of postoperative infection following sinus augmentation. J Periodontol Implant Sci 2010;40:144–149.

47. Chanavaz M. Maxillary sinus: Anatomy, physiology, surgery, and bone grafting related to implantology—Eleven years of surgical experience (1979–1990). J Oral Implantol 1990;16:199–209.

48. Zijderveld SA, van den Bergh JP, Schulten EA, ten Bruggenkate CM. Anatomical and surgical findings and complications in 100 consecutive maxillary sinus floor elevation procedures. J Oral Maxillofac Surg 2008;66:1426–1438.

49. Lindhe J, Lang NP, Karring T. Clinical Periodontology and Implant Dentistry, ed 5. Oxford: Blackwell, 2008.

50. Jensen J, Simonsen EK, Sindet-Pederson S. Reconstruction of the severely resorbed maxilla with bone grafting and osseointegrated implants: A preliminary report. J Oral Maxillofac Surg 1990;48:27–32.

51. Guibert M, Avenard M, Rose X, Cabos A, Pessey JJ, Serrano E. Major orbital complications of acute maxillary sinusitis of dental aetiology [in French]. Rev Laryngol Otol Rhinol (Bord) 2008;129(4–5):319–323.

52. Patt BS, Manning SC. Blindness from orbital complications of sinusitis. Otolaryngol Head Neck Surg 1991;104:789–795.

53. Maniglia AJ, Goodwin WJ, Arnold JE, Ganz E. Intracranial abscesses secondary to nasal, sinus, and orbital infections in adults and children. Arch Otolaryngol Head Neck Surg 1989;115:1424–1429.

54. Alrajhi AA, Enani M, Mahasin Z, Al-Omran K. Chronic invasive aspergillosis of the paranasal sinuses in immunocompetent hosts from Saudi Arabia. Am J Trop Med Hyg 2001;65:83–86.

55. Khongkhunthian P, Reichart PA. Aspergillosis of the maxillary sinus as a complication of overfilling root canal material into the sinus: Report of two cases. J Endod 2001;27:476–478.

56. Del Fabbro M, Testori T, Francetti L, Weinstein R. Systematic review of survival rates for implants placed in the grafted maxillary sinus. Int J Periodontics Restorative Dent 2004;24:565–577.

57. Pignataro L, Mantovani M, Torretta S, Felisati G, Sambataro G. ENT assessment in the integrated management of candidate for (maxillary) sinus lift. Acta Otorhinolaryngol Ital 2008;28:110–119.

58. Weingart D, Bublitz R, Petrin G, Kälber J, Ingimarsson S. Combined sinus lift procedure and lateral augmentation. A treatment concept for the surgical and prosthodontic rehabilitation of the extremely atrophic maxilla [in German]. Mund Kiefer Gesichtschir 2005;9:317–323.

59. Tatum OH, Lebowitz MS, Tatum CA, Borgner RA. Sinus augmentation: Rationale, development, long-term results. N Y State Dent J 1993;59(5): 43–48.

PART 5 # Pharmacology:
Prevention and Management
of Pain, Infection, and Drug-Related
Complications

Complications

Introduction

The success of a dental implant procedure often is perceived by the patient in relation to the number of intraoperative and postoperative complications experienced. The two types of complications that will most strongly affect a patient's perception are occurrences of infection and pain during and following the surgical and prosthetic appointments. The use of sound pharmacologic principles can aid in preventing these complications. Practitioners have a responsibility to their patients to follow a proper protocol when prescribing medications. The improper use of analgesics can leave the patient overmedicated or with undue discomfort. The inappropriate use of antibiotics can lead to the development of bacterial resistance, overgrowth of microorganisms, the development of gastrointestinal (GI) disturbances (including pseudomembranous colitis), and/or immunologic problems.[1]

The intent of part 5 is to aid the implant dentist in effectively preventing and managing intra- and postoperative infection and pain using pharmacology. Brief discussions on the management of patients receiving oral bisphosphonates, anticoagulants, and/or antiplatelet agents also are presented.

Intra- and Postoperative Infection

Antibiotic therapy

Antibiotics should be used to manage orofacial infections and as prophylaxis when surgical and/or prosthetic manipulations are performed. Antibiotics are effective when the serum concentration will inhibit 90% of the species of the target microorganisms (MIC-90).[2] To achieve this, the clinician must be aware of the half-life elimination, peak serum level, and time-to-peak serum level of the antibiotic of choice (Table 5-1).

The problem implant dentists face is that there are more than 400 known and chemically distinct bacterial groups that colonize the oral cavity's ecologic niche.[4,5] Whether or not these bacterial groups will present a problem for the patient is based on the nature of the procedure and the patient's ability to withstand the presence of a transient bacteremia. Anaerobic bacteria normally outnumber aerobic bacteria by 10:1 or 100:1. The clinician should remember that infectious microorganisms usually are made of the host's normal flora.[6]

When prescribing antibiotics for a patient, it is important that one understands that microorganisms adapt to environmental factors. Their response to exogenous antibiotic therapy is no exception. Overuse and inappropriate use of antibiotics have led to an alarming increase in the prevalence of multidrug-resistant bacteria.[7] This is not only an issue for dental implant treatment but also a global concern for the effectiveness of antibiotic therapy against all infectious diseases known to mankind.[8]

Antimicrobial therapy, when used properly, demonstrates powerful and specific activity against bacteria. The bacteria most often implicated in periodontal disease and bone loss are *Actinobacillus actinomycetemcomitans* (gram-negative, aerobic coccobacilli) and *Porphyromonas intermedia* (gram-negative, anaerobic bacilli). The most often recovered organism from patients with severe odontogenic infection is *Fusobacterium nucleatum* (gram-negative, anaerobic bacilli). The rate of recovery from infections by various organisms implicated in oral infections is influenced by age, underlying systemic disease, and local factors. The pathogens involved are usually indigenous to the oral cavity, but in the immunocompromised patient, other bacteria such as *Escherichia coli* (gram-negative, anaerobic bacilli) or *Bacteroides fragilis* (gram-negative, anaerobic bacilli) may be found.[2]

A universal side effect of antibiotics is GI irritation. Research has shown that several strains of probiotics are helpful in the prevention and treatment of antibiotic-associated diarrhea. The most commonly studied probiotics are *Lactobacillus GG* and *Saccharomyces boulardii*.[9] Patients should be advised to take probiotics along with antibiotics to help prevent GI irritations, including pseudomembranous colitis.

Table 5-1	Antibiotic half-life eliminations, time-to-peak serum levels, and peak serum levels*		
Antibiotic	**Half-life elimination (h)**	**Time-to-peak serum level (h)**	**Peak serum level (µg/mL)**
Penicillin G	0.5–1.0	0.5–1.0	2
Penicillin V	0.5–1.0	0.5–1.0	4
Ampicillin	1.0–1.8	1–2	7.8
Amoxicillin	0.7–1.4	2	7.5
Amoxicillin + clavulanic acid	0.7–1.4	2	7.5
Erythromycin	1.5–2.0	4	1.09
Clarithromycin	2–3	1	4
Azithromycin	68	2.3–4.0	4.5
Ciprofloxacin	3–5	0.5–2.0	1.22
Clindamycin	2–3	1	2.44
Metronidazole	6–8	1–2	20

*Data from Brunton[2] and Lexi-Comp.[3]

The antibiotic groups of interest to the implant dentist are the β-lactam antibiotics (penicillins and cephalosporins), tetracyclines, macrolides, lincosamides, and fluoroquinolones. The antibacterial and antiprotozoal agent metronidazole also has applications in the prevention of infection in implant dentistry.[2] Table 5-2 presents a summary of the classification of the antibiotics described in the following sections.

Table 5-2 Antibiotic classification

Antimicrobial drug classification	Mechanism of action	Examples	Spectrum
Penicillins	Interference with bacterial cell wall synthesis	Narrow-spectrum penicillins —Penicillin G (IV) —Penicillin V potassium (oral)	• Bactericidal • Gram-positive organisms • Gram-negative cocci • Non–β-lactamase-producing anaerobes • Gram-negative rods (little activity)
		Extended-spectrum penicillins —Ampicillin (IM, IV, oral) —Amoxicillin (oral) —Amoxicillin + clavulanic acid (oral)	• Spectrum similar to penicillin G but greater activity against gram-negative bacteria because of their superior ability to penetrate the gram-negative outer membrane • Inactivated by β-lactamases
Cephalosporins	Interference with bacterial cell wall synthesis	First-generation cephalosporins —Cephalexin (oral) —Cephradine (oral) —Cefadroxil (oral) —Cefazolin (IM, IV)	• Bactericidal • More stable than penicillins to bacterial β-lactamases • Gram-positive cocci (pneumococci, streptococci, staphylococci)
		Second-generation cephalosporins —Cefaclor (oral) —Cefprozil (oral) —Cefuroxime (oral, IM, IV)	• Similar to first-generation cephalosporins with extended activity against gram-negative but less activity against gram-positive bacteria
		Third-generation cephalosporins —Cefotaxime (IM, IV) —Ceftazidime (IM, IV)	• Extended gram-negative coverage (except cefoperazone) • Crosses blood-brain barrier
		Fourth-generation cephalosporins —Cefepime (IV only)	• Similar to 3rd generation, but more resistant to chromosomal β-lactamases
β-lactamase inhibitors	Potent inhibitors of many β-lactamases Protect hydrolysable penicillins from inactivation by β-lactamases	Clavulanic acid	• Bactericidal • Very weak antibacterial action • Effective against amber class A β-lactamases produced by staphylococci, *Bacteroides*, *E coli*
Tetracyclines	Inhibit protein synthesis by binding reversibly to the 30S subunit of the bacterial ribosome	Tetracycline Demeclocycline Doxycycline Minocycline	• Broad spectrum • Bacteriostatic for many gram-positive and gram-negative bacteria, including anaerobes • Effective against tetracycline-resistant strains
Macrolides	Inhibit protein synthesis by binding reversibly to the 50S subunit of the bacterial ribosome	Natural —Erythromycin Semisynthetic —Clarithromycin —Azithromycin	• Effective against gram-positive bacteria, especially pneumococci, streptococci, and staphylococci, and gram-negative strains such as *Neisseria* • Bacteriostatic at lower concentrations • Bactericidal at higher concentrations
Lincosamides	Inhibit protein synthesis by binding to the 50S subunit of the bacterial ribosome	Clindamycin	• Bacteriostatic • Effective against staphylococci, streptococci, pneumococci, *Bacteroides,* and other anaerobes (gram-positive and gram-negative) • Ineffective against enterococci, gram-negative aerobes, *Clostridium difficile*
Fluoroquinolones	Inhibit DNA gyrase, thereby blocking DNA synthesis	Ciprofloxacin Levofloxacin	• Broad spectrum • Effective against a variety of gram-positive cocci and gram-negative bacteria • Especially effective against *Pseudomonas aeruginosa* or methicilllin-resistant *Staphylococcus aureus* • Should not be used for routine upper and lower respiratory tract, skin, or soft tissue infections
Miscellaneous	Reactive reduction; the nitro group of metronidazole is chemically reduced in anaerobic bacteria	Metronidazole	• Bactericidal • Effective against anaerobes, including *Bacteroides* and *Clostridium*

IM—intramuscularly; IV—intravenously.

Penicillins

Penicillins are a broad category of β-lactam antibiotics (cell wall inhibitors rendered ineffective by bacteria that produce the enzyme β-lactamase) that includes, among others, narrow-spectrum antibiotics such as pencillin G, penicillin V, penicillin VK, ampicillin, and amoxicillin.

Penicillin

The term *penicillin* in this context refers to a class of narrow-spectrum antibiotics, in particular, penicillin G; however, penicillin V potassium is the first choice in the treatment of many orofacial infections.

Indications
Penicillin is no longer recommended for dental prophylaxis, and it is indicated for only minor dental infections. Orofacial infections treatable by penicillin may include cellulitis, periapical abscess, periodontal abscess, acute suppurative pulpitis, oronasal fistula, pericoronitis, osteitis, osteomyelitis, and postsurgical and posttraumatic infection. Penicillin is useful for infections by certain bacteria, such as streptococci, enterococci, *Listeria*, *Neisseria meningitidis*, many anaerobes, spirochetes, *Actinomyces*, *Erysipelothrix* species, and *Pasteurella multocida*.

Administration
Penicillin should be taken on an empty stomach 1 hour before or 2 hours after meals because food decreases the drug absorption rate and serum concentration.[3]

Ampicillin

Ampicillin is better able to penetrate the cell membrane of gram-negative bacteria (gram-positive bacteria do not have a cell membrane) compared with penicillin G. Ampicillin also has better oral bioavailability because of its acid resistance and ease of absorption.[2]

Indications
Ampicillin is used to treat a variety of infections, such as those caused by susceptible bacteria (non–β-lactamase-producing organisms), streptococci, pneumococci, non–penicillinase-producing staphylococci, *Listeria,* meningococci, and some strains of *Haemophilus influenzae, Salmonella, Shigella, E coli, Enterobacter,* and *Klebsiella.*

Contraindications
Patients with infectious mononucleosis should not be given ampicillin because it may cause a rash.[2,3]

Administration
Ampicillin should be taken on an empty stomach 1 hour before or 2 hours after meals.[3] Ingesting food prior to taking ampicillin will decrease the drug's absorption rate and may decrease serum concentration.[2,3]

Amoxicillin

Amoxicillin is a moderate-spectrum antibiotic. It is used more often than other penicillins because it is absorbed more rapidly and completely from the GI tract. Peak plasma concentrations of amoxicillin are two to four times greater than those of ampicillin after oral administration of the same dose.

Indications
In dental practice, amoxicillin is used as antibiotic prophylaxis for patients who are at risk of infective endocarditis or those who have had total joint replacement. It also is used to treat orofacial infections.

Administration
Taking amoxicillin with food does not interfere with absorption.

Amoxicillin plus clavulanic acid

Amoxicillin may be given with clavulanic acid to expand its spectrum of activity. However, some bacterial strains have developed resistance to this combination.[2]

Indications
In dental use, amoxicillin plus clavulanic acid is used to treat orofacial infections when β-lactamase-producing staphylococci and *Bacteroides* are present. It also is used to treat sinusitis. It can treat β-lactamase-producing *Moraxella (Branhamella) catarrhalis, H influenzae, Neisseria gonorrhoeae*, and non–methicillin-resistant *S aureus* (non-MRSA). This treatment is useful when a patient has amoxicillin resistance and cannot tolerate alternative treatments.[2] The UK Committee on the Safety of Medicines (CSM) recommends that treatments such as amoxicillin plus clavulanic acid preparations should be reserved for bacterial infections likely to be caused by amoxicillin-resistant β-lactamase-producing strains and that treatment normally should not exceed 14 days.

Contraindications
The use of clavulanic acid with penicillins has been associated with an increased incidence of cholestatic jaundice and acute hepatitis during therapy or shortly after, especially in men and those aged 65 years and older. The associated jaundice is usually self-limiting and rarely fatal.[10] Based on the number of treated subjects and reported cases, the risk of developing hepatitis with the amoxicillin plus clavulanic acid combination is estimated at below 1 in 100,000. The association of hepatitis and signs of hypersensitivity may suggest an immunoallergic mechanism of hepatotoxicity in some patients.[11]

Patients should not take amoxicillin plus clavulanic acid if they have a hypersensitivity to amoxicillin, clavulanic acid, penicillin, or any component of the formulation; history of cholestatic jaundice; or hepatic dysfunction with amoxicillin plus clavulanic acid therapy. Do not use in patients with phenylketonuria (PKU). Use with caution in patients with hepatic or renal impairment.

The dosage should be adjusted in patients with renal deficiency.[2] Women who are pregnant should only be given amoxicillin plus clavulanic acid with caution when clearly indicated. This medication passes into breast milk and caution should be used when given to nursing mothers. The risk of adverse events in the infant may be increased when compared to the use of amoxicillin alone.

Administration

Amoxicillin plus clavulanic acid should not be taken with a high-fat meal because this can decrease the absorption of the drug. Food will increase the absorption and decrease GI upset; however, it also may be taken without food.[2] It may be mixed with milk, formula, or juice. Extended-release tablets should be taken with food.

Warnings and adverse effects associated with all penicillins

Patients who have a hypersensitivity to penicillins or any component within the formulation should not take this class of antibiotic. Patients with renal impairment, asthma, or seizure disorders should use this drug with caution. In pregnant women, penicillin is considered safe; however, there are no controlled tests to confirm this.[12] Women who are nursing may be given penicillin with caution because it is absorbed through the breast milk and may cause diarrhea or allergic responses in nursing infants.

The most common adverse effects with penicillins are hypersensitivity reactions; penicillins are the most common cause of drug allergy.[2] The incidence of these allergies may vary from 0.7% to 10% and may include rash, urticarial rash, fever, bronchospasm, vasculitis, serum sickness, exfoliative dermatitis, Stevens-Johnson syndrome, and anaphylaxis.[2] Other side effects may include angioedema, urticaria, diarrhea, nausea, vomiting, erythema, dermatitis, black hairy tongue, glossitis, sore mouth or tongue, tooth discoloration, stomatitis, heartburn, agranulocytosis, anemia, eosinophilia, leukopenia, thrombocytopenia purpura, laryngeal stridor, seizures, cardiovascular events, and central nervous system symptoms. Fungal or bacterial superinfections, including *C difficile*–associated diarrhea (CDAD) and pseudomembranous colitis, may result from prolonged use; CDAD has been observed more than 2 months after antibiotic treatment.[3]

Cephalosporins

Cephalosporins are bactericidal β-lactam antibiotics with a structure similar to that of the penicillins; however, they are more stable to β-lactamase activity and have a broader spectrum than the penicillins.[2]

First-generation cephalosporins

First-generation cephalosporins (eg, cephalexin, cephalothin, cefazolin) are predominantly active against gram-positive bacteria; successive generations have increased activity against gram-negative bacteria (albeit often with reduced activity against gram-positive organisms). Most anaerobes found in the oral cavity are sensitive to first-generation cephalosporins; however, *B fragilis* is resistant.

Second-generation cephalosporins

Second-generation cephalosporins include cefuroxime, cefprozil, and cefmetazole. They have increased gram-negative activity compared to first-generation cephalosporins, but less than third-generation cephalosporins. Some second-generation cephalosporins (eg, cefoxitin, cefotetan, cefmetazole) are active against *B fragilis* bacteria.

Third-generation cephalosporins

Third-generation cephalosporins have less activity than first-generation agents against gram-positive cocci but possess greater activity against Enterobacteriaceae, including the β-lactamase-producing strains. A subset of these agents (eg, ceftazidime, cefoperazone) have activity against *P aeruginosa*.

Fourth-generation cephalosporins

Fourth-generation cephalosporins are reserved for serious infections in hospitalized patients when Enterobacteriaceae and *Pseudomonas* are of concern.

Tetracyclines

Tetracyclines are broad-spectrum bacteriostatic agents for many gram-positive and gram-negative aerobic and anaerobic bacteria. Unfortunately, the widespread use and often misuse of tetracyclines has resulted in the development of many resistant bacterial strains, which has diminished their clinical usefulness. The various derivatives exhibit differences in absorption, protein binding, metabolism, and degree of activity against susceptible microorganisms. For example, tetracyclines in general are adequately absorbed orally, but there are significant differences in bioavailability with the various derivatives.

Indications and contraindications

The use of tetracyclines in the management of orofacial infections is considered inappropriate because of their bacteriostatic activity and extensive bacterial resistance. Long-term systemic administration in the management of adult periodontitis must involve evaluation of the risk-benefit ratio because of questionable clinical efficacy.[13]

Interestingly, tetracyclines are used to treat *Helicobacter pylori* in combination with other antibiotics. *H pylori* has been found to exist in chronic maxillary sinus infections for patients with gastric *H pylori* infections, which is important to the implant dentist performing subantral augmentations.[14]

Adverse effects

Tetracyclines bind to developing teeth and bones. The two main complications seen with tetracyclines are the development of opportunistic *Candida albicans* infections and photosensitivity. Tetracyclines also cause multiple adverse side effects including blood dyscrasia, liver dysfunction, *C albicans* overgrowth, GI irritation, and multiple allergic reactions.[15]

Administration

These antibiotics should not be administered with calcium-containing products (dairy) because they bind to calcium and will not be absorbed.

Macrolides

Macrolide antibiotics include erythromycin, clarithromycin, and azithromycin. These antibiotics contain a many-membered lactone ring as a core, which improves tissue penetration and broadens the spectrum of activity.

Erythromycin

Erythromycin has gram-positive and gram-negative activity. At a low dose it is bacteriostatic, but at higher doses it is bactericidal.

Indications

Erythromycin can be used to treat bacterial infections, including those with some strains of *Streptococcus pyogenes, Streptococcus pneumoniae, S aureus, Moraxella pneumoniae,* and *Legionella pneumophila.* It is a suitable alternative for penicillin-allergic patients.[2] Erythromycin and clarithromycin potentiate the effects of carbamazepine, corticosteroids, cyclosporine, digoxin, ergot alkaloids, theophylline, triazolam, valproate, and warfarin.

Contraindications

Erythromycin is excreted at low concentrations in breast milk; therefore, alternative antibiotics may be preferred for nursing mothers.

Adverse effects

Erythromycin has several adverse effects. The main side effect related to dental treatment is oral candidiasis. Other effects include a prolonged Q-T interval, torsades de pointes, ventricular arrhythmia, ventricular tachycardia, seizures, pruritus, rash, abdominal pain, anorexia, diarrhea, infantile hypertrophic pyloric stenosis, nausea, pancreatitis, psuedomembranous colitis, and vomiting. Cholestatic jaundice, hepatitis, abnormal liver function tests, thrombophlebitis, weakness, hearing loss, allergic reactions, anaphylaxis, hypersensitivity reactions, and urticaria also may occur.[3]

Administration

The absorption of erythromycin, 18% to 45%, is variable and better with salt forms. When taking erythromycin, alcohol consumption should be avoided because it can decrease the absorption of erythromycin or the erythromycin can enhance the effects of alcohol. Food and St John's wort also can alter erythromycin levels. Because the antibiotic may induce GI irritation, some formulations should be taken with food. In fact, the ethylsuccinate is better absorbed when taken with food.

Clarithromycin

Clarithromycin is a later generation of erythromycin that demonstrates greater acid stability and oral absorption. It requires only twice daily dosing, as opposed to the four times daily dosing of erythromycin. Clarithromycin has a major metabolite that demonstrates antibacterial activity. Clarithromycin has decreased GI intolerance compared to erthromycin; however, it is expensive and it is involved in multiple important clinical drug interactions.[2]

Indications
The main dental use of this antibiotic is prevention of infective endocarditis and for treatment of orofacial infections.

Contraindications
As with erythromycin, clarithromycin is excreted in breast milk; therefore, caution should be taken when giving this antibiotic to nursing mothers. It also should be prescribed with caution to patients with coronary artery disease, myasthenia gravis, or renal impairment.

Adverse effects
Adverse effects are similar to those of erythromycin but also include abnormal taste, headache, rash, behavioral changes, hepatitis, dizziness, hallucinations, hypoglycemia, insomnia, Stevens-Johnson syndrome, tremor, vertigo, and decreased white blood cell count. With prolonged use, superinfections can develop.

Administration
Food delays the rate of absorption. St John's wort should not be taken with clarithromycin because it may decrease clarithromycin levels in the blood.

Azithromycin

Azithromycin is the newest macrolide and has less activity against staphylococci and streptococci compared with the other macrolides. However, it does have greater activity against H pylori. It penetrates tissues better and therefore is released slowly from tissues. The most attractive aspect of azithromycin is that it is free of the multiple drug interactions associated with clarithromycin.

Indications
Azithromycin has the same dental indications as clarithromycin.

Contraindications
Caution should be taken when giving this antibiotic to patients with hepatic impairment, myasthenia gravis, or renal impairment.[2]

Adverse effects
Adverse effects include diarrhea, nausea, pruritus, rash, abdominal pain, anorexia, cramping, vomiting, vaginitis, acute renal failure, angioedema, chest pain, increased cough, dermatitis, facial edema, fungal infections, hyperkinesia, nervousness, pancreatitis, smell perversion, taste perversion, and tongue discoloration. It is possible that this antibiotic can hide the symptoms of incubation gonorrhea or syphilis.

Administration
Azithromycin should be administered 1 hour before or 2 hours after meals. However, if GI upset is an issue, it may be administered with food.

Lincosamides

Like macrolides, lincosamides are bacteriostatic at low concentrations and bactericidal at higher concentrations.

Clindamycin

Clindamycin is the primary lincosamide. It has activity against streptococci, staphylococci, and pneumococci. However, enterococci and gram-negative aerobes are resistant because clindamycin does not penetrate the outer membrane. Therefore, C difficile is resistant to clindamycin, which increases the patient's susceptibility to pseudomembranous colitis.

Indications
Dental use includes prevention of endocarditis and treatment of orofacial infections. It often is used in patients with a penicillin allergy.

Contraindications
Clindamycin can transfer into breast milk in small amounts; however, it is usually considered to be compatible with breastfeeding.[2] Use caution when administering to patients with hepatic impairment.[2,3]

Adverse effects
Adverse effects include cardiac arrest, hypotension, erythema multiforme, exfoliative dermatitis, pruritus, rash, Stevens-Johnson syndrome, urticaria, abdominal pain, diarrhea, esophagitis, nausea, pseudomembranous colitis, vomiting, vaginitis, agranulocytosis, eosinophilia, neutropenia, thrombocytopenia, jaundice, abnormal liver function test, polyarthritis, renal dysfunction, anaphylactoid reactions, and superinfections.

Administration
Clindamycin is well absorbed orally, but peak concentrations can be delayed when it is taken with food.

Fluoroquinolones

Fluoroquinolones have excellent gram-negative aerobic activity and little gram-positive activity, although newer agents have been improved in this regard. They are well absorbed and have a wide volume of distribution. Most dental infections have high concentrations of anaerobes, and most fluoroquinolones, with the exception of the newer agents, demonstrate no activity against anaerobes. Therefore, their use in dental infections is rarely a good option. Fluoroquinolones are associated with few adverse side effects, the most common involving the GI tract: nausea, vomiting, and/or abdominal pain.[2] Other side effects may include dizziness and headaches.[2]

Ciprofloxacin

Ciprofloxacin is a synthetic chemotherapeutic antibiotic and a second-generation fluoroquinolone antibacterial.[2]

Indications
Ciprofloxacin may be used alone or in combination with metronidazole for the management of rapidly progressive or refractory periodontitis associated with Enterobacteriaceae. It also may be used for treatment of bone and joint infections.[3]

Contraindications
Patients who have a hypersensitivity to quinolones or any component of the formulation should not take ciprofloxacin.

Administration
The manufacturer recommends that the immediate-release tablet be taken 2 hours after meals and the extended-release tablet be taken with meals. Dairy products or calcium-fortified juices may decrease ciprofloxacin serum levels. Caffeine should be limited because serum levels of caffeine may be increased when taken with ciprofloxacin. Patients taking this drug are cautioned against taking certain herbs and nutraceuticals, such as dong quai and St John's wort.[2,3]

Levofloxacin

Levofloxacin is broad-spectrum fluoroquinolone with activity against streptococci.[2]

Indications
Levofloxacin is used to treat bacterial infections of the bones, joints, and sinuses.[3]

Contraindications
Patients who are pregnant should take this drug only if the benefit justifies the risk to the fetus. The manufacturer recommends that breast-feeding women not take this drug.[3]

Adverse effects
Levofloxacin may prolong the Q-T interval and is considered to have a risk of causing torsades de pointes. A medical consult is suggested because it is not known what effect vasoconstrictors in the local anesthetic regimen will have in patients with a known history of congenital prolonged Q-T interval or in patients taking any medication that prolongs the Q-T interval. Non–dose-related side effects could include modification of bowel flora.

Metronidazole

Metronidazole has extensive anaerobic activity and is well absorbed and widely distributed. It is almost always bactericidal and is effective against obligate anaerobes. Bacterial resistance is limited because of its limited clinical use.[15]

Indications
Metronidazole is highly effective against gram-negative bacteria, which can be found in acute orofacial infections and adult periodontitis. However, it should not be used as the sole primary treatment for adult periodontitis. Rather, it is often used in combination with a β-lactam antibiotic.

Drug interactions
Metronidazole is metabolized by the liver; therefore, it has multiple drug interactions that must be taken into consideration. Barbiturates and phenytoin (eg, Dilantin, Pfizer) may decrease the efficacy of metronidazole; however, cimetidine may increase metronidazole blood levels. Metronidazole may increase lithium phenytoin serum concentrations. Metronidazole potentiates warfarin anticoagulants and therefore should be avoided in patients who are taking them. It is important that patients do not consume alcohol when taking metronidazole because of a possible acute psychosis and a disulfiram-like reaction (flushing, tachycardia, nausea, and vomiting), although for most individuals the risk is minor.[16] Patients should be cautioned not to drink alcohol during or within 3 days of cessation of metronidazole therapy.[2]

Empiric antibiotic therapy for suspected infections

When a patient presents with a suspected infection, empiric antibiotic therapy should be carried out through the selection of the most appropriate antibiotic based on the suspected organism(s). Empiric therapy is justified by the hope that early intervention will improve the outcome. This therapeutic concept has been proven acceptable by placebo-controlled, double-blinded prospective clinical trials. The decision to use empiric therapy should be based on scientific knowledge and clinical experience.

Before initiating empiric antimicrobial therapy, the clinician should make certain that it is necessary. The following questions should be addressed:

- Is an antibiotic indicated on the basis of clinical findings, or would it be more prudent to wait until such clinical findings become apparent?
- What are the most likely pathogens responsible for the infection?
- Is there a clinical basis for instituting therapy?
- Is it possible to obtain a culture so that the causative pathogen(s) can be identified?

Positive answer(s) to the above should be followed up with the questions below to determine selection of the appropriate antibiotic:

- If a specific pathogen has been identified, is it possible to use a narrow-spectrum antibiotic in place of the empirically prescribed agent?
- Is one agent sufficient or are more needed?
- What would be the optimal dosage, route of administration, and duration of therapy?

Anaerobic organisms (predominantly gram-positive facultative) were found in the overwhelming majority (81.1%) of patients in a study by Matijevic et al,[17] and when aerobic organisms were present, they were mostly gram-positive. Thus, it would be prudent to start with a bactericidal antibiotic that is effective against anaerobic and gram-positive aerobic organisms.

Suggested empiric antibiotic regimen

Step 1
A penicillin-like antibiotic meets the criteria for activity against anaerobic gram-negative and aerobic gram-positive bacteria. Amoxicillin would be a logical first choice except that it is susceptible to degradation by β-lactamase-producing bacteria.

This leads one to consider amoxicillin plus clavulanic acid. However, cephalexin, which demonstrates greater stability than the penicillins against β-lactamase-producing anaerobes, would provide suitable coverage with less expense than amoxicillin plus clavulanic acid.

Therefore, a good first-line antibiotic prescription would be cephalexin 1,000 mg initially, followed by 500 mg every 6 hours for a total of 7 to 10 days. This should represent 3 to 5 days beyond the last signs of infection. For more severe infections, it may be necessary to administer 1,000 mg every 6 hours for the first 2 days, followed by 500 mg every 6 hours for a total of 7 to 10 days.

Step 2
If the β-lactam antibiotic (eg, cephalexin) fails to bring considerable resolution in 48 to 72 hours after the onset of infection, then one of the following should be considered:

1. Institute superior anaerobe coverage by adding metronidazole 1,000 mg initially followed by 500 mg every 6 to 8 hours. This is continued for 7 to 10 days, which should represent 3 to 5 days beyond the last signs of infection.
2. Discontinue the cephalexin and begin clindamycin 300 mg initially followed by 150 mg every 6 hours for 7 to 10 days. For more severe infections, it may be necessary to administer 300 mg every 6 hours for the first 48 hours then 150 mg every 6 hours for 7 to 10 days.

Notes
For patients who are allergic to penicillins or cephalosporins, one should consider using clindamycin or azithromycin initially. Azithromycin would be prescribed as 500 mg initially then 250 mg daily for 4 days or 500 mg daily for 3 days.

Initial doses normally are twice the subsequent doses so an initial blood level may be obtained quickly. For severe infections and antibiotics with 6-hour dosages, it would be prudent to administer the second dose 4 hours after the initial dose to achieve a more constant blood level. It normally takes four to five half-lives of a medication to reach a steady blood level.[10] Incision and drainage always should be used when they would be of value. Moist heat applied either intraorally or extraorally is a must to accelerate vasodilation and tissue concentrations of the antibiotic. When the above therapy fails to resolve the infection, perform aerobic and anaerobic cultures with sensitivity testing. More severe infections should be treated with parenteral antibiotics. Table 5-3 provides a summary of recommended therapeutic adult dosages of antibiotics.

Table 5-3 Recommended adult dosages for antibiotics commonly used in implant dentistry

Generic name	Proprietary name	Recommended dosage*
Penicillin V potassium	Generic; sold as penicillin VK	1,000 mg initially followed by 500 mg every 6 hours for 7 to 10 days
Amoxicillin	Amoxil (GlaxoSmithKline)	1,000 mg initially followed by 500 mg every 8 hours for 7 to 10 days
Amoxicillin + clavulanic acid	Augmentin (GlaxoSmithKline)	1,000 mg amoxicillin + 125 mg clavulanic acid initially followed by 500 mg every 8 hours for 7 to 10 days
Cephalexin	Keflex (Victory Pharma)	1,000 mg initially followed by 500 mg every 6 hours for 7 to 10 days
Cefaclor	Ceclor (Eli Lilly)	1,000 mg initially followed by 500 mg every 8 hours for 7 to 10 days
Tetracycline	Sumycin (Par Pharmaceutical)	250–500 mg initially followed by 250 mg every 6 hours
Erythromycin base Erythromycin stearate Erythromycin ethylsuccinate	Erythrocin (stearate) (Abbott) E.E.S. 400 (ethylsuccinate) (Abbott)	Base or stearate: 500 mg initially followed by 250–400 mg every 6 to 12 hours (maximum 4 g/day) Ethylsuccinate: 800 mg initially, followed by 400–800 mg every 6 to 12 hours (maximum 4 g/day)
Clarithromycin	Biaxin (Abbott) Biaxin XL (Abbott)	500 mg initially followed by 250–500 mg every 12 hours 500 mg every 12 hours for 7 to 14 days
Azithromycin	Z-Pak (six 250-mg tablets) (Pfizer) Zithromax Tri-Pak (three 500-mg tablets) (Pfizer)	500 mg the first day, then 250 mg daily for 4 days 250–500 mg daily for 3 days
Clindamycin	Cleocin (Pfizer)	300 mg initially followed by 150 mg every 6 hours for 7 to 10 days Severe infections: 600 mg initially followed by 300 mg every 6 hours for 48 hours, then 150 mg every 6 hours for a total of 10 days
Ciprofloxacin	Cipro (Bayer)	Sinusitis: 500 mg every 12 hours for 10 days
Levofloxacin	Levaquin (Ortho-McNeil-Janssen)	Sinusitis: 500 mg every 24 hours for 10 to 14 days or 750 mg every 24 hours for 5 days
Metronidazole	Flagyl (Pfizer)	250–500 mg initially followed by 250–500 mg every 6 to 8 hours (maximum 4 g/day)

*For adults with no hepatic or renal disease.

Antibiotics for surgical prophylaxis

Prospective clinical trials have demonstrated that a single dose of antibiotics prior to implant surgery is effective in preventing infection.[2] During lengthy oral surgical procedures, it often is difficult to maintain strict aseptic conditions, which offers further justification for surgical prophylaxis. Moreover, surgical antibiotic prophylaxis is indicated for patients with medical conditions such as bacterial endocarditis infection, compromised immune function, poorly controlled type 1 diabetes, renal failure with dialysis, significant malnutrition or alcoholism, symptomatic HIV, inflammatory arthropathies, prosthetic joints, or infections. When using antibiotic prophylaxis, an adequate serum concentration should be established within 2 hours of the time of surgical incision and should not be continued for more then 24 hours. Prolonged use may encourage the growth of resistant organisms; avoiding this outcome is of particular importance with implant placement. Table 5-4 presents recommended antibiotic prophylactic adult doses based on patient conditions.

Table 5-4 Preoperative antibiotic adult doses based on patient condition

Patient condition	Agent	Adult dose*
No special needs	Amoxicillin or cephalexin[†]	2 g oral
Unable to take oral medication	Ampicillin or cefazolin	2 g IM or IV
Allergic to penicillins or ampicillin	Clindamycin Azithromycin Clarithromycin	2 g oral 600 mg oral 500 mg oral
Allergic to penicillins or ampicillin and unable to take oral medications	Clindamycin Azithromycin	2 g IM or IV 600 mg IM or IV

IM—intramuscularly; IV—intravenously.
*Single dose 30 to 60 minutes before procedure.
[†]Or other first- or second-generation oral cephalosporin. Cephalosporins should not be given to patients with a history of anaphylaxis, angioedema, or urticaria associated with the administration of penicillins or ampicillin.

COMPLICATION 73 | Intra- and Postoperative Pain

Local anesthetics

Patients undergoing dental implant procedures will require some form of pain management. Immediate postoperative pain can be controlled with the use of local anesthetics. For more invasive procedures, use of the local anesthetic bupivacaine with epinephrine 1:200,000 should be considered because it will give prolonged (6- to 12-hour) anesthesia.

Analgesics

Pain control should be specific, and an agent with the fewest possible side effects should be chosen. Nonopioid analgesic agents should be used initially, and then opioid agents should be added as needed. Careful operative techniques should be used to minimize tissue trauma and therefore diminish postoperative pain. All patients should leave the dental implant appointment with written postoperative instructions that include directions for pain control.

Nonopioid analgesics

Nonopioid analgesics should be the first-line drugs for controlling postoperative pain because they lack the unwanted side effects of opioids (eg, constipation, respiratory depression, and physical dependence). Nonopioid analgesics can be either centrally acting (acetaminophen) or peripherally acting (nonsteroidal anti-inflammatory drugs [NSAIDs]). All these agents achieve pain control by interrupting the synthesis of prostaglandins that lead to inflammation and pain.[18] NSAIDs have the additional advantage of not changing the perception of sensory modalities other than pain.

NSAIDs
Traditional NSAIDs do not inhibit the formation of leukotrienes, which are synthesized by lipooxygenases and contribute to inflammation.[2] A buildup of leukotrienes can result in NSAID intolerance, which may be manifested by bronchospasm, anaphylaxis, urticaria, rash, and hives that are not autoimmune in nature.[19] If this severe reaction occurs, NSAIDs should not be used.

The most commonly used NSAIDs include ibuprofen, naproxen, fenoprofen, flurbiprofen, and ketoprofen. These NSAIDs all have similar analgesic efficacy and similar side effect profiles.

Enolic acids (oxicams) such as meloxicam (Mobic, Boehringer Ingelheim) demonstrate approximately a 10-fold cyclooxygenase-2 (COX-2) selectivity in ex vivo studies, although this is somewhat variable.[20] Having this COX-2 selectivity translates into fewer GI side effects at lower dosages (7.5 mg/day), but not higher dosages (15 mg/day).[21] Another COX-2 selective inhibitor is celecoxib (Celebrex, Pfizer). Celecoxib has been approved for postextraction dental pain and therefore would be of benefit in dental implant procedures.

Both traditional and COX-2 selective NSAIDs, especially with high-dose and long-term use, inhibit renal prostaglandin production, which can lead to hemodynamic deterioration of renal function or tubulointerstitial nephritis. The result may be salt and water retention that can evolve into edema and hypertension.[22] There appears to be little effect on renal function in patients with disease-free kidneys, especially with short-term use. These effects are more likely to occur in patients with decreased renal flow as a result of congestive heart failure, cirrhosis, chronic renal disease, hypovolemia, edema, and increased blood pressure.

Studies suggest that the occurrence of hypertension may be related to the degree of COX-2 inhibition and the selectivity of the various agents. Therefore, the risk of thrombosis, hypertension, accelerated atherogenesis, and stroke are mechanistically integrated and can be possible side effects.[23] Patients at risk for cardiovascular or cerebrovascular disease must use these agents with caution, especially with prolonged usage. For this group of patients, it would be prudent, even for a short course of therapy, to record the patient's baseline blood pressure and recheck it at days 3 and 5, then daily thereafter. All NSAIDs and antihypertensive agents, with the exception of calcium channel blockers, have been implicated in a potential drug interaction that diminishes the antihypertensive agent's efficacy. It is best to discontinue NSAID therapy if an increase in blood pressure is noted.

NSAIDs typically demonstrate more analgesic efficacy than oral opioids while causing fewer side effects. Aspirin 650 mg was shown to be more effective than codeine 30 mg oral.[24] Ibuprofen 400 mg was demonstrated to be superior to the combination of aspirin 650 mg (or acetaminophen 1,000 mg) with codeine 60 mg.[25,26] Ibuprofen 400 mg has been shown to be superior to dihydrocodeine 30 mg and was found to be comparable to all other NSAIDs.[27]

Traditional NSAIDs
Ibuprofen Ibuprofen, like all NSAIDs, controls pain at lower dosages (200 to 400 mg every 6 hours) but demonstrates anti-inflammatory activity at higher dosages (600 to 800 mg every 6 hours).[27,28] Ibuprofen is supplied as tablets ranging from 200 to 800 mg. The 200-mg tablets are available without a prescription. Ibuprofen 600 mg every 6 hours usually controls most dental pain.

Ibuprofen generally is better tolerated than aspirin and has been used with some success in patients with a history of GI intolerance to other NSAIDs.[2] Despite this finding, 5% to 15% of patients taking ibuprofen experience GI side effects.[7] Other side effects occurring with less frequency include thrombocytopenia, rashes, headache, dizziness, blurred vision, fluid retention, edema, and toxic amblyopia. When ocular disturbances are observed, ibuprofen should be discontinued immediately.[2]

Ibuprofen has been found to cross the placenta in animal studies.[2] There is positive evidence of fetal risk that outweighs any analgesic benefits when ibuprofen is taken during the third trimester of pregnancy.[29] There are no known controlled studies examining the effects of ibuprofen on the fetus during the first two trimesters.

For patients taking immediate-release aspirin 81 mg daily for stroke prevention and cardioprotective effects, ibuprofen 400 mg or greater may interfere with aspirin's antiplatelet effect, with its greatest effect occurring if it is administered less than 8 hours prior to aspirin.[30,31] Patients should be informed concerning the proper timing of ibuprofen dosing in relationship to aspirin therapy: With routine or long-term administration, ibuprofen should be taken at least 8 hours before taking aspirin or 30 to 120 minutes after taking aspirin.[30] The clinical significance of this interaction is not fully understood; however, the occasional use of ibuprofen is unlikely to significantly interfere with aspirin's antiplatelet activity.

Naproxen Naproxen is well absorbed; food delays the rate but not the extent of absorption.[2] Peak plasma concentrations of naproxen are achieved in 2 to 4 hours, while the sodium formulation (naproxen sodium) will achieve these levels in less time, therefore decreasing the time for onset of action. Concomitant administration of sodium bicarbonate will accelerate the rate of absorption.[2] The plasma half-life is variable and ranges from 14 hours in the young to approximately twice this in the elderly because of decreased renal function. Naproxen and its metabolites are eliminated by the kidneys; therefore, renal disease may be exacerbated with its long-term use. It is 99% plasma-protein bound.

Naproxen is available as either naproxen sodium (200-, 250-, or 500-mg tablets) or as naproxen (250-, 375-, or 500-mg tablets; 125 mg/5 mL suspension; 375 or 500 mg controlled-release). When naproxen sodium is prescribed, the dosage is 550 mg initially followed by 550 mg every 12 hours or 275 mg every 6 to 8 hours. The total daily dose on day 1 should not exceed 1,375 mg and thereafter the total daily dose should not exceed 1,100 mg. For naproxen, the dosage is 500 mg initially, followed by 500 mg every 12 hours or 250 mg every 6 to 8 hours. The total daily dose on day 1 should not exceed 1,250 mg and thereafter the total daily dose should not exceed 1,000 mg. When the controlled-release formulation is used, the total daily dose is 1,000 mg, but for patients requiring greater analgesic benefit, 1,500 mg/day may be used for a limited period.[32]

Naproxen crosses the placenta, and approximately 1% is found in breast milk. GI side effects occur at approximately the same frequency as they do with indomethacin, but with less severity. Drowsiness, headache, dizziness, sweating, fatigue, depression, and ototoxicity have been observed. Pruritus and other dermatologic problems are observed less often. Rarely observed are jaundice, impairment of renal function, angioedema, thrombocytopenia, and agranulocytosis; all are seemingly associated with prolonged treatment.

Fenoprofen Fenoprofen, taken orally, is rapidly absorbed, but only about 85% reaches the bloodstream. Food impairs absorption but may reduce GI side effects. Peak plasma concentrations are achieved within 2 hours.[2] Concomitant use of antacids does not alter plasma concentrations. It is highly plasma-protein bound and extensively metabolized and excreted by the kidneys. The plasma half-life is approximately 3 hours.[2] Approximately 15% of patients experience GI side effects. Other side effect profiles are similar to other propionic acid–derived traditional NSAIDs. The usual daily dosage is 200 to 600 mg three to four times per day. Total daily dose should not exceed 3,200 mg.[33]

Ketoprofen Ketoprofen has a pharmacologic profile similar to that of the other propionic acid derivatives. Its plasma half-life is approximately 2 hours, except in the elderly, in whom it may demonstrate a longer half-life.[2] Ketoprofen is conjugated in the liver and excreted in the urine. First-day dosage is 75 mg every 8 hours or 50 mg every 6 hours followed by 25 to 50 mg every 6 to 8 hours daily. The initial dose should be decreased in patients older than 75 years even if they demonstrate normal serum creatinine or blood urea nitrogen (BUN) levels. It is available in normal-release tablets or capsules (12.5, 25, 50, and 75 mg) or extended-release capsules (100, 150, and 200 mg).

Total daily dose of regular formulations should not exceed 300 mg, while the total daily dose of the extended-release forms should not exceed 200 mg. For patients with mildly impaired renal function, the maximum recommended total daily dose is 150 mg. For patients with more severe renal impairment (glomerular filtration rate < 25 mL/min) or end-stage renal impairment, the maximum total daily dose should be 100 mg. For patients with impaired liver function and serum albumin concentration < 3.5 g/dL, the maximum initial daily dose should be 100 mg. Patients with hypoalbuminemia and/or reduced renal function have an increased fraction of free drug available and therefore would be at a greater risk of adverse effects and should be given lower doses and monitored closely.[32]

The side effect profile is similar to that of the other propionic acid derivatives. Approximately 30% of patients experience GI side effects. Severity of GI side effects can be reduced if ketoprofen is taken with food or antacids. It has been known to increase plasma creatinine, especially in the elderly and/or those taking diuretics. Renal function studies should be performed routinely on patients requiring long-term therapy.

Flurbiprofen Flurbiprofen shares a similar pharmacologic profile with the other propionic acid derivatives. Flurbiprofen is available as 50- and 100-mg tablets. The initial recommended total daily dose is 200 to 300 mg. This total dose should be divided over two to four doses for the first day. Subsequent daily doses should not exceed 100 mg at any one time and are usually divided over three or four doses per day. The total routine daily dose should not exceed 300 mg.[32]

COX-2 selective NSAIDs

The clinically used COX-2 inhibitors are referred to as *coxibs*. Celecoxib was the first of these to be cleared by the FDA in December of 1998.[34] Rofecoxib and valdecoxib showed greater COX-2 selectivity than celecoxib but have been removed from the market by the FDA because of increased cardiovascular complications associated with the use of these two agents.

Celecoxib is lipophilic, so it concentrates in fat and readily crosses the blood-brain barrier. Because of this, celecoxib has a central analgesic effect along with a prostaglandin-inhibiting peripheral effect.[2,31] Celecoxib is well absorbed, reaches peak plasma level in 2 to 4 hours with 97% plasma protein binding, and has a plasma half-life of 6 to 12 hours. Celecoxib is metabolized predominantly by the enzyme CYP2C9 and inhibits CYP2D6, which is responsible for metabolizing approximately 20% of all drugs. Poor metabolizers may develop high concentrations of celecoxib, while fast metabolizers may be prone to drug interactions. Celecoxib inhibits the metabolism of the selective β-blocker metoprolol and therefore allows for its accumulation. Coxibs do not pharmacodynamically enhance the bleeding risk of warfarin, but valdecoxib and rofecoxib may have affected the disposition of warfarin, leading to increased international normalized ratio (INR) and the risk of bleeding. Interactions of significance are known to occur with fluconazole and lithium.

Ketoconazole does not appear to interact with celecoxib.[6] Awareness of potential interactions is important when administering celecoxib with drugs that either inhibit CYP2C9 or drugs that are metabolized by CYP2D6. COX-2 selective and traditional NSAIDs may limit the effectiveness of some antihypertensives. These drugs must be used with good judg-

ment in patients with secondary hyperaldosteronism due to hepatic, cardiac, or renal insufficiency.[2] Renal insufficiency produces a clinically insignificant decrease in plasma concentration. Patients with mild to moderate hepatic impairment may experience a 40% to 180% increase in plasma concentrations. Patients with moderate hepatic disease should have their dosages reduced by at least 50%.[33]

Celecoxib's recommended dose for acute pain is 400 mg initially with a follow-up dose of 200 mg 12 hours later. Subsequent dosages should be 100 to 200 mg twice daily. The dose should be reduced by 50% in patients with moderate hepatic impairment (Child-Pugh Class B). It should be remembered that coxibs have not been shown to have greater clinical efficacy compared with traditional NSAIDs.[2] Celecoxib has not demonstrated superiority over traditional NSAIDs in decreasing adverse GI effects. Celecoxib is cleared for use in the United States only for the treatment of osteoarthritis and rheumatoid arthritis. It may be beneficial in treating postoperative dental pain, but it has not been proven to be superior to the less expensive traditional NSAIDs. Research does not support the use of celecoxib as a first choice over traditional NSAIDs in treating dental pain.

Conclusion

Traditional NSAIDs are effective agents in the treatment of postoperative dental pain and should be considered the first line of treatment for patients not presenting with contraindications to NSAID use. NSAIDs should not be used in patients with nephropathy, erosive ulceration of the GI tract, anticoagulant therapy, hemorrhagic disorders, a history of NSAID (or aspirin) intolerance or hypersensitivity, or uncontrolled cardiovascular disease. The concurrent use of antihypertensive therapy represents a relative contraindication. Recommended dosages of specific NSAIDs are provided in Table 5-5.

Table 5-5 | Recommended NSAID dosages

Generic name	Trade name	Adult dosage
Aspirin	Bayer (Bayer Healthcare)	325–650 mg every 4 hours
Diflunisal	Dolobid (Merck)	100 mg initially, then 500 mg two to three times per day
Ibuprofen	Advil (Wyeth), Motrin (McNeil)	200–600 mg every 6 hours
Naproxen sodium	Aleve (Bayer), Anaprox (Roche)	275–550 mg twice daily
Naproxen	Naprosyn, Naprosyn suspension (Roche), Naprelan (Elan)	375–500 mg twice daily
Fenoprofen	Nalfon (Pedinol)	200–600 mg three to four times daily
Ketoprofen	No US trade name	50–75 mg three to four times daily (maximum 300 mg/day)
Flurbiprofen	Ansaid (Pfizer)	50–75 mg two to four times daily
Oxaprozin	Daypro (Pfizer) Celebrex (Pfizer)	600–1,200 mg once daily 200 mg/day
Celecoxib	Mobic (Boehringer Ingelheim)	7.5–15 mg once daily
Meloxicam	Relafen (GlaxoSmithKline)	1,000 mg initially followed by 1,500–2,000 mg/day
Nabumetone	No US trade name	1,000 mg daily; may increase to 1,000 mg twice daily

Acetaminophen

Acetaminophen (eg, Tylenol, McNeil) is the active metabolite of phenacetin, a drug that was removed from the market in 1984 because of its association with nephropathy and hemolytic anemia. Acetaminophen is a suitable alternative to aspirin because it lacks the unwanted GI side effects. In potency and efficacy, it is equal to aspirin but inferior to traditional NSAIDs. Acetaminophen demonstrates weak anti-inflammatory effects because it partially inhibits COXs. It has been determined that it is a COX-3 inhibitor with slight inhibition of COX-1 and COX-2.[35,36] COX-3 is found in sites of low peroxide formation such as the hypothalamus, not in inflammatory sites, which have high peroxide concentrations.[2] Oral absorption of acetaminophen is excellent with little irritation. The peak plasma concentration is achieved in 30 to 60 minutes, and the plasma half-life is approximately 2 hours.

Single or multiple therapeutic doses of acetaminophen do not seem to affect the cardiovascular or respiratory systems, platelets, or coagulation. Toxic doses of acetaminophen are 10 to 15 grams (150 to 250 mg/kg), with 20 to 25 grams being potentially fatal in normal, healthy individuals.[2,37–39] The toxic dose is lower if the patient is experiencing depleted glycogen levels. Glycogen levels may be depleted as a result of dieting, anorexia, primary liver dysfunction, or more than 1,000 hepatotoxic medications such as sulfonamides, dapsone, ketoconazole, isoniazid, rifampin, and phenytoin.[40,41] In patients with chronic liver disease or alcoholism, the maximum daily dose is 2.0 g versus the normal 4.0 g. Patients who consume alcohol on a routine daily basis should be instructed to continue consuming their normal daily intake of alcohol while taking acetaminophen and only use half the normal acetaminophen dosage. For alcoholics, the sudden cessation of ethanol consumption creates a major risk of enhanced acetaminophen toxicity. This is a drug interaction that has been given a severity rating of *major* because it is established, probable, or suspected. Alcoholic patients may have more fat in the liver and suffer from malnutrition, which may further predispose them to acetaminophen toxicity.

Conventional oral dosage of acetaminophen is 325 to 1,000 mg every 6 hours (maximum 4.0 g/day). For patients unable to use the oral route of administration, the rectal recommended dosage is 650 mg every 6 hours (2.6 g/day). Epidemiologic studies imply that therapeutic dosages of acetaminophen demonstrate fewer adverse GI effects than therapeutic dosages of traditional NSAIDs.[42] Higher dosages of acetaminophen, which may achieve complete COX inhibition, begin to approach the adverse side effect rate of traditional NSAIDs.

Opioid analgesics

Patients given therapeutic dosages of opioids for pain predictably experience reduced discomfort, decreased intensity of pain, and/or complete remission of pain. Drowsiness and euphoria or dysphoria often occur along with the analgesic response. Patients also may experience nausea and occasionally vomiting, difficulty in cognition, apathy, a decreased desire for physical activity, constipation, and urinary retention; however, these side effects are seen more frequently in the elderly and in those not accustomed to routine use of opioids. The other side effects listed in Box 5-1 tend to occur with longer-term use.

Patients frequently state that the pain is still present but more tolerable with opioid treatment. At therapeutic dosages, continuous dull pain is relieved more effectively than sharp intermittent pain, although higher dosages can relieve more severe pain. Pain caused by activation of nociceptors and transmitted over intact neural pathways (nociceptive pain) is responsive to opioid analgesics, but pain that is caused by damage to neural structures causing neural supersensitivity (neuropathic pain) is poorly responsive to opioids.[2,43] The analgesic effect of opioids can be summarized as altering the sensation of pain and also decreasing the usual secondary responses such as anxiety, fear, panic, and suffering that a patient may experience when pain is induced.

Most opioids are rapidly absorbed from the GI tract but are then subject to first-pass metabolism in the liver. Therefore, the oral dosage required to elicit a therapeutic effect may be much higher than parenteral dosages. Hepatic enzyme activity responsible for first-pass metabolism varies considerably individually; therefore, the effective oral dosage in one particular patient is difficult to predict.[44]

Two commonly prescribed opioid analgesics used in dentistry, codeine and oxycodone, have greater oral efficacy than morphine; however, the required oral dosage still is significantly greater compared with the parenteral dosage.[2,44] Transdermal administration of fentanyl has become important for patients suffering from chronic pain because it provides stable blood levels of the drug and better pain control while avoiding the need for repeated parenteral injections. Other routes of administration are intranasal (butorphanol) and buccal transmucosal (fentanyl), both of which prevent repeated parenteral injections and avoidance of first-pass metabolism.[44] However, for dental implant procedures, the oral route is the principle administration route.

Fortunately, most analgesic needs for dental implant surgeries are short term. Some patients may present with a medical history of current or chronic opioid use, which must be considered when making management decisions. One concern is the development of tolerance and dependence with chronic use of these drugs. Development of tolerance begins with the initial dose of an opioid but is not clinically manifested until after 2 to 3 weeks of routine exposure to therapeutic dosages. Cross-tolerance from one opioid to another can occur.[44]

Box 5-1	Adverse effects of opioids

- Respiratory depression
- Nausea
- Vomiting
- Constipation
- Urinary retention
- Behavioral restlessness, tremulousness, hyperactivity
- Dysphoria
- Euphoria
- Postural hypotension
- Sedation
- Histamine release (parenteral administration)
- Tolerance
- Physical dependence

Tolerance is minimized by giving smaller doses with longer intervals between doses.

The chemical classes of opioids that are of interest in dentistry are the phenanthrenes, phenylheptylamines, and phenylpiperidines. Each of these classes is divided into groups based on their relative agonist potency. Table 5-6 provides the chemical classifications and relative potencies of several opioids. If a patient has a history of true immunoglobulin-induced allergic reaction to one agent in the class, he or she potentially will demonstrate a similar reaction to other drugs in the same

Table 5-6 Classification of opioids

Chemical class	Relative agonist potency	Agent	Source (natural or synthetic)	Trade name	Combination drugs (oral)*	Controlled drug schedule
Phenanthrenes	Strong (full agonist)	Morphine	Natural	MS-Contin (Purdue)	None	II
		Hydromorphone	Natural	Dilaudid (Purdue)	None	II
		Oxymorphone	Natural	Numorphan (DuPont)	None	II
	Mild to moderate (partial agonist)	Codeine	Natural	Multiple generic	Acetaminophen/codeine (generic) 300/15, 300/30, 325/30 mg; Tylenol w/codeine 15/300, 30/300, 60/300 mg (also contains sodium metabisulfite)	III
		Oxycodone	Natural	Multiple generic	Oxycodone/acetaminophen (generic) 5/325 mg or 5/500 mg; Percocet (Endo) 5/500 mg; Roxicet (Roxane) 5/500 mg; Endocet (Endo) 5/500 mg; Tylox (McNeil) 5/500 mg (also contains sodium metabisulfite)	III
		Hydrocodone	Natural	NA	Hydrocodone/acetaminophen (generic) 5/500, 7.5/500, 7.5/650, 10/650 mg; Vicodin (Abbott) 5/500 mg; Vicodin ES 7.5/750 mg; Vicodin HP 10/650 mg; Lorcet HD (UAD) 5/500 mg; Lorcet Plus 7.5/650 mg; Lorcet 10/650 mg; Lortab (UCB) 5/500, 7.5/500, 10/500 mg; Vicoprofen (Abbott) (hydrocodone 7.5 mg plus ibuprofen 200 mg)	III
Phenylheptylamines	Strong (full agonist)	Methadone, levomethadyl acetate	Synthetic	Not used in dentistry	None	II
	Mild to moderate (partial agonist)	Propoxyphene	Synthetic	Darvon-N (Xanodyne); Darvon Pulvules	Propoxyphene HCl w/acetaminophen (generic) 65/650 mg; Propoxyphene napsylate w/acetaminophen (generic) 50/325, 100/650 mg; Darvocet-N 50 (Xanodyne) 50/325 mg; Darvocet-N 100 100/650 mg	IV
Phenylpiperidines	Strong (full agonist)	Meperidine	Synthetic	Demerol (Hospira)	Meperidine w/acetaminophen (generic) 50/100 mg; Demerol 50/100 mg (liquid 50 mg/5 mL)	II
		Fentanyl	Synthetic	Sublimaze (Taylor); Duragesic (Ortho-McNeil-Janssen) (transdermal)	None	II
Benzomorphans	Weak antagonist (μ-opioid receptor) or partial agonist (μ- and κ-opioid receptors)	Pentazocine	Synthetic	Talwin (Hospira)	Talwin NX (pentazocine 50 mg w/naloxone 0.5 mg)	NA
Miscellaneous	Weak	Tramadol	Synthetic	Ultram (PriCara)	None	NA

NA—not applicable.
*Many combination products are available; only a few of the more commonly prescribed ones are listed.

class. If opioid analgesia is needed and such an allergy exists, it would be prudent to use an agent from a different chemical classification.

Morphine is a strong agonist and should be used only to treat severe pain. Rarely does it have a use in implant dentistry. MS-Contin (sustained-release oral morphine) has great abuse potential and should be used only in patients with terminal disease and intractable pain.

Meperidine is typically prescribed in medicine for the hospitalized patient or those with severe pain induced by cancer. Meperidine, like morphine, is rarely needed in implant dentistry.

Codeine and its derivatives (ie, oxycodone and hydrocodone) are all less effective than morphine. These compounds are rarely used alone but rather in combination with aspirin or acetaminophen.[26] Codeine demonstrates greater oral efficacy than morphine. It should be noted that codeine has a low affinity for opioid receptors and the majority of its analgesic effect is due to its conversion to morphine. The conversion of codeine to morphine is affected by the genetic polymorphisms of the cytochrome enzyme CYP2D6, which may lead to the inability of the patient to convert codeine to morphine. Codeine is ineffective as an analgesic for about 10% of the white population.[43,45] An enhanced metabolism by other polymorphisms leads to an increased sensitivity to codeine's effects. Various ethnic groups appear to have varying metabolic efficiency. For example, Asians metabolize less morphine from codeine than do Caucasians and are less sensitive to morphine's side effects.

Tramadol is a synthetic codeine analog. Onset of action occurs within 1 hour with peak analgesia in 2 to 3 hours. The duration of action is 6 hours. Common side effects are nausea, vomiting, dizziness, dry mouth, sedation, and headache. Respiratory depression and constipation are less common than that observed with codeine.[2] The efficacy of tramadol is equivalent to the combination of aspirin and codeine. Due to the inhibition of serotonin by tramadol, it should not be prescribed for patients who are also taking monoamine oxidase inhibitors (MAOIs) such as selegiline or phenelzine; the combination may lead to mania or hypertension. Seizures have been reported with tramadol use and tramadol possibly can exacerbate seizure in patients with predisposing factors.[2]

Acetaminophen-opioid combinations

For pharmacologic reasons, ease of administration, and patient compliance, the combination of acetaminophen and an opioid narcotic often is prescribed. Such combination formulations are varied in concentration with respect to each of the ingredients. Dosages of opioids should be adjusted according to the severity of pain and the patient's reaction to the medication. Adult doses of codeine greater than 60 mg fail to provide additional pain relief but instead merely prolong analgesia and are associated with a marked increase in side effects. For a healthy patient with no contraindications, the analgesic dosage for combination drugs is 30 to 60 mg of codeine per dose every 4 to 6 hours, with the acetaminophen dosage not exceeding 4,000 mg per day. When contraindications to either medication are present, dosages must be adjusted accordingly or not prescribed. It is the practitioner's responsibility to review each patient's medical history to assure proper prescribing of analgesic medications and dosages.

Many of the acetaminophen-opioid combinations (eg, Vicodin ES, Vicodin HP, Lorcet Plus) and some generics contain 650 or 750 mg of acetaminophen per tablet, which does not permit the prescribing of two tablets every 6 hours (or more frequently) because this would exceed the total recommended daily dose of acetaminophen. The acetaminophen total daily dose should be reduced to 2,000 mg in the presence of decreased liver function or chronic alcohol use (see acetaminophen section). Lortab is available in combinations of 5, 7.5, and 10 mg hydrocodone per 500 mg of acetaminophen, allowing the prescription of one or two tablets every 6 hours in the healthy patient. Table 5-7 presents recommended combination opioid dosages.

Table 5-7	Combination opioid dosages
Drug and strength	**Dosages**
Acetaminophen/codeine 300/15 or 300/30 mg	One or two every 4 hours
Acetaminophen/codeine 300/60 mg	One every 4 hours
Oxycodone/acetaminophen 5/325 or 5/500 mg	One every 6 hours
Hydrocodone/acetaminophen 5/500 or 7.5/500 mg	One or two every 4 to 6 hours; up to eight per day
Hydrocodone/acetaminophen 7.5/650 or 10/650 mg	One every 4 to 6 hours; up to six per day
Hydrocodone/acetaminophen 7.5/750 mg	One every 4 hours; up to four per day
Propoxyphene napsylate/acetaminophen 50/325 mg	One or two every 4 hours
Propoxyphene HCl/acetaminophen 65/650 mg Propoxyphene napsylate w/acetaminophen 100/650 mg	One every 4 hours; up to six per day
Hydrocodone/ibuprofen 7.5/200 mg	One every 4 to 6 hours; up to eight per day

Anesthetic-analgesic pain-management algorithm

Controlling intra- and postoperative pain is of great importance for perceived and actual success of the dental implant surgical and prosthetic appointments. It is best to have a logical, science-based pain-management plan. Pain management that does not interfere with the patient's subsequent daily activities is desirable. Considering the side effects of opioids, it therefore is prudent to use them only as a last resort. Most pain can be managed well with traditional NSAIDs. Provided the patient is healthy and does not present with contraindications, the following is a suggested science- and evidence-based pain-management algorithm:

Step 1

Most postoperative pain reaches a peak within 2 to 6 hours after surgical completion. Using a long-acting local anesthetic, such as bupivacaine 0.5% with epinephrine 1:200,000, provides prolonged anesthesia and helps manage immediate postoperative discomfort. The patient must be made aware of the prolonged numbness and instructed to be careful that lips, cheeks, or tongue are not traumatized while talking or masticating.

Step 2

The patient should be given a first dose of a traditional NSAID 30 to 60 minutes prior to surgery. If the patient is receiving sedation and has had nothing by mouth, then administration of the NSAID can resume immediately postoperatively. It would be best to give a dosage of an NSAID that would be anti-inflammatory, eg, ibuprofen 600 mg every 6 hours postoperatively for 3 to 5 days and continued as needed thereafter.

Step 3

If the ibuprofen (or other traditional NSAID) does not control the pain adequately, then acetaminophen 500 to 1,000 mg every 6 hours should be added. In this case, the patient will be taking ibuprofen 600 mg and acetaminophen 500 to 1,000 mg every 6 hours. The drugs may be alternated every 3 hours to lessen irritation to the stomach, particularly if the patient is not eating. These dosages are within the therapeutic range and should not be misinterpreted as being excessive.

Step 4

If steps 2 and 3 do not control the pain adequately (eg, if there are breakthrough episodes of pain), a narcotic should be added to the regimen. Usually a combination formulation of acetaminophen and codeine, hydrocodone, or oxycodone is added. For every combination tablet given, the prescribing practitioner must confirm that the total acetaminophen dose for 24 hours does not exceed 4,000 mg (2,000 mg in patients with compromised liver functions). An ideal narcotic-acetaminophen combination to use is one that contains 500 mg of acetaminophen. In such cases, for each narcotic-acetaminophen combination tablet given, the patient should drop 500 mg acetaminophen from step 3.

Conclusion

The above algorithm uses three separate mechanisms of analgesic action to alleviate the patient's discomfort. Each step logically adds another mechanism that is synergistic to the previous step. It has been found that this regimen is acceptable to the majority of patients. If a patient feels that a narcotic is necessary from the beginning, a brief explanation of the effectiveness of traditional NSAIDs and acetaminophen versus oral narcotics may increase patient acceptance of the above algorithm.

Steroids

Steroids often are used in dentistry to help control postoperative discomfort caused by inflammation, although there is some controversy surrounding their use. The steroids frequently used in dentistry are glucocorticoid in nature and usually are derivatives or synthetic analogs of the endogenous hormone *cortisol*.

Exogenously administered corticosteroids are categorized by their relative potencies in sodium retention, effects on carbohydrate metabolism, and anti-inflammatory effects. Each of these effects reflects selective actions at distinct receptors in the various tissues or organs. Table 5-8 provides the relative anti-inflammatory and sodium-retaining potencies, equipotent doses, durations of action, and available forms of various corticosteroids.

Table 5-8 **Comparison of corticosteroids**					
Corticosteroid	Relative anti-inflammatory potency (cortisol = 1)	Relative sodium-retaining potency (cortisol = 1)	Equipotent dose (mg)	Duration of action (hours)	Available forms
Cortisol	1	1	20	8	Oral, injectable, topical
Cortisone	0.8	0.8	25	8	Oral, injectable, topical
Prednisone	4	0.8	5	16–36	Oral
Triamcinolone	5	0	4	12–36	Oral, injectable, topical
Betamethasone	25	0	0.75	36–54	Oral, injectable, topical
Dexamethasone	25	0	0.75	36–54	Oral, injectable, topical

Preventive and therapeutic applications

The proper use of glucocorticoid steroids to prevent inflammation will lead to decreased swelling and postoperative pain. Glucocorticoid steroids also will help reduce local congestion caused by the inflammation process due to the increased migration of the anti-inflammatory monocytes to the site, where they will have the enhanced ability to clear debris.

If the inferior alveolar, mental, or infraorbital nerves were violated iatrogenically during the surgical procedure, and the offending dental implant was removed or the injury was not overly severe, the use of a glucocorticoid may diminish the damage by keeping the inflammatory response to a minimum. Additionally, it may be of benefit in accelerating recovery of normal sensory perception. Multicenter trials have revealed significant decreases in neurologic defects in patients with acute spinal cord injury if treatment with large dosages of methylprednisolone (30 mg/kg initially followed by an infusion of 5.4 mg/kg/hour for 23 hours) is begun within 8 hours of injury. There was no increase in the rate of infection with this short-term high steroid dosage.[18]

Adverse effects

Glucocorticoids may aggravate glycemic control in patients with overt diabetes and can precipitate hyperglycemia in patients who are otherwise predisposed.[2] The use of glucocorticoids in diabetic patients is therefore controversial and rightly so. Glucocorticoids should only be used in life-threatening situations for the patient with uncontrolled diabetes; there does not appear to be a valid reason for using these agents in the dental implant arena for a patient with uncontrolled diabetes. Patients with controlled diabetes may be administered glucocorticoids for a short time period at reduced dosages and with careful monitoring of blood glucose levels. Most patients with well-controlled type 1 (insulin-dependent) diabetes are accustomed to adjusting their daily insulin doses based on their current blood glucose values. The patient's physician should be consulted for the advisability of glucocorticoid use for these individuals.

Higher dosages of glucocorticoids often produce behavioral changes that include insomnia and euphoria initially, followed by depression. Other effects at high dosages include increased intracranial pressure (pseudotumor cerebri), peptic ulcer, fat redistribution, decreased vitamin D and calcium absorption, and an increase in platelet and red blood cell numbers.

Glucocorticoids can induce hypertension by an as-yet unknown mechanism. This hypertension persists even with decreased sodium consumption.[2] Patients receiving glucocorticoids should be monitored carefully for the development of hyperglycemia, glycosuria, and sodium retention with edema or hypertension.[2] These changes will be of little consequence with short-term therapy, provided there are no contraindications to their use. Glucocorticoids should be used with caution in patients with active peptic ulcer, heart disease, hypertension, congestive heart failure, systemic infections, psychoses, diabetes, osteoporosis, glaucoma, or herpes simplex infections.[2] Those with uncontrolled diabetes or cardiovascular disease should not be given steroids without careful monitoring and supervision by an appropriate medical specialist.

Rationale for use

Unfortunately, glucocorticoids are not used to full prophylactic benefit because of misconceptions and improper use. Cited reasons for avoiding the use of steroids are:

1. Hypothalamic-pituitary-adrenal (HPA) axis suppression
2. Increased infection
3. Occurrence of inflammation and swelling after steroids are cleared from the body (approximately 2 to 3 days)

However, the current body of knowledge regarding glucocorticoids provides evidence that short-term use will not induce HPA axis suppression nor will patients have a higher incidence of infection. Antibody production is affected by large dosages of steroids but not by moderate dosages (eg, 20 mg of prednisone per day). In addition, long-term (but not short-term) glucocorticoid use is associated with an increased susceptibility to infection and the risk for reactivation of latent tuberculosis. Therefore, in the presence of infections, steroids should be administered only if absolutely necessary and concomitantly with appropriate and effective antimicrobial or antifungal therapy.[2] With short-term use and in the absence of infection, there has not been a significant increase in reported infection.[18]

It is true that if therapy lasting less than the normal 7- to 10-day inflammatory cycle is used, the patient eventually will experience inflammation, although the severity is lessened. This eventual inflammatory response can be lessened further or eliminated by providing steroid coverage for 7 days, which would still be less than the timeline known to cause the more severe adverse reactions. Traditional NSAIDs are effective in managing any late inflammation.

Suggested protocol

Provided no contraindications are present and the patient is of normal weight and neither very young nor elderly (in which case dosages would need to be adjusted), glucocorticoid dosages should be determined according to the degree of surgical invasiveness the patient will undergo (ie, lower dosages for minor procedures and higher dosages for more aggressive procedures). Dosages should be decreased for patients who are elderly or have complications.

When injectable glucocorticoids are used, they should be administered immediately prior to surgery. A suggested dose would be dexamethasone sodium phosphate 4 to 8 mg intravenously (IV) or deep intramuscularly (IM) in a large muscle mass. After the procedure is completed, a long-acting IM glucocorticoid, such as methylprednisolone acetate suspension 20 to 60 mg, should be administered via deep IM injection. Note that the acetate suspension cannot be administered IV; it should be administered only deep IM, preferably into a large muscle. Some have advocated administration of the injectable forms into the mucobuccal fold or masseter muscle; however, this is not advisable because it may induce tissue necrosis when injected into a small muscle.

If the patient or practitioner prefers to use oral rather than injectable medication, a Medrol DosePak (Pfizer) should be taken as directed. A Medrol DosePak consists of 21 tablets of 4 mg each. The DosePak is designed with rows of tablets; the patient should take the complete row for each day. Each row represents an initial high dose then diminishing doses of methylprednisolone each day. The patient should be instructed to take the first row prior to the start of the surgical procedure.

Notwithstanding the route of administration, patients should be informed that they may experience insomnia that will pass in a few days. Medical histories should be verified to assure that there are no known contraindications to the use of glucocorticoids. Long-term use of glucocorticoids as an adjunct to dental implant surgery is not valid or indicated.

If a patient is currently taking glucocorticoids routinely for other medical conditions (eg, acute or chronic adrenal insufficiency, congenital adrenal hyperplasia, rheumatic disorders, renal disease, bronchial asthma or other pulmonary diseases, allergy, ocular diseases, some infectious diseases, gastrointestinal disease, hepatic diseases, malignancies, cerebral edema, autoimmune diseases, or chronic skin disorders), the patient's prescribing physician should be consulted as to the advisability of a temporary dosage increase. It also should be noted that dental implant surgery may be contraindicated in some of the mentioned disease states. Abrupt cessation of glucocorticoids after prolonged therapy is associated with the risk of adrenal insufficiency due to suppression of the HPA axis and may be fatal. Therefore, if a patient is receiving chronic therapy, it should not be abruptly discontinued.

Bisphosphonate-Related Osteonecrosis of the Jaw

The term *bisphosphonate* refers to a family of drugs used in the treatment of a variety of bone metabolism conditions. Bisphosphonates have proven to be highly effective in the treatment and management of osteoporotic bone diseases with considerable ease of pain and minimization of complications.[46] They have become widely prescribed drugs in different dosages, potencies, and durations in many bone conditions, including Paget disease, bone malignancies, and osteoporosis.[47] Bisphosphonates, including zoledronate (IV), pamidronate (IV), and alendronate (oral), also are used in the treatment of bone lesions of multiple myeloma in patients with breast and prostate cancer.[46] However, long-term intake of bisphosphonates has been implicated in serious medical conditions such as atrial fibrillation and osteonecrosis of the jaw (ONJ).[48]

Bisphosphonate-related ONJ (BRONJ) is a potentially harmful side effect of bisphosphonate therapy. According to recent studies, the best-known triggering event of this severe condition is dentoalveolar surgery. A wide array of extrinsic and intrinsic factors such as duration of therapy, smoking, and surgical procedures also affect the onset of BRONJ. BRONJ affects the mandible more often than the maxilla, implicating an abolition of osteoclast-mediated bone resorption rather than antiangiogenesis.[49,50]

Alveolar bone necrosis is a condition characterized by death of osseous tissue or part of a bone in mass.[49] This has been seen with IV bisphosphonate therapy for treatment of osteolytic bone diseases. Alendronate has been linked to this severe condition in patients being treated for bone malignancies. However, the low, short-term dosages of alendronate used in the treatment of osteoporosis in postmenopausal women are not known to cause bone necrosis.[51]

The prevalence of BRONJ varies from 1% to 10%; however, the frequency and reporting have increased over the past 5 years. In a 2007 Australian study, it was found that the incidence of BRONJ in patients who were taking oral alendronate and had a tooth extracted was 1 in 270. One case was reported per week following 13 weeks of 70 mg of alendronate.[52] Patients treated with bisphosphonates showed evident bone histomorphologic alterations, indicating active osteomyelitis filled with inflammatory infiltrates, acellular necrotic debris, dilated blood vessels, prominent scalloping of the bone trabeculae borders, nonnecrotic areas with large osteonic structures, and abundant deposition of interosteonic woven bone.[51]

BRONJ and toxicity

Most cases of BRONJ occur after 2 to 3 years of continuous treatment at higher dosages (70 mg/week) or 5 years at lower dosages (35 mg/week). Bisphosphonates have a tendency to accumulate in osseous tissue over time. Dental surgical procedures and local trauma may lead to the release of high concentrations of these accumulated chemicals from the bone. High levels of bisphosphonates are toxic to epithelial tissues and may cause failure in wound healing and closure, thus increasing the susceptibility of tissues to infection.[53] Toxicity to epithelial tissues may lead to osteonecrosis of the jaw. Alendronate has been found to be toxic to GI epithelial tissues at a concentration of 30 nmol, while risedronate has been known to be toxic at 10 nmol.[51]

Changes in oral flora

Bisphosphonates have been known to cause a shift in the balance of the normal oral flora. Invasion of bacteria into bone causes osteocyte death and the formation of bacterial biofilms resulting in pocket formation, bone disintegration, and bone loss.[54]

Bisphosphonate use impedes oral cavity host defenses and helps establish a niche for *Actinomyces* within the bone when it is subsequently introduced. Most affected patients show disruption in the mucous membrane lining the oral cavity as a result of dental procedures, trauma, oncologic surgery, or dental diseases.[55] Bisphosphonate inhibition of the life cycle of keratinocytes further aggravates mucosal breakdown and prevents repair. Previous disruption of bone may facilitate infection. *Actinomyces* are thought to then infect living bone without secondarily infecting already necrotic bone.[56]

Timely recognition of actinomycosis is critical. In the absence of appropriate treatment, recovery is unlikely. High dosages of antimicrobials and a prolonged course of antibiotics are needed for management of the condition. It is customary to use 2 to 6 weeks IV therapy, followed by oral therapy for 6 to 12 months for more serious infections. The optimal therapy for BRONJ remains unknown, and therefore, the best and most prudent treatment for BRONJ involves a prolonged combined IV-oral antibiotic-antimicrobial regimen for 9 to 12 months.[57] It also is reasonable to debride the affected area periodically. Stopping bisphosphonate therapy with or without debridement in the absence of appropriate management for actinomycosis is unlikely to result in improvement.

General features of this unique infection include: *(1)* combination of chronicity, progression across tissue boundaries, and masslike features that mimic malignancy; *(2)* development of sinus tracts that may spontaneously resolve and recur; and *(3)* refractory or relapsing infection after a short course of therapy.

Osteonecrosis solely due to bisphosphonates has not been described in animals or humans with normal bone. The concomitant occurrence of *Actinomyces* infection with BRONJ has been seen in an increasing number of cases. Histologic studies have shown a nearly universal presence of *Actinomy-* *ces*-like organisms from affected bone. Furthermore, *Actinomyces* can instigate bone resorption.

Trauma

A history of dentoalveolar trauma, denture use, and poor oral hygiene are risk factors for BRONJ. Ruggiero et al[58] reported 63 cases of BRONJ from their oral surgery practice over a span of 2 years, and 86% of these patients had undergone a previous dental procedure that did not heal.

Preventive measures

Because surgical trauma is the most common initiating event of BRONJ, maintenance of good oral hygiene and dental care is advisable to prevent the necessity of dental surgery. For patients on bisphosphonate treatment for 3 to 4 months, a checkup should be performed every 6 months to detect early signs of BRONJ. However, in the case of imperative dental procedures, a conservative and less traumatic dental procedure should be adopted with the use of antibiotics whenever necessary.[59] If dental surgery is necessary during bisphosphonate treatment, bisphosphonate therapy may need to be suspended for 3 to 4 months until the site of the surgical procedure has healed.

Currently, medical and dental disciplines are unable to accurately predict which patients may be susceptible to developing BRONJ following an oral surgical procedure.[60] However, the use of bone turnover markers (BTMs) and bone mineral density (BMD) studies provide some indication of the patient's overall bone metabolic stability. If BTMs such as the patient serum cross-linked N-terminal telopeptide (NTX) and serum bone-specific alkaline phosphatase (BSAP) values are within an acceptable range, the implant dentist should consult with the prescribing physician and discuss if a bisphosphonate therapy holiday would be acceptable (if the patient has been on bisphosphonates for 2 years or more). If any of the values are out of range, this may indicate that the bisphosphonate therapy is ineffective, and therefore other treatment modalities (eg, teriparatide) may be indicated. Repeating these tests annually provides guidance as to when antiresorptive bisphosphonate therapy should be reinstituted.

If the BTMs are within normal range, the implant surgeon may have reason to believe that the patient can undergo surgery successfully. However, all patients who recently have taken a bisphosphonate should be advised that the risk of BRONJ exists. The patient may be at a greater risk of developing BRONJ if BTMs are not within the acceptable range, and it may be advisable to delay implant surgery.

Treatment of patients with BRONJ

Patients showing signs of BRONJ should be treated with systemic antibiotics, oral rinses (0.12% chlorhexidine gluconate or minocycline hydrochloride), pain control, and limited debridement.[61] Microbial cultures may help identify infectious microorganisms that may require antibiotics and antiseptic mouthwash.[62]

In advanced and more severe stages, long-term IV antibiotic treatment may be necessary with aggressive surgical debridement.[46,52,63] A penicillin and metronidazole combination is useful in patients with refractory and recurrent infections. Azithromycin or a quinolone may be used instead of penicillin in allergic patients.[58,64]

Bleeding Problems in Patients Taking Anticoagulants or Antiplatelet Agents

Many implants are placed in medically compromised patients, and the implant dentist often will find that these individuals are currently taking either anticoagulants or antiplatelet agents to prevent venous or arterial thrombosis. The implant dentist will need to have a sound foundation on which to base decisions regarding whether the patient should remain on the medication or discontinue it. If a decision is made to discontinue medication, the duration of the discontinuation period must be determined. A comprehensive medical history is imperative to optimize the patient's treatment and minimize the morbidity risk. The implant dentist should follow the guidelines presented in Box 5-2 when treating patients receiving anticoagulant therapy.[65]

Box 5-2	Guidelines for dental treatment of patients receiving anticoagulants/antiplatelet agents*

1. Identify the reason the patient is receiving anticoagulation therapy.
2. Know the laboratory tests used to assess anticoagulation levels.
3. Evaluate the potential risk versus benefit of altering the drug's regimen.
4. Be familiar with local methods of obtaining hemostasis both intraoperatively and postoperatively.
5. Consult with the patient's prescribing physician and inform him or her about the type of dental treatment planned and investigate whether there is a need to alter the anticoagulant regimen.

*Based on Jeske and Suchko.[65]

For many years, it was thought that when a patient taking an anticoagulant or antiplatelet agent was to undergo a surgical procedure, the anticoagulant or antiplatelet medication should be discontinued; however, this strategy is no longer acceptable. Disproportionate activation of coagulation or inhibition of anticoagulant mechanisms may result in hypercoagulability and thrombosis. Thrombosis formation is of greater clinical concern in terms of morbidity and mortality compared with all hemorrhagic disorders combined. Thrombosis can be induced by injury to a blood vessel wall, alterations in blood flow, and changes in the composition of blood.[66]

Anticoagulants

Several studies have evaluated the adjustment of oral anticoagulant levels prior to dental procedures.[67] Devani et al[68] concluded that, because of the difficulty in predicting the decrease in INR value in any given patient, the risk of experiencing a thromboembolism overrides the risk of experiencing excessive postoperative bleeding with tooth removal.

The literature supports the idea that bleeding observed from dental surgery in patients with INR values of less than 4.0 is manageable with local measures and that it is not necessary or recommended that anticoagulant (eg, warfarin) therapy be interrupted. Local hemostatic measures may include collagen plugs, powder, or sheets; gelatin sponges with sutures; soaked sponges, mouthrinse, oral tablets, or IV forms of tranexamic acid; vasoconstrictors in local anesthetic; and atraumatic surgical techniques.[38–40]

If the INR value is beyond the acceptable range of ≤ 4.0 and dental implant treatment is deemed necessary, then the prescribing physician should be consulted to determine what the appropriate INR target value should be. Ideally, an INR value should be obtained on the day of the dental procedure, although the INR obtained within the previous 4 weeks may be acceptable. However, if any changes in warfarin therapy or in other medications were instituted since the previous INR, a new INR value should be obtained. Table 5-9 lists the recommended INR therapeutic ranges for warfarin therapies.

Table 5-9	Recommended INR therapeutic ranges		
Intensity	**INR goal**	**INR range**	**Treatment condition**

Low-intensity therapy	2.5	2.0–3.0	• Prophylaxis of venous thromboembolism associated with high-risk surgery
			• Treatment of venous thrombosis and pulmonary embolism
			• Prevention of systemic embolism for patients with:
			  —Prosthetic heart valves
			  —Acute myocardial infarction
			  —Chronic atrial fibrillation
			  —Valvular heart disease

High-intensity therapy	3.0	2.5–3.5	• Mechanical prosthetic heart valve(s) • Prevention of recurrent myocardial infarction • Treatment of thrombosis associated with antiphospholipid antibodies

*Based on Guna et al.[69]

Alteration of anticoagulation (warfarin) therapy

It is of great importance that the implant dentist recognize that anticoagulation therapy is a medical therapy carefully planned and adjusted by the prescribing physician and is not within the scope of dental practice. If it is necessary to alter the warfarin therapy, three strategies can be pursued: (1) reduce the level of anticoagulation by partially withdrawing the warfarin therapy; (2) discontinue the warfarin therapy entirely for a brief time period; or (3) substitute heparin anticoagulant therapy for warfarin.[67]

Partial reduction or interruption of anticoagulant therapy will result in a decreased INR value yet still maintain the INR within the therapeutic target range. A practical way of accomplishing this is by a 2- or 3-day warfarin withdrawal protocol.[47] Following this protocol will keep the duration of reduced anticoagulant to a minimum.[67] Usually a 2-day withdrawal is adequate, but if the patient is elderly or has an extremely high INR, a 3-day protocol may be necessary.[66] Partial reduction or interruption of warfarin therapy should not be carried out without the support of current INR values. Complete cessation of warfarin therapy for greater time periods without supportive INR values is risky and should not be done.[2]

Substitution of warfarin with heparin therapy is a complex and costly medical intervention that should be reserved for patients at greatest risk of thromboembolism (ie, those with mitral valve prostheses) and performed in consultation with the prescribing physician.[2] With the exception of cases in which patients have significantly high INR values, this option is rarely exercised.

Drug interactions

The implant dentist should be aware that many drugs affect the action of warfarin. Drugs that may be used during implant placement or restorative treatment that potentiate the anticoagulant action include acetaminophen, metronidazole, salicylates, broad-spectrum antibiotics, erythromycin, NSAIDs, and COX-2 inhibitors. Other drugs that are known to potentiate warfarin actions are cimetidine, chloral hydrate, phenytoin, propranolol, and thyroid drugs such as thyroxine (T_4) and triiodothyronine (T_3). Drugs that antagonize the effect of warfarin include carbamazepine, cholestyramine, griseofulvin, rifampin, and trazodone.[3]

Antiplatelet agents

Platelets provide the initial hemostatic plug at sites of vascular injury. They also play a part in pathologic thromboses that lead to myocardial infarction, stroke, and peripheral vascular thromboses. Antiplatelet agents include aspirin, dipyridamole, nonaspirin NSAIDs, and adenosine diphosphate (ADP) receptor inhibitors.

Aspirin

Aspirin, the prototype antiplatelet drug, is the least expensive, most often used, and best-known drug in this group.[4,5] Aspirin's maximal antithrombotic effect is achieved at dosages much lower than are required for other actions of aspirin. Higher dosages of aspirin do not prove to be more effective; in fact, they may potentially be less effective. The antiplatelet actions of other salicylates and NSAIDs are reversible, and these agents have a shorter duration of platelet-inhibitory action.[44]

Although there is long-standing concern on the part of dental practitioners about the possibility of prolonged bleeding during and after invasive dental procedures in patients taking aspirin, a prospective study of single-tooth extraction on patients randomized to aspirin versus a placebo failed to show a statistically significant difference in postoperative bleeding.[67] Aspirin use should not be discontinued for dental implant pro-

cedures in patients receiving low doses (81 mg) of aspirin or a single, conventional 325-mg dose daily. If the patient recently or traditionally has taken several adult aspirin tablets daily, the implant dentist in consultation with the patient's physician can consider evaluating platelet function with a platelet function analyzer or an Ivy bleeding time test. Rarely is there significant bleeding (ie, lasting longer than 20 minutes) during or following oral surgical procedures. The risk of excessive bleeding with aspirin is increased by the concurrent use of anticoagulants or alcohol and conditions such as advanced age, liver disease, and coexisting coagulopathies.[66]

Dipyridamole

Dipyridamole is a vasodilator that is used in combination with warfarin. When used as a single agent it has little effect as an antithrombotic drug.[2] Aggrenox (Boehringer Ingelheim) is a formulation containing 200 mg of an extended-release dipyridamole and 25 mg of aspirin. The only current recommended use of dipyridamole is in combination with warfarin for postoperative primary prophylaxis of thromboemboli in patients with prosthetic heart valves.[2] Alteration of dipyridamole-warfarin therapy would only be warranted if the INR is above 4.0 and then only in consultation with the patient's physician.

NSAIDs

NSAIDs are covered extensively in the section on analgesics, but they do merit mention as antiplatelet agents. NSAIDs, such as ibuprofen and indomethacin, have limited clinical use as antiplatelet agents. Salsalate and COX-2 inhibitors, such as celecoxib, do not significantly affect platelet activity when used at a therapeutic dosage.[66] When these are used alone, it is not necessary to discontinue therapy prior to dental implant procedures. Excessive bleeding, if observed, should be controlled by local measures. If the NSAID is being taken for analgesic purposes and not antiplatelet effects, the implant dentist may discontinue it for three half-lives of the NSAID to allow sufficient elimination of the drug and thus allow normal platelet function to return. The risk of excessive bleeding with NSAIDs is increased by the simultaneous use of anticoagulants or alcohol and circumstances such as advanced age, liver disease, and coexisting coagulopathies.[2]

ADP receptor inhibitors

ADP receptor inhibitors are the thienopyridines ticlopidine and clopidogrel. Thienopyridine therapy in combination with aspirin is the principal antiplatelet treatment strategy for the prevention of stent thrombosis. Inappropriate discontinuation of antiplatelet therapy markedly increases the risk of stent thrombosis, a catastrophic event that frequently leads to myocardial infarction and/or death. There have been several reports of mortalities resulting from stent thrombosis that occurred after the discontinuation of thienopyridine antiplatelet therapy for noncardiac surgery among patients recently treated with coronary stents.[24,26,28,29] Implant practitioners concerned about bleeding during and after the procedure must be aware of these potential risks associated with premature discontinuation of thienopyridine therapy. There are no prospective studies of invasive dental procedures on patients taking a thienopyridine alone or in combination with aspirin, but there are also no well-documented cases of clinically significant bleeding after dental procedures, including multiple dental extractions, for this group of patients. The implant practitioner should discuss concerns regarding the patient's thienopyridine therapy and the nature of the implant procedure with the patient's cardiologist to assure optimal patient management.[24]

Because of the predictability with which the incidence and severity of oral bleeding can be reduced with local measures during surgery and the unlikely occurrence of bleeding once an initial clot has formed, there is little or no indication to interrupt the use of these antiplatelet drugs for dental procedures.[30] However, the concurrent use of NSAIDs or salicylates with thienopyridines may increase the risk of bleeding and should therefore be avoided. Cases of thrombotic thrombocytopenic purpura may occur during the first 2 weeks of thienopyridine therapy or after 2 years of therapy in the elderly. For these individuals, a platelet count and bleeding time values can be referenced.

Conclusions

A risk-benefit assessment must be made for each patient currently undergoing anticoagulant or antiplatelet therapy. It should be recognized that dental implant procedures safely can be performed on these patients without the need for altering these therapies. The risk of unwanted thrombosis often-times is of greater consequence than the localized bleeding that may be experienced. However, practitioners should not be cavalier with concerns posed by the use of these medications in their patients and should develop a treatment strategy that addresses all possible risks mentioned in this section.

References

1. McFarland LV. Evidence-based review of probiotics for antibiotic-associated diarrhea and *Clostridium difficile* infections. Anaerobe 2009;15:274–280.

2. Brunton LL (ed). Goodman and Gilman's the Pharmacological Basis of Therapeutics, ed 11. New York: McGraw-Hill Medical, 2006.

3. Lexi-Comp. Lexi-Comp Drug Information Handbook, ed 16. Hudson, OH: Lexi-Comp, 2007.

4. Siqueira JF Jr, Rocas IN. Diversity of endodontic microbiota revisited. J Dent Res 2009;88:969–981.

5. Kolenbrander PE, Andersen RN, Blehert DS, Egland PG, Foster JS, Palmer RJ Jr. Communication among oral bacteria. Microbiol Mol Biol Rev 2002;66:486–505.

6. Brook I. Microbiology of polymicrobial abscesses and implications for therapy. J Antimicrob Chemother 2002;50:805–810.

7. Chastre J. Evolving problems with resistant pathogens. Clin Microbiol Infect 2008;14(suppl 3):3–14.

8. McDonnell Norms Group. Antibiotic overuse: The influence of social norms. J Am Coll Surg 2008;207:265–275.

9. Jones K. Probiotics: Preventing antibiotic-associated diarrhea. J Spec Pediatr Nurs 2010;15:160–162.

10. Joint Formulary Committee. British National Formulary, ed 47. London: British Medical Association and Royal Pharmaceutical Society of Great Britain, 2004.

11. Larrey D, Vial T, Micaleff A, et al. Hepatitis associated with amoxycillin-clavulanic acid combination report of 15 cases. Gut 1992;33:368–371.

12. Mycek MJ, Harvey RA, Champe PC. Pharmacology, ed 2. Philadelphia: Lippincott-Raven, 1997.

13. Olsvik B, Tenover FS. Tetracycline resistance in periodontal pathogens. Clin Infect Dis 1993;16(suppl 4):S310–S313.

14. Morinaka S, Ichimiya M, Nakamura H. Detection of *Helicobacter pylori* in nasal and maxillary sinus specimens from patients with chronic sinusitis. Laryngoscope 2003;113:1557–1563.

15. Yagiela JA, Dowd FJ, Neidle EA. Pharmacology and Therapeutics for Dentistry, ed 5. St Louis: Mosby, 2004.

16. Tatro DS (ed). Drug Interaction Facts: Herbal Supplements and Food. St Louis: Facts and Comparisons, 2002.

17. Matijevic S, Lazic Z, Kuljic-Kapulica N, Nonkovic Z. Empirical antimicrobial therapy of acute dentoalveolar abscess. Vojnosanit Pregl 2009;66:544–550.

18. Becker DE, Phero JC. Drug therapy in dental practice: Nonopioid and opioid analgesics. Anesth Prog 2005;52:140–149.

19. Greenberger PA. 8. Drug allergy. J Allergy Clin Immunol 2006;117(2 suppl mini-primer):S464–S470.

20. Panara MR, Renda G, Sciulli MG, et al. Dose-dependent inhibition of platelet cyclooxygenase-1 and monocyte cyclooxygenase-2 by meloxicam in healthy subjects. J Pharmacol Exp Ther 1999;290:276–280.

21. Patoia L, Santucci L, Furno P, et al. A 4-week, double-blind, parallel-group study to compare the gastrointestinal effects of meloxicam 7.5 mg, meloxicam 15 mg, piroxicam 20 mg and placebo by means of faecal blood loss, endoscopy and symptom evaluation in healthy volunteers. Br J Rheumatol 1996;35(suppl 1):61–67.

22. White WB. Cardiovascular risk, hypertension, and NSAIDs. Curr Rheumatol Rep 2007;9:36–43.

23. Rainsford KD. Anti-inflammatory drugs in the 21st century. Subcell Biochem 2007;42:3–27.

24. Cooper SA, Beaver WT. A model to evaluate mild analgesics in oral surgery outpatients. Clin Pharmacol Ther 1976;20:241–250.

25. McQuay HJ, Carroll D, Guest PG, Robson S, Wiffen PJ, Juniper RP. A multiple dose comparison of ibuprofen and dihydrocodeine after third molar surgery. Br J Oral Maxillofac Surg 1993;31:95–100.

26. Forbes JA, Barkaszi BA, Ragland RN, Hankle JJ. Analgesic effect of fendosal, ibuprofen and aspirin in postoperative oral surgery pain. Pharmacotherapy 1984;4:385–391.

27. Bradley JD, Brandt KD, Katz BP, Kalasinski LA, Ryan SI. Comparison of an antiinflammatory dose of ibuprofen, an analgesic dose of ibuprofen, and acetaminophen in the treatment of patients with osteoarthritis of the knee. N Engl J Med 1991;325:87–91.

28. Brune K, Furst DE. Combining enzyme specificity and tissue selectivity of cyclooxygenase inhibitors: Towards better tolerability? Rheumatology (Oxford) 2007;46:911–919.

29. Schoenfeld A, Bar Y, Merlob P, Ovadia Y. NSAIDs: Maternal and fetal considerations. Am J Reprod Immunol 1992;28:141–147.

30. Catella-Lawson F, Reilly MP, Kapoor SC, et al. Cyclooxygenase inhibitors and the antiplatelet effects of aspirin. N Engl J Med 2001;345:1809–1817.

31. Bejarano F, Herrero JF. A critical appraisal of COX-2 selective inhibition and analgesia: How good so far? Pain Pract 2003;3:201–217.

32. Wickersham RM, Novak KK (eds). Drug Facts and Comparisons. St Louis: Wolters Kluwer, 2005.

33. US Food and Drug Administration. Science Background Paper: Concomitant Use of Ibuprofen and Aspirin: Potential for Attenuation of the Anti-Platelet Effect of Aspirin, 9/8/06. http://www.fda.gov/Drugs/DrugSafety/PostmarketDrugSafetyInformationforPatientsandProviders/ucm110510.htm. Accessed 23 August 2010.

34. Silverstein FE, Faich G, Goldstein JL, et al. Gastrointestinal toxicity with celecoxib vs nonsteroidal anti-inflammatory drugs for osteoarthritis and rheumatoid arthritis: The CLASS study: A randomized controlled trial. Celecoxib long-term arthritis safety study. JAMA 2000;284:1247–1255.

35. Ishida T, Sato T, Irifune M, Tanaka K, Nakamura N, Nisikawa T. Effect of acetaminophen, a cyclooxygenase inhibitor, on Morris water maze task performance in mice. J Psychopharmacol 2007;21:757–767.

36. Courad JP, Besse D, Delchambre C, et al. Acetaminophen distribution in the rat central nervous system. Life Sci 2001;69:1455–1464.

37. Bessems GM, Vermeulen NP. Paracetamol (acetaminophen)-induced toxicity: Molecular and biochemical mechanisms, analogues and protective approaches. Crit Rev Toxicol 2001;31(1):55–138.

38. Moynihan R. FDA fails to reduce accessibility of paracetamol despite 450 deaths a year. BMJ 2002;325:678.

39. Ostapowicz G, Fontana RJ, Schiodt FV, et al. Results of a prospective study of acute liver failure at 17 tertiary care centers in the United States. Ann Intern Med 2002;137:947–954.

40. Lee WM. Acetaminophen and the U.S. Acute Liver Failure Study Group: Lowering the risks of hepatic failure. Hepatology 2004;40:6–9.

41. Lazarou J, Pomeranz BH, Corey PN. Incidence of adverse drug reactions in hospitalized patients: A meta-analysis of prospective studies. JAMA 1998;279:1200–1205.

42. García Rodríguez LA, Hernández-Díaz S. Risk of uncomplicated peptic ulcer among users of aspirin and nonaspirin nonsteroidal antiinflammatory drugs. Am J Epidemiol 2004;159:23–31.

43. McQuay HJ. Pharmacological treatment of neuralgic and neuropathic pain. Cancer Surv 1988;7:141–159.

44. Katzung BG. Basic and Clinical Pharmacology, ed 8. New York: Lange, 2001:516.

45. Eichelbaum M, Evert B. Influence of pharmacogenetics on drug disposition and response. Clin Exp Pharmacol Physiol 1996;23:983–985.

46. Yamaguchi T, Sugimoto T. New development in bisphosphonate treatment. When and how long should patients take bisphosphonates for osteoporosis? [in Japanese]. Clin Calcium 2009;19:38–43.

47. Nishizawa Y, Nakamura T, Ohta H, et al. Guidelines for the use of biochemical markers of bone turnover in osteoporosis (2004). J Bone Miner Metab 2005;23:97–104.

48. Goss A, Bartold M, Sambrook P, Hawker P. The nature and frequency of bisphosphonate-associated osteonecrosis of the jaws in dental implant patients: A South Australian case series. J Oral Maxillofac Surg 2010;68:337–343.

49. de Papp A, Bone HG, Caulfield MP, et al. A cross-sectional study of bone turnover markers in healthy premenopausal women. Bone 2007;40: 1222–1230.

50. Edwards BJ, Hellstein JW, Jacobsen PL. Updated recommendations for managing the care of patients receiving oral bisphosphonate therapy: An advisory statement from the American Dental Association Council on Scientific Affairs. J Am Dent Assoc 2008;139:1674–1677 [erratum 2009;140:522].

51. Dannemann C, Grätz KW, Riener MO, Zwahlen RA. Jaw osteonecrosis related to bisphosphonate therapy: A severe secondary disorder. Bone 2007;40:828–834.

52. Mavrokokki T, Cheng A, Stein B, Goss A. Nature and frequency of bisphosphonate-associated osteonecrosis of the jaws in Australia. J Oral Maxillofac Surg 2007;65:415–423.

53. Chapurlat RD. Treatment of osteoporosis with annual IV zoledronic acid: Effects on hip fracture. Ther Clin Risk Manag 2009;5:169–175.

54. Chesnut III CH, Skag A, Christiansen C, et al. Effects of oral ibandronate administered daily or intermittently on fracture risk in postmenopausal osteoporosis. J Bone Miner Res 2004;19:1241–1249.

55. Twiss IM, Pas O, Ramp-Koopmanschap W, Den Hartigh J, Vermeij P. The effects of nitrogen-containing bisphosphonates on human epithelial (CaCo-2) cells, an in vitro model for intestinal epithelium. J Bone Miner Res 1999;14:784–791.

56. Szeto CC, Chow KM. Nephrotoxicity related to new therapeutic compounds. Ren Fail 2005;27:329–333.

57. Naik NH, Russo TA. Bisphosphonate-related osteonecrosis of the jaw: The role of *Actinomyces*. Clin Infect Dis 2009;49:1729–1732.

58. Ruggiero S, Gralow J, Marx RE, et al. Practical guidelines for the prevention, diagnosis, and treatment of osteonecrosis of the jaw in patients with cancer. J Oncol Pract 2006;2:7–14.

59. Lo JC, O'Ryan FS, Gordon NP, et al. Prevalence of osteonecrosis of the jaw in patients with oral bisphosphonate exposure. J Oral Maxillofac Surg 2010;68:243–253.

60. Tucci JR. Effect of inappropriate and continuous therapy with alendronate for ten years on skeletal integrity—Observations in two elderly patients. J Endocrinol Invest 2008;31:251–254.

61. Reid IR, Bolland MJ, Grey AB. Is bisphosphonate-associated osteonecrosis of the jaw caused by soft tissue toxicity? Bone 2007;41:318–320.

62. Sayed-Noor AS, Sjödén GO. Case reports: Two femoral insufficiency fractures after long-term alendronate therapy. Clin Orthop Relat Res 2009; 467:1921-1926.

63. Knapen MH, Schurgers LJ, Vermeer C. Vitamin K_2 supplementation improves hip bone geometry and bone strength indices in postmenopausal women. Osteoporos Int 2007;18:963–972.

64. Goh SK, Yang KY, Koh JS, et al. Subtrochanteric insufficiency fractures in patients on alendronate therapy: A caution. J Bone Joint Surg Br 2007; 89:349–353.

65. Jeske AH, Suchko GD. Lack of a scientific basis for routine discontinuation of oral anticoagulation therapy before dental treatment. J Am Dent Assoc 2003;134:1492–1497 [erratum 2004;135:28].

66. Little JW, Miller CS, Henry RG, McIntosh BA. Antithrombotic agents: Implications in dentistry. Oral Surg Oral Med Oral Pathol Oral Radiol Endod 2002;93:544–551.

67. Valerin MA, Brennan MT, Noll JL, et al. Relationship between aspirin use and postoperative bleeding from dental extractions in a healthy population. Oral Surg Oral Med Oral Pathol Oral Radiol Endod 2006;102:326.

68. Devani P, Lavery KM, Howell CJ. Dental extractions in patients on warfarin: Is alteration of anticoagulant regime necessary? Br J Oral Maxillofac Surg 1998;36:107–111.

69. Guna R, Kumar, R, McKinney WP. Long-term oral anticoagulant therapy: Update on indications, therapeutic ranges, and monitoring. Am J Med Sci 1994;307:128–132.

Appendices

Appendix A Implant Treatment Protocol

Implant dentistry is a complex discipline. Proper implant treatment planning requires the collection and analysis of a great amount of diagnostic data, and implant surgical, prosthetic, and follow-up procedures involve many steps. For these reasons, it is very important to develop within the dental office a protocol, such as the one presented in this appendix, to which all staff members adhere. This will standardize the flow of all potential implant cases and help to eliminate miscommunication with patients, laboratories, and referring dentists, as well as among members of the staff. However, the steps are too complicated, in particular during the learning curve, to be summed up so succinctly and left to the memory of the dentist and staff. Therefore, the basic implant treatment protocol presented here is supplemented with checklists, step-by-step protocols, and adjunct information to help clinicians avoid complications that may be caused by missing crucial steps of the diagnostic, surgical, prosthetic, and postoperative implant procedures.

Basic implant treatment protocol

1. Perform initial consultation (see *Diagnostic data collection*).
2. Perform comprehensive examination (see *Diagnostic data collection*).
3. Order diagnostic wax-up (see *Diagnostic wax-up*).
4. Order radiographic template.
5. Provide radiographic template to the patient with a referral to a computed tomography (CT) imaging center for scanning with the template in place (see *CT scans*).
6. Import the CT data into a computer-based implant planning software program.
7. Analyze the data and develop a treatment plan (*see Implant treatment planning*, *Risk factors*, and *Contraindications to implant placement*).
8. Make case presentation to patient (see *Case presentation*).
9. Order surgical guides if needed (see *Surgical guides*).
10. Place implant(s) (see *Basic implant placement*, *Guided bone regeneration using particulate bone graft and a barrier membrane*, *Guided bone regeneration using rhBMP-2/ACS and titanium mesh*, *Lateral window sinus elevation*, *Block grafting procedure*, *Bleeding control*, and *Nerve injury*).
11. Provide postoperative instructions (see Appendix C).
12. Remove sutures.
13. Place provisional prosthesis.
14. Perform stage-two surgery (if necessary).
15. Take impressions and obtain jaw relationship record, facebow transfer, and shade match in preparation for definitive restoration.
16. Fabricate definitive restoration.
17. Try in definitive restoration and make any necessary adjustments.
18. Deliver definitive restoration.
19. Provide patient with home care protocol.
20. Recall patient for routine professional maintenance.

Diagnostic data collection

At initial consultation:
- Main concern/complaint
- Patient goals

At comprehensive examination:
- Medical history
- Medications (history, current, and allergies)
- Dental history (restorations, missing teeth, fractures, caries, etc)
- Periodontal charting
- Soft tissue evaluation (adequacy of facial support with and without existing prostheses, amount of dentition and gingiva revealed during full smile and in repose, adequacy of attached keratinized gingiva, soft tissue biotype)
- Oral cancer evaluation
- Full-mouth radiographs
- Panoramic radiograph
- Photographs
- Impressions and jaw relationship record for diagnostic casts, diagnostic wax-up, and radiographic template
- Facebow transfer using semi-adjustable articulator
- Shade selection
- Determination of ideal shape and size of planned restorations

Diagnostic wax-up

Benefits
Benefits to the dentist, surgeon, and patient
- Facilitates determination of final gingival contours and emergence profile
- Aids in the determination of the amount of bone to be replaced (in case of bone loss)
- Allows patients to visualize their current situation and compare it to ideal restored situation
- Enables occlusal relationships to be reestablished
- Allows determination of the ideal number, position, and angulation of implants
- Facilitates evaluation of retained natural teeth and their role in the overall treatment plan
- Provides means for fabrication of provisional restorations
- Simplifies case presentations
- Enhances patient understanding of proposed treatment
- Fulfills medicolegal obligations for proper and complete pretreatment planning

Benefits to the laboratory technician
- Clarifies communication between the dentist and the laboratory
- Simplifies fabrication of provisional restorations
- Provides means for determining and gaining approval for shape and contour of definitive prosthesis

Requirements

Items to be provided by the dentist
- Two sets of maxillary and mandibular impressions
- Facebow record
- Jaw relationship record
- Shade selections and/or color photographs
- Proposed treatment plan

Items to be provided by the laboratory
- Preoperative cast
- Wax-up showing optimal hard and soft tissue contours, including tooth shapes and shade, according to the dentist's instructions

CT scans

Advantages of CT scans
- *Very high geometric and contrast resolution.*[1] *Geometric resolution* is the ability to distinguish between closely positioned objects; *contrast resolution* is the ability to distinguish between objects that are similar anatomically and chemically, such as neural tissue and fat.
- *Three-dimensional images.* The dentist can view and evaluate the cross-sectional dimensions of the area to be treated with implants, including the buccolingual dimension of the jaw, which cannot be assessed on two-dimensional images such as panoramic radiographs.[2]
- *Life-size images.* The dentist can perform accurate measurements on the CT film or on the computer screen when viewing digital CT files, making implant surgery more efficient and precise. The inconsistent magnification of panoramic radiographs makes accurate measurements impossible.[3,4]
- *Bone density measurement.* Periapical or panoramic radiographs are not helpful in detecting the density of the bone because the cortical plates often obscure the trabecular density. CT scans provide exact density measurements. Each axial image has 260,000 pixels, and each pixel has a CT number (Hounsfield unit) related to the density of the tissues within the pixel. The higher the CT number, the denser the tissue.
- *Anatomy and pathology detection.* Certain anatomical landmarks, such as the submandibular fossa and maxillary sinus septa, and certain pathologies, such as thickening of the sinus membrane, polyps, and mucoceles in the maxillary sinuses, cannot be detected on panoramic radiographs but can be easily viewed and evaluated on CT scans.
- *Computer-guided treatment planning.* The use of computer-guided treatment planning gives the dentist the ability to transfer the desired angle and location of the implants from the working cast to the computer screen and then, using surgical guides, to the mouth successfully.

Parameters to evaluate on the CT scan
Maxilla
- Subnasal and sub-buccal fossae
- Available alveolar bone height below the nasal floor
- Available alveolar bone height below the sinus floor
- Location of the greater palatine foramen
- Location of the incisive foramen
- Shape and size of the incisive canal
- Bone density
- Width and height of the alveolar ridge in the cross-sectional slices at the proposed implant locations

Mandible
- Submandibular fossa
- Sublingual fossa
- Inferior alveolar canal
- Mental foramen
- Anterior loop of the mental nerve
- Mandibular incisive canal
- Accessory lingual foramina of the mandible
- Bone density
- Width and height of the alveolar ridge in the cross-sectional slices at the proposed implant locations

Implant treatment planning

- Analyze all photographs and radiographs.
- Assess the diagnostic wax-up in relation to occlusion, arch relationship, soft tissue, and the available vertical and horizontal restorative spaces.
- On the CT scan, evaluate the volume and density of the bone available for implant placement, anatomical landmarks, bone density, and any pathologies, including bone or soft tissue defects that may require augmentation.
- Consider risk factors and contraindications.
- Determine factors such as type of surgical guide; immediate or staged treatment protocol; prosthesis type; implant type, number, length, diameter, position, and angulation; provisional prosthesis; and prognosis.
- Consult with surgeon and/or laboratory.
- Develop a goal-oriented treatment plan, narrowing the options to two or three.

Risk Factors Checklist *

General risk factors
- Age (very young or elderly)
- Compromised medical condition
- Compromised psychologic condition
- High esthetic demands
- Low scheduling availability
- Tobacco use
- Alcohol abuse
- Temporomandibular disorders
- Periodontal disease
- Occlusal trauma
- Small jaw opening
- Poor oral hygiene
- Low bone density
- Buccal concavity
- Narrow alveolar ridge
- Vertical bone resorption
- Excessive or inadequate vertical restorative space
- Excessive or inadequate horizontal restorative space

*The presence of one risk factor is not necessarily a contraindication to implant treatment; however, the presence of several risk factors is cause for concern.

- Acute lesions
- Chronic lesion distant from the implant zone

Esthetic risk factors
- Gingival smile line
- Thin and/or scalloped gingiva
- Crestal bone height deficiency
- Bone infection at the crest
- Reduced height of the keratinized gingiva
- Long and thin papillae between adjacent teeth
- Triangular tooth form
- Position of interdental contact point relative to the crestal bone level (distance of < 5 mm represents less of a risk than distance of > 5 mm)
- Amount of interdental contact (a small area of contact represents a higher risk than a large area of contact)
- Absence of a bony papilla (septum) between two implants
- Unstable provisional restoration

Functional risk factors
- Bruxism
- Clenching
- Tongue thrusting
- Large tongue size
- Compromised position of the planned implant in the mouth
- Prosthesis in opposing arch (opposing fixed prosthesis represents a higher risk than a removable appliance)

Occlusal risk factors
- Unfavorable direction of load
- Wide occlusal table
- Lateral occlusal contact on the implant-supported prosthesis only

Biomechanical risk factors
- Fewer implants than number of roots replaced
- Small implant diameter
- Short implant
- Connection of prosthesis to natural teeth
- Unsplinted implant crowns
- Straight (rather than tripod) configuration of implants
- Excessive pontic
- Use of cantilever
- Implants offset from the center of the prosthesis
- Excessive restoration height
- Unsatisfactory primary implant stability
- Lack of passive prosthetic fit
- Cemented prosthesis
- Use of intermediate abutment
- Mandibular flexure
- Use of a cylindric implant
- Immediate loading

Contraindications to implant placement

Absolute contraindications to implant placement*
- Recent myocardial infarction
- Cerebrovascular accident
- Valvular prosthesis surgery
- Bleeding issues
- Drug abuse
- Psychiatric illness
- Intravenous bisphosphonate use
- Terminal illness (evolving cancer)
- Tumoricidal radiation to implant site (active treatment of malignancy)
- Unrealistic expectations
- Surgeon's lack of experience
- Inability to prosthodontically restore the implant(s)
- Collagen and bone diseases (osteomalacia, osteogenesis imperfecta, Paget disease)
- Immunosuppressive disorders/AIDS
- Hyperactive involuntary muscle movements (Parkinson disease, Huntington chorea)
- Patient younger than 16 years

Relative contraindications to implant placement†
- Blood dyscrasia (anemia, sickle cell anemia, polycythemia vera, purpura, granulocytopenia)
- Pulmonary problems (asthma, bronchitis, emphysema)
- Anticoagulant therapy
- Psychiatric or psychologic disorders
- Mental retardation
- Chemotherapy
- Tobacco use
- Osteoporosis
- Diabetes
- Human immunodeficiency virus (HIV)
- Hypothyroidism
- Immunosuppression therapy
- Positive interleukin-1 genotype
- Lupus
- Renal insufficiency
- Scleroderma
- Pregnancy
- Elderly patients
- Cervicofacial irradiation

Case presentation
- Present treatment options using the diagnostic wax-up and treatment planning computer software.
- Discuss limitations and risk factors.
- Provide estimate of treatment duration.
- Present provisional prosthesis options.
- Discuss maintenance requirements.

*Placement of implants in patients with absolute contraindications may result in patient mortality.[3,5] Hence, it is essential to select patients who do not possess local or systemic contraindications to therapy. The list presented is not exhaustive.
†Illnesses that impair the normal healing cascade worsen surgical results. The mere presence of a disease, however, does not necessarily preclude implant therapy or significantly affect long-term outcomes. Certain disorders, when controlled, and other compromised situations allow implant survival rates that match those in healthy patients.[6] The list presented is not exhaustive.

- Inform the patient of possible complications.
- Explain fees and financial options.

When the patient accepts a treatment plan:
- Have the patient sign informed consent forms (see appendix B).
- Provide the patient with preoperative and postoperative instructions and a prescription for any required medication.
- Mail a confirmation letter indicating the treatment plan chosen.

Surgical guides

Laboratory-fabricated guides
- The laboratory technician fabricates the guides using the diagnostic wax-up.
- Not always accurate because the laboratory technician is unable to see the thickness of the soft tissue, detect any undercuts on the buccal plate, or know the exact dimensions of the alveolar ridge.
- Often sufficient for implant placement in posterior areas with adequate bone and soft tissue volume and no undercuts.

Types of laboratory-fabricated guides
- In the first type, only the buccal aspects of the teeth are reproduced in the guide, which provides good access and visibility but insufficient orientation for optimal esthetics.
- In the second type, teeth are fully reproduced in the guide based on the wax-up. Access holes are created along the ideal implant axes. These are sometimes bulky and provide limited visibility.

Computer-generated guides
- The fabrication of computer-generated surgical guides is based on the dentist's treatment plan created using surgical planning software. These guides are more precise than laboratory-fabricated guides and are recommended for use when esthetics is important and/or there is a high risk of complications.

Types of computer-generated guides
- Bone-supported
- Mucosa-supported
- Tooth-supported

Basic implant placement: Step-by-step surgical protocol

1. Verify that consent forms are signed.
2. Verify that medications have been taken as directed.
3. Administer the anesthetic.
4. Perform flap elevation.
5. Verify that vertical and horizontal restorative space is adequate.
6. Measure the thickness of soft tissue.
7. Place surgical guide.
8. Create the initial implant osteotomy using a pilot drill.
9. Take a radiograph to verify the position and angulation of the implant osteotomy.
10. Enlarge the osteotomy to the desired diameter.
11. Perform bone tapping if needed.
12. Irrigate the osteotomy.
13. Place the implants.
14. Take a postoperative radiograph.
15. Place the cover screw (for two-stage protocol) or the healing abutment (for one-stage protocol).
16. Suture.
17. Provide postoperative and home care instructions.
18. Schedule an appointment for a follow-up visit.

Guided bone regeneration using particulate bone graft and a barrier membrane: Step-by-step protocol

1. Verify that consent forms are signed.
2. Verify that medications have been taken as directed.
3. Administer the anesthetic.
4. Make a crestal and two releasing incisions one to two teeth away from the graft site on each side. Blade no. 12C is the blade of choice in most cases. Because the palatal flap cannot be stretched, in the maxilla, place the crestal incision slightly toward the palate rather than midcrestal.
5. Clean the bone of periosteum and muscle attachments using a back-action chisel.
6. Place the implant (if implant placement is to be performed simultaneously). Place the implant in the optimal position buccolingually and coronoapically despite the deficient bone volume. Always make sure the apical 2 to 3 mm of the implant is completely in bone.
7. Verify that the implant is stable.
8. Create about 10 bleeding points with a small round diamond bur around and apical to the implant.
9. Place tenting screws on the buccal plate and on the crest if needed (when a gain in width greater than 2 mm is required). Usually two to three tenting screws are adequate.
10. Harvest autogenous bone (eg, from the tuberosity) using a rongeur or trephine drill.
11. If you are using a nonresorbable membrane, fix the membrane buccally using screws or tacks before adding the graft material.
12. Add the autogenous bone layer.
13. Add the bone grafting material (eg, Bio-Oss, Geistlich). If an autogenous bone layer was not placed, use freeze-dried bone allograft with the Bio-Oss in a 1:1 ratio.
14. Fix the membrane on the crest or on the lingual/palatal side if you are using a nonresorbable membrane. When using a resorbable membrane, place it in two layers; there is no need for fixation in most cases. In case of a nonresorbable membrane, the border of the membrane should be well under the flap and 1 mm from adjacent teeth on the crest.
15. Release the flap for tension-free closure using a scalpel to score the periosteum, followed by Metzenbaum scissors, if needed, to release the muscle layer.

16. Close the flap without tension. Gore-Tex (W. L. Gore) is the author's suture material of choice. Use 4-0 or 5-0 depending on the thickness of the tissue. Leave the sutures for 2 weeks; during this time the patient should not wear a provisional prosthesis in the grafted area. The waiting period for bone to mature is 9 to 12 months.

17. Provide postoperative and home care instructions.

18. Schedule an appointment for a follow-up visit.

Guided bone regeneration using rhBMP-2/ACS and titanium mesh: Step-by-step protocol

1. Verify that consent forms are signed.
2. Verify that medications have been taken as directed.
3. Administer anesthetic.
4. Make a crestal and two releasing incisions one to two teeth away from the graft site on each side. Blade no. 12C is the blade of choice in most cases. Because the palatal flap cannot be stretched, in the maxilla, place the crestal incision slightly toward the palate rather than midcrestal.
5. Clean the bone of periosteum and muscle attachments using a back-action chisel.
6. Place the implant (if implant placement is to be performed simultaneously). Place the implant in the optimal position buccolingually and coronoapically despite the deficient bone volume. Always make sure the apical 2 to 3 mm of the implant is completely in bone.
7. Verify that the implant is stable.
8. Create about 10 bleeding points with a small round diamond bur around and apical to the implant.
9. Apply the rhBMP-2/ACS material per the manufacturer's guidelines; Bio-Oss can be added as well.
10. Fix the titanium mesh using fixation screws. The border of the titanium mesh should be well under the flap and 2 mm away from adjacent teeth on the crest.
11. Release the flap for tension-free closure using a scalpel to score the periosteum, followed by Metzenbaum scissors, if needed, to release the muscle layer.
12. Close the flap without tension. Gore-Tex is the author's suture material of choice. Use 4-0 or 5-0 depending on the thickness of the tissue. Leave the sutures for 2 weeks; during this time the patient should not wear a provisional prosthesis in the grafted area. The waiting period for bone to mature is 6 to 8 months.
13. Provide postoperative and home care instructions
14. Schedule an appointment for a follow-up visit.

Lateral window sinus elevation: Step-by-step protocol

1. Verify that consent forms are signed.
2. Verify that medications have been taken as directed.
3. Administer anesthetic. Maxillary, infraorbital, and greater palatine nerve blocks are recommended. Infiltration anesthesia in the labial mucosa, buccal mucosa, and palatal region is also recommended. Oral sedative medications are optional but highly recommended to guarantee optimal patient comfort during surgery.

4. Perform incision and flap reflection. A midcrestal incision is made from the maxillary tuberosity forward to the canine area, where an anterior vertical oblique releasing incision is made. Full-thickness reflection is achieved using a periosteal elevator. If the tuberosity is not to be included in the flap, then a second distal beveled releasing incision should be made.

5. Perform the osteotomy. The lateral window's location and size are outlined on the lateral wall of the maxillary bone based on measurements made from the CT scan. The osteotomy should be performed under copious irrigation with cooled sterile saline to avoid overheating the bone, using a paintbrush stroke with a no. 6 or 8 diamond round bur on a surgical straight handpiece to outline the window until a bluish hue is visible or hemorrhage occurs. The inferior osteotomy should be created approximately 2 to 3 mm superior to and parallel with the floor of the sinus. The anterior vertical line is scored 5 mm distal to the anterior vertical wall of the antrum. The posterior vertical line should be made 15 to 20 mm distal to the anterior one. The superior osteotomy connects the two vertical osteotomies, completing the window. The corners of the access window should be rounded to facilitate the introduction of the surgical curette into the corners without risk of tearing the membrane.

6. Perform window infracture or removal. In the presence of good surgical access, no septa, and a wide sinus, the bony window can be gently infractured, ie, lifted into the sinus and used as the future sinus floor using bone tampers and a mallet. Under less ideal circumstances, the window can be completely removed.

7. Elevate the sinus membrane. A sinus elevation curette of appropriate offset angle is slid along the bone 360 degrees around the margin of the access window, and then the sinus membrane is carefully separated from the anterior and medial walls of the sinus to a height at least 15 mm from the crest of the ridge. Distally, the elevation is limited to the extent needed to place implants. When the sinus membrane is pushed superiorly with the sinus freer and other sinus membrane instruments, it is important that the sharp edges of these instruments remain on the bone and that the curved portion is placed against the window. If needed, a Kerrison rongeur can be used to enlarge the access window.

8. Place the resorbable collagen membrane on the new ceiling of the sinus cavity (on the sinus membrane). The corners of the collagen membrane are cut and rounded, and 1-cm releasing incisions are made to ease the manipulation of the membrane. To prevent infection, further ease manipulation, and improve adherence, the collagen membrane must be moistened with blood or sterile saline with antibiotics such as tetracycline prior to placement. The collagen membrane is then placed on the medial and superior walls of the sinus. The author recommends the BioMend membrane (Integra LifeSciences) because it is long lasting and has the ideal level of memory for easy handling inside the sinus cavity.

9. Place the bone graft materials. Packing should be accomplished by placing only a small amount of the graft material at a time in the least accessible areas first and working in an inferior and anterior direction. The sinus should be packed until the graft material reaches the bone flap superiorly and reconstitutes the maxillary wall contour laterally. Packing should be firm but not excessive. Overfilling may increase the amount of time required for the graft to mature. Placement of an autogenous bone layer at the bottom third of the elevated sinus cavity is highly recommended. Autogenous bone remains the best grafting material; however, it is important to add xenograft to the autogenous bone, especially if it is cancellous, because the osteoconductive material increases bone density and helps to maintain the volume of the graft during the faster remodeling and resorption processes of the cancellous bone.

10. Place the implants(s) (optional). Implants can be placed simultaneously with the bone graft if the alveolar bony ridge will allow the placement of stable implants. Usually 5 mm or more of alveolar height is required for simultaneous implant placement. After the implant sites are prepared, the bone graft is placed in the sinus and packed against the intact medial and anterior walls. The implants then are placed, and the bone is packed against the posterior maxillary wall and in between the implants, leaving no voids. During this part of the procedure, it is important to maintain the implant in the proper position so that subsequent prosthetic restoration is not compromised. Next, the lateral portion of the surgical site should be firmly packed with the bone graft material.

11. Place the second resorbable collagen membrane to cover the bony window. If the membrane is nonresorbable, it should be secured with two titanium tacks or screws. However, the author recommends the Bio-Gide membrane (Geistlich) for its pliability, ease of handling, and adherence capacity that allows it to be placed without fixation screws. Placement of this membrane is important because it delays the invasion of fibrous tissue into the graft and permits the lateral bony wall to be restored.

12. Close the incision. Good surgical technique dictates wound closure over intact bone without tension. Releasing the periosteum for passive closure is necessary only if a ridge augmentation procedure is performed simultaneously with the sinus graft surgery. However, in the maxilla, the crestal incision should always be made a little more toward the palatal side (to lengthen the buccal flap as much as possible) because the palatal flap cannot be released and pulled. The first suture should be placed at the corner between the crestal incision and the oblique releasing incision, then the operator can proceed to close the crestal and the releasing incisions. PTFE (eg, Gore-Tex) is the author's preferred suture material because it has minimal elastic memory, making it easy to handle.

13. Take postoperative radiographs and deliver the provisional restoration. It is highly recommended to delay placement of a provisional prosthesis for 2 weeks or longer, if possible; however, if a removable denture must be worn during the healing period, the flanges need to be adjusted in the areas of the surgical/bone grafting sites to avoid applying any pressure to these areas during the healing period.

14. Provide postoperative and home care instructions. See Appendix C for postoperative patient instructions.

15. Schedule an appointment for a follow-up visit.

Block grafting procedure: Step-by-step protocol

1. Verify that consent forms are signed.
2. Verify that medications have been taken as directed.
3. Evaluate the anatomy of the recipient and donor sites.
4. Administer anesthetic at recipient and donor sites.
5. Prepare recipient site.
6. Perform incision and flap reflection of the donor site.
7. Execute block graft osteotomies and harvest the graft.
8. Fixate the block graft.
9. Close the recipient site.
10. Close the donor site.
11. Take postoperative radiographs and deliver the provisional restoration.
12. Provide postoperative and home care instructions.
13. Schedule an appointment for a follow-up visit.

Bleeding control*

Hematoma due to excessive bleeding in the floor of the mouth can contribute to an injury from the lingual of facial arteries or from one of their branches. The following steps can be followed to control the bleeding.

1. At the first sign of swelling in the floor of the mouth, call 911.
2. Using one hand, press with the thumb intraorally and with the index finger extraorally on the suspected perforation site.
3. Calmly explain to the patient the nature of the complication.
4. If the bleeding is from the lingual artery or any of its branches, pull the tongue out and press it against the hyoid bone to reduce bleeding.
5. If the injury is from the facial artery, press the common carotid against C4 to help reduce bleeding.
6. Avoid making incisions in the floor of the mouth to relieve the hematoma.
7. Do not remove the implant.
8. If, after the steps above have been followed, a hematoma of large size develops along with signs of respiratory distress, insert a flexible nasal airway; emergency tracheotomy or cricothyrotomy may be necessary.
9. Transfer the patient to a nearby hospital for monitoring.

*More details on this topic can be found in complication 15, part 2.

Nerve injury*

If nerve injury is suspected following implant placement, the following steps should be taken:

1. Document the dysfunction level of the nerve injury, preferably the day after surgery when the effects of the anesthetic have worn off.
2. Obtain a postoperative CT scan to determine if the alteration in sensation is due to the presence of the implant in the nerve area or is the result of soft tissue manipulation or edema.
3. If it is believed that the implant is the cause of altered sensation, remove it. However, if the problem is compression of the bone above the nerve placing pressure on the nerve, withdraw the implant 1 to 2 mm.
4. Because the alteration in sensation may be caused by an inflammatory reaction, prescribe ibuprofen (800 mg) for 3 weeks. If improvement is noted, prescribe an additional 3 weeks of anti-inflammatory drug treatment.
5. If, after 1 month, there is complete loss of sensation, diminishing sensation, or spontaneous pain, refer the patient to a microneurosurgeon. The goal of early referral is to allow the patient to undergo nerve repair within 4 months of the injury, thereby minimizing distal degeneration of the nerve.
6. Contact your malpractice insurance carrier for guidance.

References

1. Rothman SLG. Dental Applications of Computerized Tomography: Surgical Planning for Implant Placement. Chicago: Quintessence, 1998.
2. Truhlar RS, Morris HF, Ochi S. A review of panoramic radiography and its potential use in implant dentistry. Implant Dent 1993;2:122–130.
3. Chanavaz M. Screening and medical evaluation of adults: Contraindications for invasive dental procedures. J Indiana Dent Assoc 1999;78(3):10–17.
4. Klinge B, Petersson A, Maly P. Localization of the mandibular canal: Comparison of macroscopic findings, conventional radiography, and computed tomography. Int J Oral Maxillofac Implants 1989;4:327–332.
5. Hwang D, Wang HL. Medical contraindications to implant therapy. Part I: Absolute contraindications. Implant Dent 2006;15:353–360.
6. Hwang D, Wang HL. Medical contraindications to implant therapy. Part II: Relative contraindications. Implant Dent 2007;16:13–23.

*More details on this topic can be found in complication 8, part 2.

Appendix B Consent Forms

CONSENT FORM FOR IMPLANT SURGERY AND ANESTHESIA

Instructions to Patient: Please take this document home and read it carefully. Note any questions you have in the area provided in Paragraph 15. Bring this back to our office at your next appointment, and the doctor will review it with you before signing the last page.

1. My doctor has explained the various types of implants used in dentistry, and I have been informed of the alternatives to implant surgery for replacement of my missing teeth. I have also been informed of the foreseeable risks of those alternatives. I understand what procedures are necessary to accomplish the placement of the implant(s) either on, in, or through the bone, and I understand that the most common types of implants available are subperiosteal (on), endosteal (in), and transosteal (through). The implant type recommended for my specific condition is *circled above*. I also understand that endosteal implants (more commonly known as *root-form*) generally have the most predictable prognosis. I further understand that subperiosteal implants, if an option for me, are not as widely used as root-form implants but will negate the necessity of bone grafting and other surgical procedures that would be necessary for the placement of root-form implants. I understand that the risk associated with the use of a subperiosteal implant is failure and loss of the implant, which could further reduce the minimal amount of existing bone that I now have, requiring more extensive bone grafting and other surgical procedures at some future time. I also understand that other dental practitioners may not be familiar or experienced in the use of subperiosteal implants, including their placement, maintenance, and treating any problems that might arise involving the subperiosteal implant. I agree to, and accept responsibility for failing to, return to this office for examinations and any recommended treatment, at least every 6 months. My failure to do so, for whatever reason, can jeopardize the clinical success of the implant system. Accordingly, I agree to release and hold my dentist harmless if my implant(s) fail as a result of my failure to maintain an ongoing examination and preventive maintenance routine as stated above.

2. I have further been informed that if no treatment is elected to replace the missing teeth or existing dentures, the nontreatment risks include, but are not limited to:
   (a) Maintenance of the existing full or partial denture(s) with relines or remakes every 3 to 5 years or as otherwise may be necessary because of the likely gradual and progressive dissolution of the underlying denture-supporting jawbone
   (b) Persistence or worsening over time of any present discomfort or chewing inefficiency with the existing partial or full denture
   (c) Drifting, tilting, and/or extrusion of remaining teeth
   (d) Looseness of teeth and periodontal disease (gum and bone), possibly followed by extraction(s)
   (e) A potential jaw joint problem (TMJ) caused by a deficient, collapsed, or otherwise improper bite

3. I am aware that the practice of dentistry and dental surgery is not an exact science, and I acknowledge that no guarantees have been made to me concerning the success of my implant surgery, the associated treatment and procedures, or the postsurgical dental procedures. I am further aware that there is a risk that the implant placement may fail, which might require further corrective surgery associated with the removal. Such a failure and remedial procedures could also involve additional fees being assessed.

4. I understand that implant success is dependent upon a number of variables, including but not limited to: operator experience, individual patient tolerance and health, anatomical variations, my home care of the implant, and habits such as grinding my teeth. I also understand that implants are available in a variety of designs and materials and the choice of implant is determined in the professional judgment of my dentist.

———
Initial

Continued on next page

5. I have further been informed of the foreseeable risks and complications of implant surgery, anesthesia, and related drugs, including but not limited to: failure of the implant(s), inflammation, swelling, infection, discoloration, numbness (exact extent and duration unknown), inflammation of blood vessels, injury to existing teeth, bone fractures, sinus penetration, delayed healing, or allergic reaction to the drugs or medications used. No one has made any promises or given me any guarantees about the outcome of this treatment or these procedures. I understand that these complications can occur even if all dental procedures are done properly.

6. I have been advised that smoking and alcohol or sugar consumption may affect tissue healing and may limit the success of the implant. Because there is no way to accurately predict the gum and bone healing capabilities of each patient, I know I must follow my dentist's home care instructions and report to my dentist for regular examinations as instructed. I further understand that excellent home care, including brushing, flossing, and the use of any other device recommended by my dentist, is critical to the success of my treatment, and my failure to do what I have been instructed to do at home will be, at minimum, a partial cause of implant failure, should that occur. I understand that the more I smoke, the more likely it is that my implant treatment will fail, and I understand and accept that risk.

7. I have also been advised that there is a risk that the implant may break, which may require additional procedures to repair or replace the broken implant.

8. I authorize my dentist to perform dental services for me, including implants and other related surgery such as bone augmentation. I agree to the type of anesthesia—local, IV sedation, or general—that he or she has discussed with me (circled above) and have been informed of any potential side effects. I agree not to operate a motor vehicle or other device that may be hazardous to my or others' safety for at least 24 hours and until fully recovered from the effects of the anesthesia or drugs given for my care. My dentist has also discussed the various types of bone augmentation material, and I have authorized him or her to select the material that he or she believes to be the best choice for my implant treatment.

9. If an unforeseen condition arises in the course of treatment that calls for the performance of procedures in addition to or different from those now contemplated and I am under general anesthesia or IV sedation, I further authorize and direct my dentist and his or her associates or assistants to do whatever they deem necessary and advisable under the circumstances, including the decision not to proceed with the implant procedure(s).

10. I approve any reasonable modifications in design, materials, or surgical procedures if my dentist, in his or her professional judgment, decides it is in my best interest to do so.

11. To my knowledge, I have given an accurate report of my health history. I have also reported on my medical history questionnaire any past allergic or other reactions to drugs, food, insect bites, anesthetics, pollens, or dust; blood diseases; gum or skin reactions; abnormal bleeding; or any other condition relating to my physical or mental health or any problems experienced with any prior medical, dental, or other health care treatment. I understand that certain mental and/or emotional disorders may contraindicate implant therapy and have therefore expressly circled either YES or NO to indicate whether or not I have had any past treatment or therapy of any kind for a mental or emotional condition.

12. I authorize my dentist to make photographs, slides, x-rays, or any other visual records of my treatment to be used for the advancement of implant dentistry in any manner my dentist deems appropriate. However, no photographs or other records that identify me will be used without my express written consent.

13. I realize and understand that the purpose of this document is to evidence the fact that I am knowingly consenting to the implant procedures recommended by my dentist.

14. I agree that if I do not follow my dentist's recommendations and advice for postoperative care, my dentist may terminate the dentist-patient relationship, requiring me to seek treatment from another dentist. I realize that postoperative care and maintenance treatment is critical for the ultimate success of dental implants. I accept responsibility for any adverse consequences that result from not following my dentist's advice.

Initial

Continued on next page

15. Questions I have for my dentist: _____

_____

_____

_____

16. I certify that I have read and fully understand the above authorization and informed consent to implant placement and surgery and that all my questions, if any, have been fully answered. I have had the opportunity to take this form home and review it before signing it. I understand and agree that my initial on each page, along with my signature below, will be considered conclusive proof that I have read and understand everything contained in this document and I have given my consent to proceed with implant treatment and related surgery, including any ancillary bone grafting procedures.

_____   _____
Signature of dentist   Signature of patient

_____   _____
Signature of witness   Signature of witness

_____
Signature of parent or guardian (if patient is a minor)

Date _____

_____
Initial

BLOCK GRAFT CONSENT FORM

For: _____

Diagnosis: Insufficient available bone in _____.

Procedure: Taking a block of bone from _____ and placing this graft _____.

Anesthetic (circle one):   Topical   Local N_2O/O_2 IV   General

Dr _____ has explained the proposed surgery noted above, including the expected benefits and the alternatives to treatment, if any. I have also been advised of the associated potential risks and possible complications of the proposed procedures, including, but not limited to: allergic or other unexpected reaction to medications; bleeding; infection; swelling; pain; bruising; limited opening; jaw joint (TMJ) pain/dysfunction; involvement of the maxillary sinus; damage to other teeth or dental work; alveolar osteitis (dry socket or loss of the clot formed in the extracted tooth socket requiring treatment by irrigation and dressing placement); numbness of the tongue, lips, or face; nausea/vomiting; unplanned laceration, tear, burn, or abrasion of intraoral mucosa or skin with the need for additional treatment or surgical repair; and the possibility of the need for other surgery or hospitalization.

I understand that if the planned procedure is performed by laser, a risk of burns to the mucosa, skin, or eyes could exist.

If I am to receive medicines to relax me (IV sedation, general anesthetic, nitrous oxide–oxygen analgesic, or oral sedative), I have been advised that although well-monitored anesthesia is generally very safe, comfortable, and well-tolerated, there are additional associated risks and possible complications, which include nausea; vomiting; an allergic or unexpected reaction that, if severe, might cause more serious respiratory (lung) or cardiovascular (heart) problems that may require treatment; pain, swelling, inflammation, or infection of the area of the injection; injury to nerves or blood vessels in the area; disorientation, confusion, or prolonged drowsiness after surgery; and/or cardiovascular or respiratory responses that could lead to heart attack, stroke, or death. I have been encouraged to ask questions, and all questions I have asked have been answered to my satisfaction.

I also have been advised of the possible risks of nontreatment and understand that I have the option of seeking additional opinions from other providers if desired.

I understand I am to:

- Have nothing to eat or drink 8 hours prior to surgery
- Have a responsible adult drive me to the appointment, stay in the waiting room, and drive me home after my surgery

I understand that I am to follow the oral and written instructions given to me, realizing failure to do so may result in less than optimal results of the procedure, and that I am to present myself for postoperative appointments as scheduled.

I request the performance of the procedure named above and such additional procedures as may be found necessary in the judgment of my doctor during the course of this treatment. I understand unforeseen circumstances may necessitate a change in the procedure, or, in rare cases, prevent completion of the planned procedure.

_____
Initial

Continued on next page

I request the administration of anesthetic as considered necessary or advisable in the judgment of the doctor.

Exceptions to surgery and/or anesthetic, if any, are: _____.

I request the disposal of any tissues that may be necessary to remove.

I authorize photographs, slides, x-rays, or any other visual records of my care and treatment during or after its completion to be used for the advancement of dentistry and for reimbursement purposes. However, my identity will not be revealed to the general public without my permission.

I understand that there may be additional laboratory charges for specimens taken for analysis.

I have read and understand the consent for surgery above and desire to proceed as planned. I acknowledge that no guarantees have been made to me concerning the outcome or results of the surgery or procedure. I have no unanswered questions concerning the proposed treatment.

Signature of patient _____ Date _____ Time _____

Signature of doctor_____ Date _____ Time _____

_____
Initial

BONE GRAFTING AND BARRIER MEMBRANE CONSENT FORM

For: _____

I understand that bone grafting and barrier membrane procedures include inherent risks, including but not limited to the following:

1. *Pain*. Some discomfort is inherent in any oral surgery procedure. Grafting with materials that do not have to be harvested from the body is less painful because they do not require donor site surgery. If the necessary bone is taken from the chin or wisdom tooth area, there will be more pain, which can be largely controlled with pain medications.
2. *Infection*. No matter how carefully surgical sterility is maintained, it is possible, because of the existing nonsterile oral environment, for infections to occur postoperatively. At times, these may be serious in nature. Should severe swelling occur, particularly if it is accompanied with fever or malaise, professional attention should be sought as soon as possible.
3. *Bleeding, bruising, and swelling*. Some moderate bleeding may last several hours. If bleeding is profuse, the office should be contacted as soon as possible. Likewise, some swelling is normal, but if it is severe, the office should be notified. Swelling usually starts to subside after about 48 hours. Bruises may persist for a week or more.
4. *Loss of part or all of the graft*. Success with bone and membrane grafting is high. Nevertheless, it is possible that the graft could fail. A block bone graft taken from somewhere else in the mouth may not adhere or could become infected. Despite meticulous surgery, particulate bone graft materials can migrate out of the surgical site and be lost. A membrane graft could start to dislodge. If so, the doctor should be notified. Patient compliance is essential for success.
5. *Types of graft material*. Some bone graft and membrane materials commonly used are derived from human or other mammalian sources. These grafts are thoroughly purified to be free of contaminants. Signing this consent form signifies my approval for the doctor to use materials according to his or her knowledge and clinical judgment of my situation.
6. *Injury to nerves*. A possible consequence of the surgical procedures or anesthetic administration is injury causing numbness of the lips and tongue as well as any tissues of the mouth, cheeks, and/or face. This numbness may be of a temporary nature, lasting a few days, weeks, or months, or could possibly be permanent.
7. *Sinus involvement*. In some cases, the root tips of upper teeth lie in close proximity to the maxillary sinus. Occasionally, with extractions and/or grafting near the sinus, the sinus can become involved. If this happens, special medications will be necessary. Should sinus penetration occur, it may be necessary to later have the sinus surgically closed.

I understand that it is my responsibility to seek attention should any undue circumstances occur postoperatively and that I should diligently follow any preoperative and postoperative instructions.

Informed Consent

As a patient, I have been given the opportunity to ask questions regarding the nature and purpose of surgical treatment and have received answers to my satisfaction. I voluntarily assume any and all possible risks, including the risk of harm, if any, that may be associated with any phase of this treatment in hopes of obtaining the desired results, which may or may not be achieved. No guarantees or promises have been made to me concerning my recovery and results of the treatment to be rendered to me. The fees for this service have been explained to me and are satisfactory. I authorize photographs, slides, x-rays, or any other visual records of my care and treatment during or after its completion to be used for the advancement of dentistry and for reimbursement purposes. However, my identity will not be revealed to the general public without my permission. By signing this form, I am freely giving my consent to allow and authorize Dr _____ and his or her associates to render any treatments necessary or advisable to my dental conditions, including any and all anesthetics and/or medications.

Patient name _____

Signature of patient _____ Date _____

_____
Initial

BIOPSY AND SOFT TISSUE CONSENT FORM

For: _____

Section I: Patient Information

1. I hereby authorize and direct Dr _____ and assistants of his or her choice to perform the following operation(s) or procedure(s): _____.

2. I hereby authorize and direct the above surgeon or other physician and/or associates and assistants to provide or arrange for the provision of such additional services or related procedures that are deemed necessary or advisable, including but not limited to pathology and radiology services.

3. I have been informed of my following rights as a patient: All operations and procedures may involve risks of unsuccessful results, complications, injury, or even death from known and unforeseen causes. I have the right to be informed of such risks, as well as the nature of the operation or procedure, the expected benefits or effects of such operation or procedure, and the available alternative methods of treatment and their risks and benefits. I also have the right to be informed as to whether my physician has any independent medical research or economic interests related to the performance of the proposed operation or procedure. Except in cases of emergency, I have the right to receive this information and to give my consent before operations or procedures are performed. I have the right to consent to or to refuse any proposed operation or procedure at any time prior to its performance. No warranty or guarantee is made as to the result or cure.

4. My signature below confirms that I authorize the pathologist to use his or her discretion in the disposition or use of any member, organ, or other tissue removed from my person during the operation or procedure identified above.

My signature below indicates: *(1)* I have read and understood the information contained herein; *(2)* I have been verbally informed about this operation or procedure; *(3)* I have had the opportunity to ask questions regarding this operation or procedure; *(4)* I have received all of the information I desire; and *(5)* I authorize and consent to the performance of the operation or procedure.

Signature of patient _____ Date _____Time _____

Signature of witness _____ Date _____Time _____

My signature below indicates that: *(1)* I have read and discussed the risks, benefits, and options for anesthesia with a representative of the anesthesia department; *(2)* I have received answers to all of my questions; and *(3)* I authorize and consent to the anesthesia plan discussed.

Signature of patient _____ Date _____Time _____

Signature of witness _____ Date _____Time _____

Section II: Patient Declines to Be Informed

Although I have been given an opportunity to be advised as to the nature and purpose of the operation or procedure and the risks, benefits, and alternatives, I specifically decline to be so advised, but I do give my consent to the operation. No warranty or guarantee has been made as to the result or cure.

Signature of patient _____ Date _____Time _____

Signature of witness _____ Date _____Time _____

_____
Initial

EMAIL CONSENT FORM

For: _____

1. Risk of Using Email

Provider offers patients the opportunity to communicate by email. Transmitting patient information by email, however, has a number of risks that patients should consider. These include but are not limited to the following risks:

(a) Email can be circulated, forwarded, and stored in numerous paper and electronic files.

(b) Email can be immediately broadcast worldwide and be received by many intended and unintended recipients.

(c) Email senders can easily misaddress an email.

(d) Email is easier to falsify than handwritten or signed documents.

(e) Backup copies of email may exist even after the sender or the recipient has deleted his or her copy.

(f) Employers and online services have a right to archive and inspect emails transmitted through their systems.

(g) Email can be intercepted, altered, forwarded, or used without authorization or detection.

(h) Email can be used to introduce viruses into computer systems.

(i) Email can be used as evidence in court.

2. Conditions for the Use of Email

Provider will use reasonable means to protect the security and confidentiality of email information sent and received. However, because of the risks outlined above, Provider cannot guarantee the security and confidentiality of email communication and will not be liable for improper disclosure of confidential information that is not caused by Provider's intentional misconduct. Thus, Patient must consent to the use of email for the transmittal of patient information. Consent to the use of email includes agreement with the following conditions:

(a) All emails to or from Patient concerning diagnosis or treatment will be printed out and made part of Patient's medical record. Because they are a part of the medical record, other individuals authorized to access the medical records, such as staff and billing personnel, will have access to those emails.

(b) Provider may forward emails internally to Provider's staff and agents as necessary for diagnosis, treatment, reimbursement, and other handling. Provider will not, however, forward emails to independent third parties without Patient's prior written consent, except as authorized or required by law.

(c) Although Provider will endeavor to read and respond promptly to email from Patient, Provider cannot guarantee that any particular email will be read and responded to within any specified period of time. Thus, Patient should not use email for medical emergencies or other time-sensitive matters.

(d) If Patient's email requires or invites a response from Provider and Patient has not received a response within a reasonable time period, it is Patient's responsibility to follow up to determine whether the intended recipient received the email and when the recipient will respond.

(e) Patient should not use email for communication regarding sensitive medical information, such as information regarding sexually transmitted diseases, AIDS/HIV, mental health, developmental disability, or substance abuse.

(f) Patient is responsible for informing Provider of any type of information Patient does not want to be sent by email in addition to those listed in 2(e) above.

(g) Patient is responsible for protecting his or her password or other means of access to email. Provider is not liable for breaches of confidentiality caused by Patient or any third party.

(h) Provider shall not engage in email communication that is unlawful, such as unlawfully practicing medicine across state lines.

(i) It is Patient's responsibility to follow up and/or schedule an appointment, if warranted.

_____
Initial

Continued on next page

3. Instructions

To communicate via email, Patient shall:

(a) Limit or avoid use of his or her employer's computer.

(b) Inform Provider of changes in his or her email address, including his or her name in the body of the email.

(c) Include the category of the communication in the email's subject line for routing purposes (eg, billing question).

(d) Review the email to make sure it is clear and that all relevant information is included before sending to Provider.

(e) Inform Provider when Patient receives an email from Provider.

(f) Take precautions to preserve the confidentiality of emails, such as using screen savers and safeguarding his or her computer password.

(g) Withdraw consent only by email or written communication to Provider.

4. Patient Acknowledgment and Agreement

I acknowledge that I have read and fully understand this consent form. I understand the risks associated with the communication by email between Provider and me and consent to the conditions outlined herein. In addition, I agree to the instructions outlined herein, as well as any other instructions that Provider may impose to communicate with patients by email. Any questions I had were answered.

Patient name _____

Signature of patient _____ Date _____

_____
Initial

TRIAZOLAM INFORMATION AND CONSENT FORM

For: _____

Taking triazolam 1 hour prior to your dental appointment is an excellent way to minimize or eliminate anxiety that may be associated with going to the dentist. However, even though it is safe, effective, and wears off rapidly after the dental visit, you should be aware of some important precautions and considerations.

1. This consent form and the dental treatment consent form should be signed before you take the medication. They are invalid if signed after you take the pills.
2. After you have taken the medication, do not drive. Onset of triazolam occurs within 15 to 30 minutes, and the peak effect occurs between 1 to 2 hours after taking the medication. After that, the effects begin to subside, and most people feel back to normal after 6 to 8 hours. However, for safety reasons and because people react differently, you should not drive or operate machinery the remainder of the day.
3. This medication should not be used if:
   (a) You are hypersensitive to benzodiazepines (eg, diazepam [Valium], lorazepam [Ativan]).
   (b) You are pregnant or breastfeeding.
   (c) You have liver or kidney disease.
   (d) You are taking nefazodone antidepressant (Serzone, Nefadar), cimetidine (Tagamet, Tagamet HB, Novo-Cimetine, Peptol), or levodopa (Dopar, Larodopa) for Parkinson disease. The following substances may prolong the effects of triazolam: diphenhydramine (eg, Benadryl), promethazine (Phenergan, Promacot, Promethegan), verapamil (Calan, Covera, Isoptin, Verelan), diltiazem (Cardizem, Cartia, Dilacor, Dilt, Diltia, Taztia, Tiazac), erythromycin, HIV drugs indinavir (Crixivan) and nelfinavir (Viracept), and alcohol. There may be unusual and dangerous reactions if you are currently taking illegal drugs.
4. Side effects may include light-headedness, headache, dizziness, visual disturbances, amnesia, and nausea. In some people, oral triazolam may not work as desired.
5. Patients who smoke are likely to notice a decrease in the medication's ability to achieve desired results.
6. You should not eat heavily prior to your appointment. You may take the medication with a small amount of food such as juice or toast. Taking it with too much food can make absorption into your system unpredictable.
7. N_2O/O_2 (laughing gas) may be used in conjunction with triazolam and local anesthetic.
8. On the way home from your appointment, your car seat should be in the reclined position. When at home, lie down with the head slightly elevated. Someone should stay with you for the next several hours because of possible disorientation and injury from falling.

I understand these considerations and am willing to abide by the conditions stated above. I have had an opportunity to ask questions and have had them answered to my satisfaction.

Patient name _____

Signature of patient _____ Date _____

_____
Initial

REQUEST AND CONSENT FOR TREATMENT

SANDWICH GRAFT SURGERY: MAXILLARY (UPPER JAW) SURGERY WITH BONE GRAFTING AND POSSIBLE IMPLANT PLACEMENT

For: _____

Dr _____ has explained to me the various steps involved in my proposed surgery. Alternative treatment plans have been discussed, and I feel comfortable in proceeding with the outlined surgery.

The following facts pertaining to my surgery have been explained to me.

I understand that surgery will be performed to place bone graft material on top of and within the crestal bone of the upper jaw. The bone graft will be "sandwiched" between the existing bone. Dr _____ has explained how this operation will be performed to my satisfaction. The graft material will consist of a bone substitute material (hydroxyapatite), tissue bank bone, or a combination of both. In approximately 5 to 6 months, after the graft has partially healed, a second procedure will be done to insert the implants into the upper jaw and the grafted material. In some cases it is possible to insert the implant and graft in the same operation. It is expected that the implants will become stable and act as anchors for fixed or fixed-detachable partial dentures. This graft is also being placed in an attempt to change the contour of the bone ridge and/or increase its width and/or height.

The graft material consists of small particles. Some of the particles may become loose during the initial healing period. However, this should not influence the success of the surgery and the particles will do no harm if swallowed.

Following the grafting surgery, it is sometimes necessary to have a second procedure called a *vestibuloplasty* to provide more tissue to cover the grafted ridge.

A custom surgical splint may need to be attached to the jaw (using surgical wire, surgical screws, or sutures) for 1 to 4 weeks to help keep the synthetic bone graft in place and to form it properly to the jaw bone. The patient's existing partial denture or full denture can sometimes be modified for this purpose.

The surgical technique has been explained to me in detail. I understand that, just as in any surgery, complications can occur, including but not limited to infection, bleeding, tissue damage, temporary or permanent numbness of the upper lip, face, or cheeks, and loss of the graft (requiring future surgical procedures).

I have been informed and understand that occasionally there are complications of surgery, drugs, and anesthesia, including but not limited to:

1. Pain, swelling, and postoperative discoloration of the face, neck, and mouth.
2. Numbness and tingling of the upper lip, teeth, gums, cheek, and palate, which may be temporary or, rarely, permanent.
3. Infection of the bone that might require further treatment, including hospitalization and surgery.
4. Mal-, delayed, or nonunion of the bone graft material to the existing bone.
5. Lack of adequate bone growth into the bone graft replacement material.
6. Bleeding that may require extraordinary hemorrhage-control measures.
7. Limitation of jaw function.
8. Stiffness of facial and jaw muscles.
9. Injury to the teeth.
10. Referred pain to the ear, neck, and head.

_____
Initial

Continued on next page

11. Postoperative complications involving the sinuses, nose, nasal cavity, sense of smell, infraorbital regions, and altered sensations of the cheek and eyes.
12. Postoperative unfavorable drug reactions, such as nausea, vomiting, and allergy.
13. Possible loss of teeth and bone segments.

It is unlikely but possible that the graft material will not attach to the existing bone. The graft may be loose, and the gum tissue may ulcerate over the graft. If this occurs, the graft material will need to be removed. Further surgery, including mucosal or skin grafts, may be needed to repair lost oral tissue.

After surgery, there will be a certain amount of discomfort and swelling. I understand that I will need to be on a liquid to very soft diet for 2 to 3 weeks.

I agree to keep my teeth and mouth meticulously clean. I also agree to keep all postoperative appointments and checkups as required by my doctor.

I give my permission for Dr _____ to photograph, video record, or use other means to take visual records of this operation for purposes of education and publication. However, my identity will not be revealed to the general public without my permission.

Knowing the above facts, I freely give my consent to Dr _____ to perform a synthetic bone graft to my upper jaw.

Signature of patient _____ Date _____

Signature of doctor or witness _____ Date _____

Initial

ORAL SURGERY AND DENTAL EXTRACTIONS INFORMED CONSENT

For: _____

I understand that oral surgery and dental extractions include inherent risks, including but not limited to the following:

1. *Injury to the nerves.* A possible consequence of surgical procedures or anesthetic administration is injury causing numbness of the lips and tongue as well as any tissues of the mouth, cheeks, and/or face. This numbness may be of a temporary nature, lasting a few days, weeks, or months, or could possibly be permanent.
2. *Bleeding, bruising, and swelling.* Some moderate bleeding may last several hours. If bleeding is profuse, the office should be contacted as soon as possible. Likewise, some swelling is normal, but if it is severe, the office should be notified. Swelling usually starts to subside after about 48 hours. Bruises may persist for a week or more.
3. *Dry socket.* Dry socket sometimes occurs when teeth are extracted and is a result of a blood clot not forming properly during the healing process. Dry socket can be extremely painful if not treated.
4. *Sinus involvement.* In some cases, the root tips of upper teeth lie in close proximity to the maxillary sinus. Occasionally during extraction or surgical procedures, the sinus membrane may be perforated. Should this occur, it may be necessary to have the sinus surgically closed. Root tips may need to be retrieved from the sinus.
5. *Infection.* No matter how carefully surgical sterility is maintained, it is possible, because of the existing nonsterile oral environment, for infections to occur postoperatively. At times, these may be serious in nature. Should severe swelling occur, particularly if it is accompanied with fever or malaise, professional attention should be sought as soon as possible.
6. *Fractured jaw, roots, bone fragments, or instruments.* Although extreme care will be used, the jaw, tooth roots, bone spicules, or instruments used in the extraction procedure may fracture, requiring retrieval and possibly referral to a specialist. A decision may be made to leave a small fragment of root, bone, or instrument in the jaw when removal may require additional extensive surgery, which could cause more harm and add to the risk of complications.
7. *Injury to adjacent teeth or fillings.* Injury to adjacent teeth or fillings may occur no matter how carefully surgical and/or extraction procedures are performed.
8. *Bacterial endocarditis.* Because of the normal existence of bacteria in the oral cavity, bacterial infection may be transmitted through blood vessels to the tissues of the heart, and bacterial endocarditis (an infection of the heart) could occur. It is the patient's responsibility to inform the dentist of any known or suspected heart problems.
9. *Adverse reactions to medications given or prescribed.* Reactions, either mild or severe, may possibly occur from anesthetics or other medications administered or prescribed. All prescription drugs must be taken according to instructions. Women using oral contraceptives must be aware that antibiotics can render these contraceptives ineffective. Other methods of contraception must be used during the treatment period.

It is my responsibility to seek attention should any undue circumstances occur postoperatively, and I shall diligently follow all preoperative and postoperative instructions.

_____
Initial

Continued on next page

Informed Consent

As a patient, I have been given the opportunity to ask any questions regarding the nature and purpose of surgical treatment and have received answers to my satisfaction. I voluntarily assume any and all possible risks, including the risk of harm, if any, that may be associated with any phase of this treatment in hopes of obtaining the desired results, which may or may not be achieved. No guarantees or promises have been made to me concerning my recovery and results of the treatment to be rendered to me. The fees for this service have been explained to me and are satisfactory. I authorize photographs, slides, x-rays, or any other visual records of my care and treatment during or after its completion to be used for the advancement of dentistry and for reimbursement purposes. However, my identity will not be revealed to the general public without my permission. By signing this form, I am freely giving my consent to allow and authorize Dr _____ and his or her associates to render any treatments necessary or advisable for my dental conditions, including any and all anesthetics and/or medications.

Signature of patient _____ Date _____

Signature of doctor or witness _____ Date _____

Initial

REQUEST AND CONSENT FOR TREATMENT

SINUS LIFT PROCEDURE WITH BONE GRAFTING AND POSSIBLE IMPLANT PLACEMENT

For: _____

I authorize and request Dr _____ to perform surgery on my upper jaw (maxilla).

I understand that surgery will be performed to place a bone graft material into the floor of the sinus to build adequate bone height for the placement of implants. The bone graft will consist of a bone substitute material (hydroxyapatite), tissue bank bone, or a combination of both. In approximately 5 to 6 months, after the graft has partially healed, a second procedure will be done to place the implant(s) in the upper jaw and the grafted material. In some cases, it is possible to place the implants and graft during the same procedure. It is expected that the implants will become stable and act as anchors for fixed or fixed-detachable dentures.

Dr _____ has explained and described the procedure to my satisfaction, including the fact that if the new bone does not incorporate into the bone graft material, alternative prosthetic measures will have to be considered.

I have been informed that the likelihood for success of the suggested treatment plan is good; however, there are risks involved. The bone graft material has produced good results when placed on top of the upper or lower jaw ridge. However, there are insufficient long-term studies to evaluate placement of the material on the sinus floor. This bone graft replacement material has previously been shown to be free from rejection or infection; however, there is no guarantee that my graft will not become infected or be rejected. There have been some cases of failure of the graft to incorporate into new bone or to sustain implants. Rarely, implants have failed and require removal; occasionally, the area can be regrafted and implants reinserted.

It is understood that although good results are expected, they cannot be and are not implied, guaranteed, or warrantable. There is also no guarantee against unsatisfactory or failed results.

I have been informed and understand that occasionally there are complications of surgery, drugs, and anesthesia, including but not limited to:

1. Pain, swelling, and postoperative discoloration of the face, neck, and mouth.
2. Numbness and tingling of the upper lip, teeth, gums, cheek, and palate, which may be temporary or, rarely, permanent.
3. Infection of the bone that might require further treatment, including hospitalization and surgery.
4. Mal-, delayed, or nonunion of the bone graft replacement material to the existing bone.
5. Lack of adequate bone growth into the bone graft replacement material.
6. Bleeding that may require extraordinary hemorrhage-control measures.
7. Limitation of jaw function.
8. Stiffness of facial and jaw muscles.
9. Injury to the teeth.
10. Referred pain to the ear, neck, and head.
11. Postoperative complications involving the sinuses, nose, nasal cavity, sense of smell, infraorbital regions, and altered sensations of the cheek and eyes.
12. Postoperative unfavorable reactions to drugs, such as nausea, vomiting, and allergy.
13. Possible loss of teeth and bone segments.

_____
Initial

Continued on next page

I understand that I am not to use alcohol or nonprescription drugs during the treatment period. Dr _____ has informed me that smoking is particularly detrimental to the success of this operation; therefore, I have been asked to abstain from smoking.

I understand that Dr _____ will give his best professional care toward the accomplishment of the desired results. I understand that I can ask for full recital of all possible risks attendant to phases of my care. I further understand that I am free to withdraw from treatment at any time.

I give permission for persons other than the doctors involved in my care and treatment to observe this operation. I authorize photographs, slides, x-rays, or any other visual records of my care and treatment during or after its completion to be used for the advancement of dentistry and for reimbursement purposes. However, my identity will not be revealed to the general public without my permission.

I understand this consent form and request Dr _____ to perform the surgery discussed.

Signature of patient _____ Date _____

Signature of doctor or witness _____ Date _____

Initial

POSTOPERATIVE INSTRUCTIONS FOR IMPLANT PLACEMENT/ GUIDED BONE REGENERATION

- Take your medications (antibiotics, analgesics, anti-inflammatory medications, and chlorhexidine rinse) as directed.
- Avoid smoking.
- Avoid sucking liquid through a straw.
- Expect swelling, pain, and ecchymosis at the surgical site.
- Rest.
- During the 24-hour period following surgery, place light pressure and ice on the surgical site: 15 minutes off, 15 minutes on.
- In case of multiple implant placement, stay on a liquid diet for 2 days (Carnation Instant Breakfast, Meritene, and Ensure are recommended); then soft foods (the consistency of mashed potatoes or scrambled eggs) may be consumed following the second day and for at least 2 weeks (until the mucosal incision has closed completely).
- Do not wear a provisional prosthesis for 2 weeks. After 2 weeks, the provisional prosthesis can be worn, but you should not eat with it or wear it overnight.
- Do not lift or pull on the lip or cheek to look at the sutures.
- Do not brush or floss near the surgical site for a few days, and then brush and floss very lightly for 4 weeks before returning to routine brushing and flossing.
- In case of immediate load, avoid mastication on the implant crown for 6 to 8 weeks.
- Sutures should be removed in 2 weeks.
- Notify the office if your medications do not relieve discomfort or if you have questions.

POSTOPERATIVE INSTRUCTIONS FOR SINUS LIFT PROCEDURE

- Take your medications (antibiotics, analgesics, anti-inflammatory medications, chlorhexidine rinse, nasal spray, and decongestant) as directed.
- Avoid smoking.
- Do not blow your nose for 2 weeks because this could create positive pressure, which could spread air though confluent soft tissue planes, creating soft tissue emphysema.
- Avoid sucking liquid through a straw because this creates negative intrasinus pressure.
- Try not to sneeze or cough; if it is unavoidable, keep the mouth open to decrease internal antral pressure.
- Some nasal bleeding (oozing of blood through the nose) may occur during the first day.
- Rest as much as possible for the first 3 to 7 days following surgery.
- During the 24-hour period following surgery, place light pressure and ice on the surgical site.
- Keep your head elevated. On the first night, your head should be elevated on two or more pillows. This will prevent airway obstruction and aspiration of blood and heavy saliva and will diminish edema.
- Maintain a liquid diet for 2 days (Carnation Instant Breakfast, Meritene, and Ensure are recommended); then soft foods (the consistency of mashed potatoes or scrambled eggs) may be consumed following the second day and for at least 2 weeks (until the mucosal incision has closed completely).
- Do not wear a prosthesis for 2 weeks.
- Do not lift or pull on the lip to look at the sutures.
- Return to the office for a postoperative checkup in 1 week.
- Notify the office if you feel granules in your nose, if your medications do not relieve discomfort, or if you have questions.

POSTOPERATIVE INSTRUCTIONS FOR VESTIBULOPLASTY

- Wear the pressure dressing for 48 hours. (A pressure dressing is placed over the chin to provide close adaptation of the mucosal flap to bone, using 0.5-inch medical tape from cheek to cheek, crossing over the chin.)
- Maintain a liquid diet for a minimum of 72 hours.
- Do not lift or pull on the lip or cheek to look at sutures.
- Use chlorhexidine rinse after each meal.
- Construction or hard reline of dentures can begin in 3 months.

INDEX

Page numbers followed by "f" indicate figures; those followed by "t" indicate tables; those followed by "b" indicate boxes

A